Advanced Practice in Nursing

Under the Auspices of the International Council of Nurses (ICN)

Series Editor
Christophe Debout, GIP-IFITS
Health Chair Sciences- Po Paris/IDS UMR Inserm 1145
Paris, France

This Series of concise monographs, endorsed by the International Council of Nurses, explores various aspects of advanced practice nursing at the international level.

The ICN definition provided in the Guidelines on Advanced Practice Nursing 2020 (ICN, 2020) has been adopted for this series to define advanced practice nursing:

"A Nurse Practitioner/Advanced Practice Nurse is a registered nurse who has acquired the expert knowledge base, complex decision-making skills and clinical competencies for expanded practice, the characteristics of which are shaped by the context and/or country in which they are credentialed to practice." (ICN, 2020, p. 6). A Master's degree is required for entry level.

At the international level, the three most common levels of advanced practice nursing include three levels of clinical practice:

Nurse practitioners (NPs) are advanced practice nurses who have integrated clinical skills associated with nursing and medicine in order to assess, diagnose and manage patients usually in primary healthcare (PHC) settings and acute care populations as well as ongoing care for populations with chronic illness (ICN, 2020). NPs usually have prescriptive authority and can make referrals to other healthcare professionals. Clinical nurse specialists (CNSs) provide expert clinical advice and care based on established diagnoses in specialized clinical fields of practice along with a systems approach in practicing as a member of the healthcare team (ICN, 2020). Nurse Anesthetists (NAs) who are defined by the 2021 ICN Guidelines: *A Nurse Anesthetist is an Advanced Practice Nurse who has the knowledge, skills and competencies to provide individualised care in anesthesia, pain management, and related anesthesia services to patients across the lifespan, whose health status may range from healthy through all levels of acuity, including immediate, severe, or life-threatening illnesses or injury (ICN, 2021).*

The scope of practice and responsibilities that define these three categories of advanced practice nurses includes five interrelated components:

- Clinical practice
- Consultation
- Education
- Leadership
- Research

The monograph Series addresses four topics associated with advanced practice nursing:

- APNs in clinical practice (NPs, CNSs, NAs)
- Education and continuous professional development for advanced practice nurses
- Coordination and implementation issues related to advanced practice nursing
- Policy and regulation for advanced practice nursing

The contributing authors represent international experts in their field along with representation from the ICN Nurse Practitioner/Advanced Practice Nurse Network.

They include clinicians, educators, policymakers and researchers.

Each book within the Series reflects the fundamentals of nursing which provides the foundation for advanced practice nursing. The aim is to promote evidence-informed advanced practice nursing.

Editorial Contact: Nathalie Lhorset-Poulain

Kathy J. Wheeler • Michelle Acorn
Editors

Health Policy for Advanced Practice Nursing: A Toolkit for Implementation and Improvement

Springer

ICN
International
Council of Nurses
The global voice of nursing

Editors
Kathy J. Wheeler
University of Kentucky College of Nursing
Lexington, KY, USA

Michelle Acorn
University of Toronto & Queen's University
Toronto & Kingston, ON, Canada

ISSN 2511-3917 ISSN 2511-3925 (electronic)
Advanced Practice in Nursing
ISBN 978-3-032-03666-7 ISBN 978-3-032-03667-4 (eBook)
https://doi.org/10.1007/978-3-032-03667-4

This Springer imprint is published by the registered company Springer Nature Switzerland AG
The registered company address is: Gewerbestrasse 11, 6330 Cham, Switzerland

Preface

This book is dedicated to all the advanced practice nurses (APNs), nurses, healthcare administrators, and policymakers involved in shaping healthcare around the world.

The editors and authors worked hard to produce something meaningful and useful. Admittedly, as a very unique piece of work, it was challenging. It would have been much easier to ask everyone to tell their personal story about policy implementation and/or improvement in their own institution or jurisdiction. Instead, everyone was asked to look at APN policy issues globally, to make broad comparisons, and to share positive outcomes as well as challenges and difficulties. The intention is to inform and share lessons learned so as to make the policy work easier and more impactful to those active in APN policy work.

This toolkit is aspirational, shining a light on potential local, national, regional, and global opportunities, options, and paths. Nothing is intended to be prescriptive, as every institution and jurisdiction has unique challenges, needs, and abilities. This is consistent with the work of the International Council of Nurses (ICN) and the ICN Nurse Practitioner/Advanced Practice Nurse Network (ICN NP/APNN), whose work in defining advanced practice nursing seeks to provide a beacon balanced against a nursing world coping with challenges of finance and support.

As much as editors and authors have tried to be comprehensive, that is an impossible feat. So, not all stories or comparisons are included. Certainly, there are great exemplars yet to share as policy success unfolds. The place and opportunity to share them is via the ICN, the ICN NP/APNN, the *International Nursing Review* journal, and the many platforms dedicated to dissemination.

Kind regards,

Lexington, KY, USA — Kathy J. Wheeler, PhD, APRN, FAANP, FNAP, FGNLI

Toronto & Kingston, ON, Canada — Michelle Acorn, DNP, FCAN, FAAN

Contents

Introduction to Health Policy for Advanced Practice Nursing: A Toolkit for Policy Implementation and Improvement

Overview of Health Policy Implementation and Improvement for Advanced Practice Nursing

Kathy J. Wheeler and Michelle Acorn

1 Introduction

A significant and growing class of professionals providing healthcare around the world are advanced practice nurses (APNs). Because healthcare is a human right and a political choice, APNs need to participate in the making of policy, not only to shape the healthcare patients receive but the policies that impact the professional life of the APN. When properly supported, APNs have the potential to impact healthcare globally, nationally, and locally.

If the world is meant to achieve the Sustainable Development Goals and Universal Health Coverage (UHC) by 2030 and advance the global goals set out by the United Nations years ago, nursing bears a particular burden and opportunity to provide more generalist nurses as well as more APNs (Eozenou et al. 2023). Progress made toward achieving UHC in terms of service delivery is encouraging and demonstrates countries can achieve high levels of coverage with the right policies. Evidence also shows it is challenging to improve access to services while reducing or keeping funding fixed. Findings from the Covid 19 pandemic era indicate that previous progress towards UHC is now at stake. It is crucial that despite heightened fiscal pressure, governments continue to support UHC-targeted social and health policy interventions (Eozenou et al. 2023).

The purpose of this toolkit is to provide an overview of policy implementation and improvement in the three pillars of healthcare that affect the ability of the APN to provide the high-quality, cost-effective healthcare they are known for, namely, governance, practice, and education. Because leadership and research are

K. J. Wheeler (✉)
University of Kentucky College of Nursing, Lexington, KY, USA
e-mail: kjwheeler623@gmail.com

M. Acorn
University of Toronto & Queen's University, Toronto & Kingston, ON, Canada

K. J. Wheeler, M. Acorn (eds.), *Health Policy for Advanced Practice Nursing: A Toolkit for Implementation and Improvement*, Advanced Practice in Nursing,
https://doi.org/10.1007/978-3-032-03667-4_1

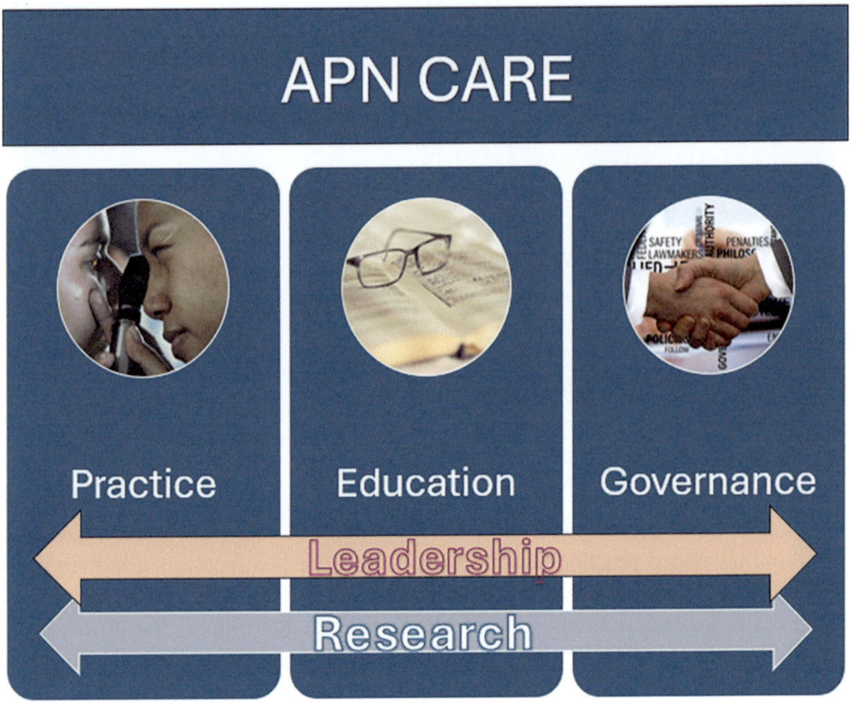

Fig. 1 Policy foundations of APN care

foundational to all APN policy development (governance, practice, and education), they will be discussed throughout. Figure 1 depicts the relationship of these policy foundations, followed by pertinent definitions.

1.1 Definition of Terms

Governance The "manner in which something is governed or regulated; method of management, system of regulation" (Oxford English Dictionary 2026, para 4). For APNs, governance is a broad term and refers to the rules, policies, and decision-making processes that affect how they practice, advocate, research, are educated, and are regulated.

Practice For an APN, the International Council of Nurses defines the nature of *practice* as (ICN 2020, p 10):

- A designated role or level of nursing that has its focus on the provision of care, illness prevention, and cure based on direct and indirect healthcare services at an advanced level, including rehabilitative care and chronic disease management. This is beyond the scope of practice of a generalist or specialized nurse

- The capability to manage full episodes of care and complex healthcare problems, including hard-to-reach, vulnerable, and at-risk populations
- The ability to integrate research (evidence-informed practice), education, leadership, and clinical management
- Extended and broader range of autonomy (varies by country context and clinical setting)
- Case-management (manages own case load at an advanced level)
- Advanced assessment, judgement, decision-making, and diagnostic reasoning skills

Education It is "the discipline that is concerned with methods of teaching and learning in schools or school-like environments as opposed to various nonformal and informal means of socialization" (Britannica 2026, para 1). For APNs, educational preparation involves (ICN 2020, p 10):

- Preparation beyond that of a generalist or specialized nurse education at a minimum requirement of a full master's degree program (master's level modules taken as detached courses do not meet this requirement). It is acknowledged that for some countries, the requirement of a master's degree may be an aspirational goal as they strive to achieve this standard. Transitional programs and bridging courses can be defined to progress to this standard.
- Formal recognition of educational programs preparing nurses specifically for advanced practice nursing (e.g., accreditation, approval, or authorization by governmental or nongovernmental agencies).
- A formal system of credentialing linked to defined educational qualifications.
- Even though some countries require clinical experience for a nurse to enter an APN education program, no evidence was found to support this requirement.

Leadership It "is the ability to influence and guide a group of people toward achieving a common goal. It encompasses a range of skills and behaviors that empower individuals to provide direction, motivate team members, make decisions, foster collaboration, and promote growth. Leadership isn't limited to formal positions of authority, and individuals at all organizational levels can exhibit it. Leadership plays a pivotal role in driving success, whether it's inspiring a team to reach new heights, facilitating effective communication, or leveraging collective knowledge and expertise. By harnessing their know-how and understanding the dynamics of a group, leaders can navigate challenges, inspire action, and unlock the full potential of their team members to achieve shared objectives" (IMD 2026, para 3–6).

Research It is the "detailed study of a subject, especially in order to discover new information about something or reach a new understanding of it" (Cambridge Dictionary 2026b, para 1). According to Kilpatrick et al. (2024, p 144–145), "There is international agreement that participation in research and research-related activities such as quality improvement (QI) and evidence-informed decision-making

(EIDM) is an essential dimension of advanced practice nursing (ICN 2020). Research includes activities where the primary goal is to generate new knowledge or strengthen existing knowledge about the phenomenon under study (Gray 2019). Nursing research has a more specific focus on investing issues that are relevant to the nursing profession…APNs are uniquely positioned to participate in research, QI, and EIDM because of their extensive knowledge of population health needs, collaboration with nurses and other healthcare providers, and detailed understanding of healthcare organisations and health systems."

Advocacy It is defined as "support for an idea, plan, or way of doing something" (Cambridge Dictionary 2026a, para 1). It usually involves activities devoted to education, issue awareness, trust building, research, and coalition building (GovFacts 2026). Sometimes it is confused with lobbying, which usually is directed at specific legislation and according to strict rules of ethics, funding, and discourse (GovFacts 2026). Advocacy customs and approaches tend to vary by country, so organizations and individual APNs must be cognizant of national laws and ethical standards. The International Council of Nurses is independent and nonpartisan and does not support any political party or candidates; examples throughout the text are illustrative of jurisdiction-specific mechanisms.

2 APN Titling and Roles

Although APN titles vary around the world, there are four types of commonly recognized APN roles—nurse practitioner (NP), nurse anesthetist (NA), nurse midwife (NM), and clinical nurse specialist (CNS). Because some blurring of roles exists between NPs and CNSs around the world, the International Council of Nurses (ICN) developed the Guidelines on Advanced Practice Nursing 2020, defining advanced practice nursing and clarifying the two roles (ICN 2020). In 2021, the ICN also developed the Guidelines on Advanced Practice Nursing: Nurse Anesthetists, providing role definition for NAs (ICN 2021). Global guidance for advanced nurse midwives, nurse midwives, and other types of midwives has been provided via the International Confederation of Midwives (ICM), via a revised definition and scope of practice as of 2024 (ICM 2024). The ICM provides standards for education, regulation, and practice for nurse and nonnurse midwives. As the ICN provides standards and guidance for nurses, all nurse midwives benefit from the guidance and support of both the ICM and ICN. It is also worth noting many countries regulate midwifery as a distinct profession. Some countries/jurisdictions use the terms nurse midwife, advanced nurse midwife, or certified nurse midwife as legally defined nursing-based roles. Table 1 presents APN definitions as provided by the above organizations. More details will be provided throughout the text.

Aside from professional titling, overlap in levels of education and roles can occur. In some jurisdictions, roles and care duties that much of the world views as *advanced* are knowingly delivered by generalist nurses who have been specifically

Table 1 APN definitions and traits

APN types/ terms	Definition	Focus and traits
Advanced practice nurse	An advanced practice nurse (APN) is a generalist or specialized nurse who has acquired, through additional graduate education (minimum of a master's degree), the expert knowledge base, complex decision-making skills, and clinical competencies for advanced nursing practice, the characteristics of which are shaped by the context in which they are credentialed to practice (adapted from ICN 2008). The two most commonly identified APN roles are CNS and NP (ICN 2020, p 6).	Blanket term generally used to describe the four common types of advanced practice nurses (nurse practitioner, clinical nurse specialist, nurse anesthetist, nurse midwife), though in some jurisdictions there may be alternative terms for any of the four roles that might be present, or the term may be the accepted term for one specific type of advanced practice nurse if present (Wheeler et al. 2022; Maier and Aiken 2016; Heale and Buckley 2015; Pulcini et al. 2010). As this text will show, variation remains for APNs, jurisdiction to jurisdiction, in terms of governance, education, and practice.
Nurse practitioner	A nurse practitioner is an advanced practice nurse who integrates clinical skills associated with nursing and medicine in order to assess, diagnose, and manage patients in primary healthcare (PHC) settings and acute care populations, as well as ongoing care for populations with chronic illness (ICN 2020, p 6).	With proper authorization, nurse practitioners: Primarily focus on direct care to patients, whether in primary care or acute care. Aside from being clinicians, NPs can be educators, researchers, legal consultants, health policy consultants, or administrators (AANP 2020). Work with nurses, doctors, physical therapists, pharmacists, and other healthcare providers (MCCMS 2023). Practice in community health clinics, hospitals, prisons, emergency rooms, urgent care clinics, private physician offices, NP practices, long-term care homes, colleges, schools, and health departments (Wheeler et al. 2022; Nursing License Map 2024).

(continued)

Table 1 (continued)

APN types/ terms	Definition	Focus and traits
Clinical nurse specialist	A clinical nurse specialist is an advanced practice nurse who provides expert clinical advice and care based on established diagnoses in specialized clinical fields of practice, along with a systems approach in practicing as a member of the healthcare team (ICN 2020, p 6).	With proper authorization, clinical nurse specialists: Primarily focus on a specialized area of practice, such as a population, setting, disease, or health specialty (Nurse License Map 2024). Works more in administration, education, or research, though does provide direct patient care according to the specialized area of practice (Johns Hopkins University School of Nursing 2020). Work with healthcare professionals, healthcare organizations, and patients of all ages, depending on role specifics (NACNS 2024). Practice in hospitals, outpatient settings, emergency departments, community health centers, and long-term care settings (ICN 2020; Bryant-Lukosius and Wong 2019; Kilpatrick et al. 2013).
Nurse anesthetist	A nurse anesthetist is an advanced practice nurse who has the knowledge, skills, and competencies to provide individualized care in anesthesia, pain management, and related anesthesia services to patients across the lifespan, whose health status may range from healthy through all levels of acuity, including immediate, severe, or life-threatening illnesses or injury (ICN 2021, p 6).	With proper authorization, nurse anesthetists: Primarily focus on providing anesthesia and pain medication to patients before, during, and after surgery and procedures (ICN 2021). Work with nurses, surgeons, doctors, dentists, and other healthcare providers (Cleveland Clinic 2024b). Practice in hospitals, surgical centers, pain clinics, outpatient clinics, obstetrical units, and other locations where anesthesia is needed (ICN 2021).

(continued)

Table 1 (continued)

APN types/ terms	Definition	Focus and traits
Nurse midwife	The definition of advanced nurse midwife draws on the definition of midwife by the International Confederation of Midwives, but with the additional requirement that the nurse midwives have additional nursing midwifery education beyond the generalist nurse. In some jurisdictions, additional education would consist of a graduate degree beyond a bachelor's degree and license as a registered nurse (ACNM 2021). According to the International Confederation of Midwives (ICM 2024, para 1): A midwife is a person who has successfully completed a midwifery education program based on the ICM Essential Competencies for Midwifery Practice and the framework of the ICM Global Standards for Midwifery Education, recognized in the country where it is located; who has acquired the requisite qualifications to be registered and/or legally licensed to practice midwifery and use the title "midwife"; and who demonstrates competency in the scope of practice of the midwife.	With proper authorization, nurse midwives: Primarily focus on care of women over the course of their reproductive lifetime, particularly before, during, and after labor. They also provide gynecological care from adolescence through menopause, and beyond (Jividen 2024). Work with obstetricians and other healthcare providers (Cleveland Clinic 2024a, Jividen 2024). Practice in hospitals, clinics, birthing centers, and health departments. Some attend home births (Jividen 2024).

educated in those duties. This has happened for a variety of reasons, some based on convenience and others based on population health needs. The demand is great and will likely be ongoing. But that does not diminish the effort to strive for education and roles as described above to advance health equity and optimize safe outcomes.

With that in mind, and because APNs are nurses who rely on nurses and nursing for every part of their work, and are the pool of professionals from which APNs evolve, it is appropriate to review a recent update of definitions by ICN, presented Table 2. It is noteworthy in this update that ICN determined both terms needed to be defined, since the term *nursing* focused on the profession (body of knowledge, regulated, practice directed at the interest of others) and the term *a nurse* focused on members of the profession. ICN also made extensive recommendations regarding the implementation of the terms *nursing* and *a nurse* at multiple policy levels. The document is available at https://www.icn.ch/sites/default/files/2025-06/ICN_Definition-Nursing_Report_EN_Web_0.pdf

Table 2 Definitions and recommendations regarding the terms nursing and a nurse

Terms	Definition
Nursing	"Nursing is a profession dedicated to upholding everyone's right to enjoy the highest attainable standard of health, through a shared commitment to providing collaborative, culturally safe, people-centred care and services. Nursing acts and advocates for people's equitable access to health and healthcare, and safe, sustainable environments. The practice of nursing embodies the philosophy and values of the profession in providing professional care in the most personal health-related aspects of people's lives. Nursing promotes health, protects safety and continuity in care, and manages and leads healthcare organizations and systems. Nursing's practice is underpinned by a unique combination of science-based disciplinary knowledge, technical capability, ethical standards, and therapeutic relationships. Nursing is committed to compassion, social justice and a better future for humanity" (ICN 2025, p 12).
A nurse	"A nurse is a professional who is educated in the scientific knowledge, skills and philosophy of nursing, and regulated to practice nursing based on established standards of practice and ethical codes. Nurses enhance health literacy, promote health, prevent illness, protect patient safety, alleviate suffering, facilitate recovery and adaptation, and uphold dignity throughout life and at end of life. They work autonomously and collaboratively across settings to improve health, through advocacy, evidence-informed decision-making, and culturally safe, therapeutic relationships. Nurses provide people-centred, compassionate clinical and social care, manage services, enhance health systems, advance public and population health, and foster safe and sustainable environments. Nurses lead, educate, research, advocate, innovate and shape policy to improve health outcomes. Further, nurses play a unique role in health and care for populations of all ages, and in all settings, building trust with individuals, families and communities and gaining valuable insights into people's experiences of health and illness. Building on a foundation of personalized direct and social care, nurses advance their capabilities through ongoing education, research and exploration of best practices. A nurse's scope of practice is defined by their level of education, experience, competency, professional standards and lawful authority. They play a key role in the coordination, supervision of, and delegation to others who may assist in the provision of health care. Often at the front line, they respond to disasters, conflicts and emergencies, demonstrating courage, dedication, adaptability and commitment to the health of individuals, communities and the environment" (ICN 2025, p 12).

(continued)

Table 2 (continued)

Terms	Definition
Recommendations	National Nursing Associations (ICN 2025, p 56): Advocate for adoption. Engage interested parties (stakeholders). Update nursing codes of ethics, practice standards, and frameworks to align with the new definitions. Develop resources, workshops, and training to help nurses integrate the definitions into their daily practice. National Regulators (ICN 2025, p 56): Harmonize regulatory frameworks. Distinguish unregulated carers from "nurses." Strengthen oversight and accountability. Promote equity. National Educators and Academic Institutions (ICN 2025, p 57): Align curricula. Support lifelong learning. Promote research and evidence-informed practice. World Health Organization (ICN 2025, p 57): Endorse the definitions as a global standard. Clarify that the role of nurses is distinct from that of Community Health Care Workers and assistants, and highlight the valuable role that nurses play in the delegation of care to non-nurses and their supervision. Support capacity building. Promote equity and inclusion. Monitor and evaluate impact. International Labour Union (ICN 2025, p 57–58): Adopt the new definitions. Support workforce planning. Protect worker rights. Promote professional mobility. International Council of Nurses (ICN 2025, p 58–59): Commit to long-term vigilance and stewardship. Promote engagement and collaboration (esp. regulation and education). Strengthen global and local methodologies. Foster ongoing scholarship and innovation. Foster inclusivity and engagement. Engage with the public.

3 APNs and Policymaking Around the World

APNs, both formally and informally, have been functioning for decades around the world. Some countries and jurisdictions have thousands of each category of APN, while others have few or no nurses in advanced nursing roles. In the past few decades, the growth has accelerated in volume, role type, and global distribution.

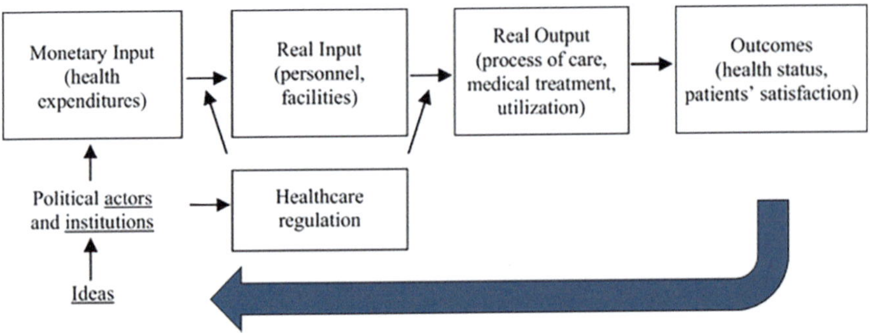

Fig. 2 Policy cycle in healthcare. (Adapted from Marmor and Wendt (2012). Adapted with permission from Elsevier)

Wheeler et al. (2022) highlighted that APNs are established in the Americas (US, Canada, Jamaica, Belize, Brazil, Chile, and Columbia, among others), much of Europe (Austria, Belgium, Czech Republic, Finland, France, Germany, Republic of Ireland, the Netherlands, Poland, Switzerland, the UK, among others), Australia, New Zealand, a few countries in Africa (Botswana, Ghana, Eswatini, Kenya, Namibia, and Zimbabwe, among others), and a few countries in Asia (Israel, Japan, Oman, Singapore, and Taiwan, among others). The same study found that the majority of the countries where APN roles were recognized reported policymaking for APNs occurred at both national and local levels.

Although there are some differences in how APNs function around the world, the process and issues of policymaking are largely the same. Figure 2 is a visual representation of the policy cycle that applies to healthcare and the professionals who deliver healthcare.

For the most part, the introduction and evolution of each of the roles where APNs are implemented has evolved along a similar continuum. Nurses are asked to do more and more. Nurses seek education to complement those added roles and responsibilities. Nurses pursue regulatory support to formally authorize what they have been doing and for which they have been educated. For that reason, a toolkit of this type is useful, not only for those with well-established roles but also for those just starting down this evolutionary path. Even countries where APNs have been functioning for some time but are lacking in what most regulators and APNs consider policy endpoints are moving along the same continuum. This has happened because lessons have been learned from working through opportunities and challenges about roles, scopes of practice, regulations, and the myriad policies that affect APN practice and quality service delivery. It has also happened because APNs now have extensive policy experiences throughout the world and are realizing the importance of sharing this information in publications and toolkits like this.

Policy work for any profession is both incremental and perpetual. To the frustration of many, the work and progress may be slow. Something will always need attention. Change is constant. Threats are always present, and a crisis creates policy window opportunities for APNs. Healthcare is one of the most dynamic, ever-changing systems in the world. For those reasons, APN policy work never goes away. It is an ever-present need that APNs, APN regulators, APN researchers, and APN educators must respond to in order to advance competencies, scopes of practice, and sustainable funding. APNs need to be mindful in order to protect patients, APN practice, and the profession.

4 This Toolkit

This toolkit is not meant to be prescriptive. It is meant to be aspirational, offering suggestions with potential paths and goals, as well as lessons learned. It is done with the recognition that all jurisdictions are going to develop their own version of nursing, based on resources and needs informed by their country's context. However, it is noteworthy that role evolution for advanced practice nursing has been more similar than dissimilar. Table 3 is offered as an introduction to a few policy implementation and improvement suggestions for APNs and the systems they serve and support.

This toolkit is composed of six sections; the first two are devoted to the basics of policy implementation and improvement, the next three are dedicated to the three pillars discussed above, and the final section is a summary. In the first section, this chapter, introduces the toolkit and provides an overview. Chapter "Changing the Game: Significance of Understanding and Implementing Health Policy Implementation and Improvement for Advanced Practice Nurses", describes the reasons APNs need to acknowledge and act on policies that affect healthcare and their profession. Chapter "Advanced Practice Nursing Health Policy: Looking Back, Looking Forward", provides a historical accounting of APN policy over the course of the profession, with an eye on what that will look like in the future. Chapter "Theoretical Foundations and Frameworks for Health Policy Implementation and Improvement", discusses the theoretical foundations of APN policy and policy making.

In the second section, chapter "The Language of Health Policy", discusses the importance of understanding the lexicon of healthcare policy and the terms, especially critical to advanced nursing practice. Chapter "Critical Building Blocks for Health Policy Implementation and Improvement", discusses the elements of policy-making from assessment, working with interested parties[1] (stakeholders) and third parties, to initiating, monitoring, and evaluating the policy project. Chapter "Building a Culture of Leadership and Advocacy", addresses the importance of instilling leadership qualities in nurses and APNs. Chapter "Creating and Sustaining an Advanced Practice Nursing Professional Organization", describes how organizations champion the policy work APNs do and the services organizations can provide. Chapter "Workforce Data Keeping as a Foundation for Policy Implementation and Improvement", discusses the importance of professional data keeping as

[1] Please note, the term interested parties will be used beside the term stakeholder throughout the toolkit in hopes of helping the transition to the more acceptable term. The term stakeholder carries a colonial or power differential connotation, but is a term used frequently in policy work.

Table 3 Pillars of advanced practice nursing care and opportunities for advanced practice nurses (APNs) and the systems they serve to improve involvement in policy implementation and improvement

Pillars of advanced practice nursing care	Opportunities for advanced practice nurses (APNs) and the systems they serve to improve involvement in policy implementation and improvement
Individual APNs and APN students can improve involvement in health policy if they…	Self-evaluate health policy knowledge and interest, particularly in areas that affect patient care and the work the APN provides Consider formal education on health policy implementation and improvement Prepare a 2-minute elevator speech and a 5-minute latte chat with a brief introduction about the APN role and a couple of key tailored points, such as positive outcomes Join nursing, APN organizations, and other organizations that work on policy implementation and improvement Serve on advisory boards, panels, and committees as leadership, thought, and technical experts Drive nursing and APN organizations to devote some portion of their efforts to policy implementation and improvement Stay informed on current events and matters that affect patient care and the work the APN provides Stay informed on applicable research and evidence-based practice Write and meet with representatives and policy makers about policy issues Collaborate with lobbyists on policy matters that affect patient care and health, as well as on practice matters Visit with legislators and policy makers who affect health policy, discussing policy issues as well as the impact of diseases and health conditions Interpret research and evidence-based practice information to policymakers Contribute and work on legislative campaigns Add to the research that contributes to APN practice, education, and governance Run for office Seek positions in agencies that affect policy implementation and improvement Attend meetings of nursing councils and nursing boards
Practice can improve involvement in health policy if they…	Create and encourage APN positions on interprofessional boards of organizations and institutions Support membership in professional organizations Support membership of APNs on advisory boards, councils, committees, and organizations that affect health policy Support APN research within the organization, as well as disseminating/implementing results Support and oversee quality improvement projects by APNs Assist APNs to disseminate/implement results from research projects

(continued)

Table 3 (continued)

Pillars of advanced practice nursing care	Opportunities for advanced practice nurses (APNs) and the systems they serve to improve involvement in policy implementation and improvement
Education can improve involvement in health policy if they…	Offer specific content and/or courses on health policy and policy implementation and improvement Encourage project/capstone/dissertation work on policy implementation and improvement Hire faculty known for their policy expertise Encourage faculty to be active in policy work Provide leadership on policy implementation and improvement to boards of nursing, nursing councils, advisory boards, panels, and committees Ask nursing boards and councils to do presentations on policy practices to students Support policy research
Governance can improve involvement in health policy if they…	Allow APNs and APN students to intern at policy offices Publish policy matters and changes via newsletters, websites, and social media platforms Offer programs on policy issues at APN conferences and APN schools Rely on APNs to inform them of practice and education issues, as well as research and evidence-based practice policies

fundamental to understanding the profession, its significance, and its needs. Chapter "Leveraging Research for the Benefit of Advanced Practice Nursing Health Policy", illuminates the importance of research to health policy.

The third section discusses health policy for APN governance, the fourth section discusses health policy for APN practice, and the fifth section discusses health policy for APN education. The last section is a summary chapter, chapter "Pearls and Parting Words: Highlights of Policy Implementation and Improvement for Advanced Practice Nursing".

References

American Association of Nurse Practitioners (AANP). The path to becoming a nurse practitioner. Author; 2020. https://www.aanp.org/news-feed/explore-the-variety-of-career-paths-for-nurse-practitioners. Accessed 1 Mar 2024.

American College of Nurse Midwives (ACNM). Comparison of certified nurse-midwives, certified midwives, and certified professional midwives. Author; 2021. https://www.midwife.org/acnm/files/acnmlibrarydata/uploadfilename/000000000268/CNM-CM-CPM%20Comparison%20Chart%20June%202021%20Final.pdf. Accessed 4 Mar 2024.

Britannica. Education. 2026. https://www.britannica.com/topic/education. Accessed 14 Mar 2026.

Bryant-Lukosius D, Wong F. International development of advanced practice nursing. In: Tracy MF, O'Grady ET, editors. Advanced practice nursing: an integrative approach. 6th ed. St. Louis: Elsevier; 2019. p. 129–41.

Cambridge Dictionary. Advocacy. 2026a. https://dictionary.cambridge.org/dictionary/english/advocacy. Accessed 10 Mar 2026.

Cambridge Dictionary. Research. 2026b. https://dictionary.cambridge.org/dictionary/english/research. Accessed 10 Mar 2026.

Cleveland Clinic. Midwife. Author; 2024a. https://my.clevelandclinic.org/health/articles/22648-midwife. Accessed 5 Mar 2024.

Cleveland Clinic. Nurse anesthetist. Author; 2024b. https://my.clevelandclinic.org/departments/health-sciences-education/careers/career-options/nurse-anesthetist. Accessed 4 Mar 2024.

Eozenou PH, Neelsen S, Florian A. Universal health coverage as a sustainable development goal. The World Bank; 2023. https://datatopics.worldbank.org/world-development-indicators/stories/universal-health-coverage-as-a-sustainable-development-goal.html. Accessed 15 Mar 2024.

GovFacts. How nonprofits shape policy: the power of advocacy vs. lobbying. 2026. https://gov-facts.org/education-family-social-services/nonprofits-philanthropy/nonprofit-organizations/how-nonprofits-shape-policy-the-power-of-advocacy-vs-lobbying/. Accessed 10 Mar 2026.

Gray M. Evidence-based practice and research. In: Tracy MF, O'Grady ET, editors. Hamric and Hanson's advanced practice nurses in hospitals: an integrative approach. 6th ed. Elsevier; 2019.

Heale R, Buckley R. An international perspective of advanced practice nursing regulation. Int Nurs Rev. 2015;62(3):421–9. https://doi.org/10.1111/inr.12193.

International Confederation of Midwives (ICM). Definition and scope of practice of the midwife. Author; 2024. https://internationalmidwives.org/resources/international-definition-of-the-midwife/. Accessed 1 Mar 2024.

International Council of Nurses (ICN). Guidelines on advanced practice nursing 2020. Author; 2020. https://www.icn.chsites/default/files/2021-04/ICN_APN%20Report_EN.pdf. Accessed 1 Mar 2024.

International Council of Nurses (ICN). Guidelines on advanced practice nursing: nurse anesthetists. Author; 2021. https://www.icn.ch/systems/files/documents/2021-05/ICN_Nurse-Anaesthetist-Report_EN_WEB.pdf. Accessed 1 Mar 2024.

International Council of Nurses (ICN). Renewing the definitions of 'nursing' and 'a nurse': final project report June 2025. 2025. https://www.icn.ch/sites/default/files/2025-06/ICN_Definition-Nursing_Report_EN_Web_0.pdf. Accessed 14 Mar 2025.

International Council of Nurses (ICN). The scope of practice, standards and competencies of the advanced nurse. Monograph, ICN Regulation Series, Geneva; 2008.

International Institute for Management Development (IMD). What is leadership and how is it evolving? 2026. https://www.imd.org/blog/leadership/what-is-leadership-how-is-it-evolving/. Accessed 14 Mar 2026.

Jividen S. What do nurse midwives do? Nurse.org. 2024. https://nurse.org/education/what-nurse-midwives-do/. Accessed 4 Mar 2024.

Johns Hopkins University School of Nursing. The NP vs. the CNS. Author; 2020. https://nursing.jhu.edu/magazine/articles/2020/11/the-np-vs-the-cns/. Accessed 3 Mar 2024.

Kilpatrick K, DiCenso A, Bryant-Lukosius D, Ritchie JA, Martin-Misener R, Carter N. Practice patterns and perceived impact of clinical nurse specialist roles in Canada: results of a national survey. Int J Nurs Stud. 2013;50(110):1524–36.

Kilpatrick K, Geese F, Zhou W, Bryant-Lukosius D. Advanced practice nurses and engagement in research, quality improvement, and evidence-informed decision-making. In: Rogers M, Lehwaldt D, Roussel J, Acorn M, editors. Advanced practice networking to enhance global health. Geneva: Springer Nature; 2024. p. 143–61. https://doi.org/10.1007/978-3-031-39740-0_8.

Maier C, Aiken L. Task shifting from physicians to nurses in primary care in 39 countries: a cross-country comparative study. Eur J Public Health. 2016;26(6):927–34. https://doi.org/10.1093/eurpub/ckw098.

Marmor T, Wendt C. Conceptual frameworks for comparing healthcare politics and policy. Health Policy. 2012;107(1):11–20. https://doi.org/10.1016/j.healthpol.2012.06.003.

Mayo Clinic College of Medicine and Science (MCCMS). Nurse practitioner. Author; 2023. https://college.mayo.edu/academics/explore-health-care-careers/careers-a-z/nurse-practitioner/. Accessed 2 Mar 2024.

National Association of Clinical Nurse Specialists (NACNS). Who are clinical nurse specialists? Author; 2024. https://nacna.org/2014/08/

who-are-clinical-nurse-specialists/#:~:text=CNSs%20work%20with%20other%20health%20care%20professionals%20and,practices%20and%20policies%20to%-20improve%20health%20care%20delivery. Accessed 4 Mar 2024.

Nursing License Map. Clinical nurse specialist. Author; 2024. https://nursinglicensemap.comadvanced-practice-nursing/clinical-nurse-specialist-cns/#:~:text=Clinical%20nurse%20specialists%20work%20within%20a%20specialty%20area,specialty%20such%20as%20pain%2C%20cardiovascular%2C%20oncology%20and%20gynecology. Accessed 2 Mar 2024.

Oxford English Dictionary. Governance. 2026. https://www.oed.com/dictionary/governance_n?tab=meaning_and_use. Accessed 14 Mar 2026.

Pulcini J, Jelic M, Gul R, Loke AY. An international survey on advanced practice nursing education, practice and regulation. J Nurs Scholarsh. 2010;43(1):31–9. https://doi.org/10.1111/j.15475069.2009.01322.x.

Wheeler KJ, Miller M, Pulcini J, Gray D, Ladd E, Rayens MK. Advanced practice nursing roles, regulation, education, and practice: a global study. Ann Glob Health. 2022;88(1):42, 1–21. https://annalsofglobalhealth.org/articles/3698/files/submission/proof/3698-1-15543-1-10-20220616.pdf.

Changing the Game: Significance of Understanding and Implementing Health Policy Implementation and Improvement for Advanced Practice Nurses

Madrean Schober

1 Introduction

The escalating costs of healthcare, an increased incidence of communicable and noncommunicable diseases, and aging populations have motivated countries worldwide to consider healthcare reform and improved approaches toward universal healthcare. These factors present an opportunity for advanced practice nurses (APNs) to contribute to strategies that could ease this burden on the provision of healthcare services internationally (Barton and East 2015; Bryant-Lukosius and Wong 2019; Harris 2023; Maier et al. 2017; Rosa et al. 2020; WHO 2020, 2021). The acknowledgment of this prospect necessitates a dynamic change in thinking and implementation of health policies that champion the APN concept. To establish supportive health policies, APNs must participate in the policy processes to ensure health policy guidelines promote optimal APN practice.

Preparing for the implementation of APNs within healthcare systems globally requires comprehending and appreciating how health policy impacts APN practice within the country or regional context. The vision of an increased presence of APNs mandates that APNs should not only understand health policy processes but should also engage in policy formation that will shape and influence effective and sustainable APN implementation. This includes health policy linked to a professional standard that adopts a clear professional identity, support for optimal clinical scope of practice, and relevant education. In addition, an understanding of hierarchical links in healthcare infrastructures that facilitate or restrict optimal potential for this level of nursing practice can ease the integration of APNs into the healthcare workforce.

Participation in health policy development necessitates that APNs acquire political know-how and leadership skills in order to meet population healthcare needs as

M. Schober (✉)
Schober Global Healthcare Consulting, Indianapolis, IN, USA
e-mail: madreans@gmail.com

K. J. Wheeler, M. Acorn (eds.), *Health Policy for Advanced Practice Nursing: A Toolkit for Implementation and Improvement*, Advanced Practice in Nursing,
https://doi.org/10.1007/978-3-032-03667-4_2

well as to advance future prospects for the profession. In addition, it is essential that educational institutions and their APN programs provide curricula that prepare the students to become active participants in health policy processes. A strong educational foundation can further ensure that the voices of APNs as participants in policymaking will be heard (Rosa et al. 2020).

In order to optimize this possibility, it is necessary for APNs to gain an understanding of the significance of how health policy decisions and relevant actions impact their practice. This chapter identifies issues of importance to APNs when considering participation in health policy development, as well as emphasizing the need for APNs to become actively involved in determining policy.

2 Background

Health policy guidelines and related actions affect institutions, organizations, and professionals that provide healthcare services and funding arrangements of the healthcare system (McGee 2019). Therefore, the context in which the term "policy" is used must be considered in order to identify the intended significance (Porche 2012). In addition, health policy is concerned not only with healthcare provision but also with environmental and socioeconomic effects on health. Health policy helps to clarify priorities; it establishes roles and expectations for different groups, whether physicians, nurses, or administrators. The health policy process also helps to build a consensus among the different participants in a community or a health system. Purposeful policy decisions represent a response to an issue that commands authority and impacts practice (Milstead 2013). Health policy decisions offer guidance in developing and evaluating regulatory systems.

Regulations and legislation, in turn, promote high-quality care by defining the scope and standard of practice, licensure, credentials, and education requirements of the nursing profession (ICN 2013). Internationally, regulations and legislation for APNs are variable and, in many cases, absent. Health policy and resulting regulatory mechanisms identifying title protection, standardized education, and competencies have been found to improve role clarity and APN implementation. Conversely, absence of regulation contributes to lack of role clarity and variability in how APNs are integrated into the healthcare workforce. Thus, the lack of health policy to acknowledge and guide APN workforce integration can have a negative impact on effective role implementation and sustainability (Bryant-Lukosius and Wong 2019).

Nurses in roles across health systems and community settings are well-positioned to assess individuals, communities, and populations; advocate for justice and equality; and partner with legislators and interprofessional leaders to identify, implement, and evaluate a "strengths-based approach" that engages communities. Health policy that influences regulations and legislation determines what nursing professionals can do, how they do it, and what they are paid. This becomes increasingly important as APNs seek to define this category of nursing.

Health policies and how they are implemented shape the direction of healthcare delivery. However, too often, data and narrative accounts confirm that health policy relevant to APNs, such as implementation of legislation, regulations, and a professional standard, are missing in national initiatives, resulting in adverse consequences. Practice environments are not always well prepared to welcome APNs. Healthcare decision-makers frequently do not understand the APN concept. APNs are struggling to be recognized, to establish appropriate practice standards, and to decide on what education is required in order to have their scope of practice legitimized and fully utilized in healthcare systems globally.

In order to align APNs as a significant solution to closing the gaps and addressing the challenges in the provision of healthcare services worldwide, supportive health policy guidance should be implemented for optimal workforce integration (Rosa et al. 2020; De Raeve et al. 2023; Schober 2016). In countries where there are policies in place, the guidelines and procedures should be reviewed to assess if there is a need for improvement. The field of advanced practice nursing is dynamic and constantly changing. Health policies that were relevant a decade ago might be considered out of date or inadequate in the current healthcare environment.

3 Establishing a Professional Identity and a Professional Standard

Advanced practice nurses are skilled in assessing individuals, families, and community health needs. Their education prepares them to provide integrated care that includes health promotion and disease management. In order to provide these services, health policies supportive of their optimal effectiveness need to be considered. This section identifies issues that significantly impact optimal APN practice and recognition of this level of nursing.

3.1 Title Protection

Designation of what title to use in reference to the nurse with advanced practice credentials is fundamental when proceeding with an APN initiative in order to reduce confusion when introducing this new professional to the healthcare workforce. A clearly identifiable and legally protected title safeguards the public from unqualified practitioners who have neither the education nor the competencies indicated by the title. The designated title refers to a certain level of confidence with respect to accountability and the healthcare services that this professional can provide. Once there is consensus on a title, the additional policies that guide the APN definition, scope of practice, competencies, and professional standards can be developed relevant to the title. A representative and legally protected title is the quickest method to communicate to other healthcare professionals, managers, administrators, clinical staff, and the public who these healthcare professionals are and what services they provide (Rosa et al. 2020; Schober 2017).

Absence of a legally protected title leads to lack of role clarity and confusion when seeking to promote the APN concept (De Raeve et al. 2023; Donald et al.

2010). This poses a barrier to role integration for a recognizable clinical position that integrates APNs into the healthcare workforce.

3.2 Scope of Practice

A defined APN scope of practice describes the range of activities related to recognized professional responsibilities that are consistent with boundaries imposed by regulations relevant to the context and setting in which the APN practices. APN scope of practice statements define what an APN can do, what population can be seen or treated, and under what circumstances the APN can provide care. The scope of practice provides guidance and direction to other healthcare professionals, educators, regulatory authorities, and the public. Once defined, the scope of practice and associated competencies are linked to a designated title and form the foundation for developing APN education and curricula.

In addition, an established APN scope of practice is one way of informing the public, administrators, and other healthcare professionals about the role in order to differentiate the qualified APN from other nurses who do not have the qualifications to be identified as an APN or have not been authorized to practice in this capacity. Specifying an APN scope of practice also assists governmental agencies, healthcare planners, and healthcare institutions with workforce planning that integrates the APN.

A scope of practice can originate from a professional association or organization as a health policy guideline or from a regulatory body as a legal requirement. In defining a scope of practice for the APN, challenges arise when there is a resistance to progress beyond the generic definition of nursing when developing a standard that emphasizes an advanced level of knowledge, competencies, clinical judgement, and decision-making that APNs bring to their practice setting.

3.3 Prescriptive Authority

Prescriptive authority is an issue that fuels animated debate when seeking health policy and regulation that supports this feature of APN practice. The discussion focuses on the changes in the boundaries of nursing practice and the impact this change has on other healthcare professions, usually a concern that it will impinge on the professional role of physicians. The degree of authority and the type of limitations placed on APN prescribing vary across jurisdictions. Approaches to APN prescriptive authority are mirrored in the wider debate on the APN role and level of practice, and reflect the confusion that surrounds APN evolution, definition, and regulation worldwide. The establishment of policies and legal authority may lag behind the reality of actual clinical practice. If advancement in nursing is to take place, prescriptive authority seems a requisite for optimal clinical practice. Consistency in criteria and education for APN prescribing, in turn, enhances credibility for APN scope of practice and requires clear health policy guidelines and regulations.

3.4 Education Criteria: Program Accreditation

Education criteria for the APN provide the basis for establishing credibility for the advancement of this nursing role and level of practice. However, a survey of European countries reported variation in entry requirements for participants of APN education programs (De Raeve et al. 2023). The integrity of APNs for the future will continue to rely on consistency for entry-level criteria to begin designated APN programs. In addition, health policy guidelines require criteria for curricula content specific and appropriate to the defined APN scope of practice. When a consistent standard for APN education is lacking, the issue of lack of role clarity and acceptance in the healthcare workforce continues to be questionable. This variability and inconsistency jeopardize the future of quality care and limit professional mobility and contributions of APN expertise (De Raeve et al. 2023). APN development would benefit from a consistent and aligned education pathway.

3.5 Credentialing the APN: Certification/Endorsement/Licensure/Registration

Health policy decisions most often guide or determine APN credentialing. Credentialing processes and procedures refer to the mechanisms that officially regulate APN practice. This can include, but is not limited to, the assignment of degrees, authorization, endorsement, certification, licensure, accreditation, and registration. The methods and processes are usually connected to a country's regulatory traditions and agency resources, in addition to what level is determined to be necessary to authorize a nurse to work within a scope of practice for an APN but beyond the scope of practice for a generalist nurse. The significance of APN participation in these health policy decisions is heightened as these topics contribute to the way advanced practice nursing is defined and put into practice (Schober 2016). The following are the ways APN credentialing occurs (Schober 2016; Hanson and Cahill 2019):

Certification enables an individual to demonstrate that specific predetermined standards have been met. Regulatory bodies may use identifiable certification processes from professional associations as well as governmental bodies to determine APN certification.

Endorsement, when used as a requirement for advanced practice, stipulates criteria that must be met to be eligible to be endorsed as an APN. Completion of the endorsement process authorizes the APN to function in an advanced clinical role.

Licensure often includes title protection, defines the qualifications, and restricts certain practice authority to nurses holding the license. It involves the application of validation processes to ensure the nurse is safe to practice in the specified scope of practice and has met predetermined standards.

Registration lists an individual's name in an official register for persons who possess specific qualifications. The register is maintained by the regulatory or other official governmental body. This is a method of identifying APNs but is not a validation of competence.

Credentialing can be considered mandatory or voluntary based on the established professional standard and requirements for the APN in the country and/or region. Whichever process is selected, identifying credentialing and professional regulation is significant in supporting the legitimacy of APNs within healthcare systems and the healthcare workforce.

4 A Rising Tide Raises All Boats

Aside from improvements in access to healthcare services (NASEM NAM Committee on the Future of Nursing 2020–2030 2021; AANP 2025), enhancing quality of care (AANP 2025; Kilpatrick et al. 2024), improved satisfaction with healthcare options (Kilpatrick et al. 2024; AANP 2025), and effective cost savings (Kilpatrick et al. 2024; Fajarini et al. 2025), the integration of APNs into healthcare systems offers additional benefits. The literature demonstrates that when nurses are educated at an advanced level to become APNs and when they receive appropriate regulatory as well as legislative support, there are beneficial outcomes to the healthcare systems where they practice. In addition, this progression benefits the nursing profession. The presence of nurses in roles or levels of practice that are considered advanced practice nursing has:

- Improved nurse recruitment and retention rates through the provision of additional career development pathways and career ladders (De Raeve et al. 2023; Buchan et al. 2013; Rakhab et al. 2021)
- Improved knowledge mobilization into systems, fostering the adherence to clinical guidelines and evidence-informed practice (McDonnell et al. 2012; Pol-Castañeda et al. 2022)
- Safeguarded patient-centered care through shared decision-making and adherence to components of a nursing model of care (Bales et al. 2025; Kinchen 2022)
- Led to innovations in healthcare delivery, such as telehealth, walk-in centers, mobile healthcare services, and implementation of quality improvement measures (Costa et al. 2025; Charalambous et al. 2024; Desborough et al. 2012; Harvard Medical School 2025; Higgins et al. 2025; Bakerjian 2022)
- Resulted in innovative teaching models, such as distance/hybrid education, utilization of simulation, and competency-based education (FNU 2025; Campbell et al. 2022; Lewis et al. 2022; ICM 2024)

Often these outcomes are unseen or unrecognized by administrations and key interested parties (stakeholders), but they align well with the recognized need for nursing to evolve and meet the increased leadership demands of evolving systems of healthcare delivery. Numerous organizations inside and outside of nursing have called on nurses to consider positions of leadership that include their skills of pivotal decision-making that could enhance healthcare services and promote the agenda for universal healthcare for the world's populations (WHO 2020; ICN 2024; PAHO, WHO, and McMaster University 2015). APNs are uniquely qualified to meet the challenge and actively contribute to the policy processes.

5 Health Policy and the Future APN

Health policy will continue to drive consumers' decisions, healthcare funding, research, and identification of professionals in the healthcare workforce. If APNs consider themselves to be an option in the provision of healthcare services for the future, they must be involved in developing and improving health policy. This will require skilled leadership and evidence-informed decisions based on research. Advocating for change requires APNs participation in the health policy process by educating themselves, supporting progressive initiatives, and promoting legislative activities that pursue health policy change that impacts their practice. In addition, this includes educating others within and outside of the healthcare arena. APNs in the future will continue to be challenged to influence health policy and actively guide development in order to respond to opposition, overcome barriers, and ensure that their scope of practice is expanded across all healthcare settings (Harris 2023; Rosa et al. 2020).

6 Conclusion

Understanding the significance and manner in which health policy impacts APN practice is fundamental for the progression of advanced practice nursing as a profession. The rapid proliferation of technology and complex global healthcare needs mandates that APNs comprehend the impact of health policy decisions and their relevance to potential and optimal clinical practice. This chapter describes the importance of this knowledge and identifies the issues that require supportive health policy decision-making. The need for APN participation in policy processes is emphasized. In addition, educational curricula for APN programs should prepare students to actively engage in health policy processes that significantly influence their future careers. The case has been made for the necessity to establish health policies to promote legislation and regulations supportive of APNs. However, the barriers and challenges are many, requiring knowledgeable and skilled APNs to participate in updating and promoting relevant health policies.

References

American Association of Nurse Practitioners (AANP). Literature of nurse practitioner cost effectiveness. AANP; 2025. https://www.aanp.org/advocacy/advocacy-resource/position-statements/nurse-practitioner-cost-effectiveness. Accessed 9 May 2025.

Bakerjian D. The advanced practice registered nurse leadership role in nursing homes: leading efforts toward high quality and safe care. Nurs Clin North Am. 2022;57(2):245–58. https://doi.org/10.1016/j.cnur.2022.02.011. Epub 2022 May 4. PMID: 35659986; PMCID: PMC9066344.

Bales G, Hasemann W, Kressig RW, et al. Scope of practice, competencies and impact of advanced practice nurses within APN-led models of care for young and middle-aged adult patients with multimorbidity and/or complex chronic conditions in hospital settings: a scoping review. BMJ Open. 2025;15:e091170. https://doi.org/10.1136/bmjopen-2024-091170.

Barton D, East L. The evolution of advanced nursing practice. In: Barton DT, Allan D, editors. Advanced nursing practice: changing healthcare in a changing world. New York: Palgrave Macmillan; 2015. p. 1–20.

Bryant-Lukosius D, Wong FKY. International development of advanced practice nursing. In: Tracy MF, O'Grady ET, editors. Advanced practice nursing: an integrative approach. 6th ed. St. Louis: Elsevier; 2019. p. 129–41.

Buchan J, Temido M, Fronteira I, Lapao L, Dussault G. Nurses in advanced roles: a review of acceptability in Portugal. Rev Lat-Am Enferm. 2013;21(Spec):38–46.

Campbell SH, Nye C, Hébert SH, Short C, Thomas MH. Simulation as a disruptive innovation in advanced practice nursing programs: a report from a qualitative examination. Clin Simul Nurs. 2022;61:79–85. https://doi.org/10.1016/j.ecns.2021.08.001.

Charalambous J, Hollingdrake O, Currie J. Nurse practitioner led telehealth services: a scoping review. J Clin Nurs. 2024;33:839–58. https://doi.org/10.1111/jocn.16898.

Costa ICP, Costa AS, Garbuio DC, Namarioli CM, Eduardo AHA, Carvalho EC, Chaves ECL. Telehealth in patient care by advanced practice nurses: a systematic review. Acta Paul Enferm. 2025;38:eAPE0003141.

De Raeve P, Davidson PM, Bergs J, Patch M, Jack SM, Castro-Ayala A, et al. Advanced practice nursing in Europe: results from a pan-European survey of 35 countries. J Adv Nurs. 2023;80(1):377–86. https://onlinelibrary.wiley.com/doi/10.1111/jan.15775.

Desborough J, Forrest L, Parker R. Nurse-led primary healthcare walk-in centres: an integrative literature review. J Adv Nurs. 2012;68:248–63. https://doi.org/10.1111/j.1365-2648.2011.05798.x.

Donald F, Bryant-Lukosius D, Martin-Misener R, Kaasalainen S, Kilpatrick K, Carter N, et al. Clinical nurse specialists and nurse practitioners: title confusion and lack off role clarity. Can J Nurs Leadersh. 2010;23(Special Issue):189–210.

Fajarini M, Setiawan A, Sung CM, Chen R, Liu D, Lee CK, Niu SF, Chou KR. Effects of advanced practice nurses on health-care costs, quality of care, and patient well-being: a meta-analysis of randomized controlled trials. Int J Nurs Stud. 2025;162:104953. https://doi.org/10.1016/j.ijnurstu.2024.104953. Epub 2024 Nov 14. PMID: 39586168.

Frontier Nursing University (FNU). History of FNU. FNU; 2025. https://frontier.edu/about-frontier/history-of-fnu/. Accessed 9 May 2025.

Hanson CM, Cahill M. Understanding regulatory, legal and credentialing requirements. In: Tracy MF, O'Grady ET, editors. Advanced practice nursing: an integrative approach. 6th ed. St. Louis: Elsevier; 2019. p. 563–84.

Harris JL. Turning health policy into practice. In: Goudreau KQ, Smolenski MC, editors. Health policy and advanced practice nursing. 3rd ed. New York: Springer Publishing Company LLC; 2023. p. 3–11.

Harvard Medical School. Mobile clinic impact tracker. Author; 2025. https://www.mobilehealthmap.org/our-impact/. Accessed 9 May 2025.

Higgins A, Tilghman M, Lin TK. Mobile health clinics in a rural setting: a cost analysis and time motion study of La Clinica in Oregon, United States. BMC Health Serv Res. 2025;25(97):1–11. https://doi.org/10.1186/s12913-024-12203-5.

International Confederation of Midwives (ICM). ICM essential competencies for midwifery practice. ICM; 2024. https://internationalmidwives.org/resources/essential-competencies-for-midwifery-practice/. Accessed 9 May 2025.

International Council of Nurses (ICN). Nursing regulation. ICN; 2013. https://www.icn.ch/sites/default/files/inline-files/B04_Nsg_Regulation.pdf#:~:text=The%20International%20Council%20of%20Nurses%20%28ICN%29%20believes%20that,through%20establishing%2C%20promoting%20and%20enforcing%20standards%20of%20practice. Accessed 9 May 2025.

International Council of Nurses (ICN). Nursing and primary health care: towards the realization of universal health coverage. ICN; 2024. https://www.icn.ch/sites/default/files/2024-09/ICN_PHC-Report-2024_EN_FINAL.pdf. Accessed 9 May 2025.

Kilpatrick K, Savard I, Audet LA, Costanzo G, Khan M, Atallah R, Jabbour M, Zhou W, Wheeler K, Ladd E, Gray DC, Henderson C, Spies LA, McGrath H, Rogers M. A global perspective of advanced practice nursing research: a review of systematic reviews. PLoS One. 2024;19(7):e0305008. https://doi.org/10.1371/journal.pone.0305008. PMID: 38954675; PMCID: PMC11218965.

Kinchen E. Holistic nurse practitioner care including promotion of shared decision-making. J Holist Nurs. 2022;40(4):326–35. https://doi.org/10.1177/08980101211062704.

Lewis LS, Rebeschi LM, Hunt E. Nursing education practice update 2022: competency-based education in nursing. SAGE Open Nurs. 2022;8:23779608221140774. https://doi.org/10.1177/23779608221140774. PMID: 36437897; PMCID: PMC9685206.

Maier C, Aiken L, Busse R. Nurses in advanced roles in primary care: policy levers for implementation. OECD Health Working Paper No. 98. OECD; 2017. https://www.oecd-ilibrary.org/docserver/a8756593-en.pdf?expires=1730501813&id=id&accname=guest&checksum=88FB4DFAF15F9DA8FBB2D5681C2B0444. Accessed 9 May 2025.

McDonnell A, Gerrish K, Kirshbaum MN, Nolan M, Tod A, Guillaume L. The perceived impact of advanced practice nurses (APNs) on promoting evidence-based practice amongst front-line nurses: findings from a collective case study. J Res Nurs. 2012;18(4):368–83. https://doi.org/10.1177/1744987112446241.

McGee P. Influences on the development of advanced nursing practice in the UK. In: McGee P, Inman C, editors. Advanced practice in healthcare: dynamics developments in nursing and allied health professions. 4th ed. Oxford: Wiley Blackwell; 2019. p. 65–84.

Milstead JA. Health policy and politics: a nurse's guide. 4th ed. Upper Saddle River: Jones & Bartlett; 2013.

National Academies of Sciences, Engineering, and Medicine (NASEM); National Academy of Medicine (NAM); Committee on the Future of Nursing 2020–2030. The role of nurses in improving health care quality. In: Flaubert JL, Le Menestrel S, Williams DR, et al., editors. The future of nursing 2020–2030. Charting a path to achieve health equity. National Academies Press (U.S.); 2021. p. 99–126. https://www.ncbi.nlm.nih.gov/books/NBK573910/. Accessed 9 May 2025.

Pan American Health Organization (PAHO), World Health Organization (WHO), and McMaster University. Report on universal access to health and universal health coverage: Advanced practice nursing summit. 2015. https://www.paho.org/sites/default/files/2023-04/150415-report-advanced-practice-nursing-summit-hamilton.pdf. Accessed 9 May 2025.

Pol-Castañeda S, Rodriguez-Calero MA, Villafáfila-Gomila CJ, et al. Impact of advanced practice nurses in hospital units on compliance with clinical practice guidelines: a quasi-experimental study. BMC Nurs. 2022;21:331. https://doi.org/10.1186/s12912-022-01110-x.

Porche DJ. Health policy: application for nurses and other healthcare professionals. 1st ed. Sudbury: Jones & Bartlett Learning; 2012.

Rakhab A, Jackson C, Butterworth T, Kane R. Factors supporting career pathway development amongst advanced practice nurses in Thailand: a cross-sectional survey. Int J Nurs Stud. 2021;117:103882. https://doi.org/10.1016/j.ijnurstu.2021.103882.

Rosa WE, Fitzgerald M, Davis S, Khanyola J, Kwong J, Moreland PJ, et al. Leveraging nurse practitioner capacities to achieve global health for all: COVID-19 and beyond. Int Nurs Rev. 2020;67(4):554–9. https://doi.org/10.1111/inr.12632.

Schober M. Introduction to advanced nursing practice: an international focus. Geneva: Springer Nature; 2016.

Schober M. Strategic planning for advanced nursing practice. Geneva: Springer Nature; 2017.

World Health Organization (WHO). State of the world's nursing 2020: investing in education, jobs and leadership. WHO; 2020. https://www.who.int/publications/i/item/9789240003279. Accessed 9 May 2025.

World Health Organization (WHO). Global strategic directives for nursing and midwifery 2021–2025. WHO; 2021. https://www.who.int/publications/i/item/9789240033863. Accessed 9 May 2025.

Advanced Practice Nursing Health Policy: Looking Back, Looking Forward

Madrean Schober

1 Introduction

Development of health policy relevant to advanced practice nursing has evolved over time, along with a transformation in the emerging professional identity of advanced practice nurses (APN). It is a paradigm shift in the perception of nursing practice for nurses themselves, other healthcare professionals, policymakers, and the public. This progression is more than a socialization process promoting expanded nursing practice. Reviewing the formation and development of a professional identity as an APN highlights the complex history of nursing and the nature of how advanced practice nursing has evolved.

Pioneer nurses ventured into advanced levels of practice prior to discussions of formal health policy. The experiences of these nurses as they carved out advanced clinical practice in diverse settings have guided contemporary APN development and provided the basis for our current thinking. An awareness of the historical perspective of APN development provides a foundation for effecting change in health policy that impacts future APN practice.

2 Background

It could be said that individuals, currently identified as nurses, have been seeking advancement as caring healthcare professionals since the time of Florence Nightingale, when she provided treatment and support for soldiers during the Crimean War (Sheer 2023). Additional early narratives provide examples of

M. Schober (✉)
Schober Global Healthcare Consulting, Indianapolis, IN, USA
e-mail: madreans@gmail.com

K. J. Wheeler, M. Acorn (eds.), *Health Policy for Advanced Practice Nursing: A Toolkit for Implementation and Improvement*, Advanced Practice in Nursing,
https://doi.org/10.1007/978-3-032-03667-4_3

individuals who identified a need and responded with the provision of healthcare that would later be described as nursing.

In the Kingdom of Saudi Arabia, Rufaida Al-Asalmiya, the daughter of a physician, born around 620 AD, is considered to be the first Islamic nurse providing care and support during the Holy Wars (Rothwell 2023). In Botswana, women took care of the sick at home as part of their household responsibilities, preceding the establishment of nursing as on-the-job hospital-based training in 1925 (Gray et al. 2023). In the USA, as early as 1893, public health models were emerging focused on disease and prevention of disease, especially to underserved and vulnerable populations (Sheer 2023). Similar stories of caring for various aspects of societal health needs resulted in establishment of nursing schools and education of nursing skills. Ultimately, this progression and advancement have led to the discussion of advanced practice nursing that we are having today.

3 Defining Categories of Advanced Nursing Practice

Advanced nursing practice and advanced practice nursing can be seen as overarching terms that embrace distinct categories of advanced nursing practice. Lacking an international consensus on terminology, titles such as advanced practice nurse (APN), nurse practitioner (NP), and clinical nurse specialist (CNS) at times are interchanged, even though country-specific descriptions vary. In addition, nurse anesthetists and nurse midwives are considered to be advanced practice nurses.

The USA identifies advanced practice registered nurses (APRN) as certified registered nurse anesthetists, certified nurse midwives, clinical nurse specialists, and certified nurse practitioners (APRN Consensus Work Group, National Council of State Boards of Nursing APRN Advisory Committee 2008). Even though some characteristics of advanced clinical practice for nurses might overlap, there are distinct differences in the history and development of these APN categories.

This section comprises select aspects of the historical origins of four established APN roles: nurse anesthetists, clinical nurse specialists, nurse midwives, and nurse practitioners.

3.1 Nurse Anesthetists

There is limited documentation of early nurse anesthesia practice and education, except in the USA. The roots of nurse anesthesia in the USA can be traced to the late nineteenth century, soon after the use of gases to induce unconsciousness was discovered (Lusk et al. 2019). Additional narratives described instances where nurses were giving anesthesia as early as the American Civil War (1861–1865). One account described a nurse ministering to the wounded using “chloroform and stimulants.” There were concerns of possible risks, but nurses typically administered anesthesia only when a physician was unavailable, often in a private house when the nurse was the only qualified person in attendance (Lusk et al. 2019).

Once early anesthesia was noted in the USA, the idea traveled quickly to Europe and worldwide (Reisen et al. 2023). Nurse anesthesia was supported by an early reluctance of physicians to engage in this practice. In addition, a shortage of qualified anesthesiologists also promoted the idea of nurses providing anesthesia in a number of countries. As the scientific and specialized nature of giving anesthesia increased and became more sophisticated, the practice became more the entitlement of physicians.

In the beginning, nurse anesthesia was not considered to be a specialty but part of nursing education. Nurse anesthesia education developed from on-the-job education progressing to a profession with a systematic, formalized, tertiary education of today. However, the beginning responsibility and documentation of anesthesia were with the surgeons, while administering anesthesia was delegated to nurses who met the requirements to fulfill this role. The progression to postgraduate education began in the mid-twentieth century (Reisen et al. 2023).

Nurse anesthesia remained invisible for a long time, but the practice developed as nurses refined their skills and knowledge, subsequently emerging as a postgraduate specialty (Reisen et al. 2023). Nurses providing anesthesia have established a credible identity measured against international education standards developed by experts in the field, imparting confidence to policymakers and the public (ICN 2021).

The International Federation of Nurse Anesthetists (IFNA) is committed to supporting the advancement of education and practices that support quality nurse anesthesia care worldwide. Founded in 1989, IFNA is the recognized international voice for nurse anesthesia and wider for all nonphysician anesthesia providers (IFNA 2021; Rod 2023). Further details and publications, including a list of member nations and country exemplars, can be accessed at https://ifna.site.

3.2 Clinical Nurse Specialists

The clinical nurse specialist (CNS) is an advanced practice nursing role that emerged to provide advanced nursing care to specialty populations. The role evolved out of the increasing complexity of nursing care, with the term specialist in nursing traced to the early twentieth century. In addition, early roots of the CNS reside in the need for improved psychiatric nursing (Lusk et al. 2019). The CNS level of practice was frequently established before a formal definition or title was used. In addition, some countries use titles such as nurse consultant or senior specialist in referring to a nurse that is similar to the CNS in reference to specialized clinical practice (Chan and Holly 2021).

In the USA, the idea of an expert clinical nurse emerged in the 1940s and further progressed to use of the term clinical nurse specialist with a minimum of master's level preparation. Nursing leaders recognized that nursing needed expert nurses at the bedside to lead the advancement of nursing. Additional countries in the late 1990s and 2000s focused on the establishment of the CNS role. In 1996, Japan began certifying CNSs with the formation of the Japanese Association for CNSs. Finland first implemented the CNS role in 2001, and the presence of the CNS is growing even though the role is not title protected or regulated (Chan and Holly 2021).

CNS practice has evolved on distinct timelines and with diverse approaches in different countries. No one definition exists globally, but all definitions require two criteria: Education is recommended at the graduate level, and the specified expertise is in a specialty area of nursing. The authority to practice is determined by professional and legal regulation (Chan and Holly 2021).

The CNS role emerged as a response to the societal need for improved and advanced nursing care usually within hospital settings. The call for expert nurses, such as the CNS, continues to exist today. As with other levels of advanced nursing practice, educational and regulatory support is essential to fully implement the role and successfully integrate CNSs into the healthcare workforce. Common concerns include title protection, defining scope of practice, and identifying core competencies and education criteria. Creating a strategic plan for health policy is viewed as imperative in creating incremental and positive change (Chan and Holly 2021).

3.3 Nurse Midwives

Midwives have practiced since the beginning of time (Lusk et al. 2019). Midwifery is considered a unique profession distinct from nursing and medicine but is combined with nursing in some countries. Over time, midwifery has evolved from individuals with limited preparation to a more sophisticated professional standard today (Avery and Saftner 2019). In many countries, midwifery may be regulated as a distinct profession; this chapter uses "nurse-midwife" only where it is a legally defined nursing-based advanced practice role. Where midwifery is distinct, ICM (International Confederation of Midwives) standards apply. Although globally midwifery and nurse-midwifery represent dissimilar definitions and preparation, the common premise is providing care for women during pregnancy and birth. Over time, practice in some countries includes a broader scope, including more comprehensive care for women over their life span (Avery and Saftner 2019).

As childbirth became more medicalized in the late nineteenth and early twentieth centuries, midwifery lost some of the public's favor. With the rise of scientific medicine and the beginning use of anesthesia with childbirth, upper- and middle-class women began to request obstetricians to deliver their babies in hospital delivery rooms, while women continued to also access the care of midwives. As a result, physicians, especially in the USA, took over the role of birth attendant, which led to a decrease in the use of midwives. Physicians in many countries continue to regulate the practice of nurse-midwifery today (Avery and Saftner 2019).

Midwifery remained part of mainstream healthcare in many European, Asian, and African countries, with a rebirth of midwifery in the USA in 1920, along with growth in nurse-midwifery practice in the 1940s and 1950s. Nurse-midwifery continues to evolve and has a broader scope of practice now than it did 90 years ago (Avery and Saftner 2019). Consistent with APN guidelines, nurse-midwives accept responsibility and accountability for their practice as primary healthcare professionals (Avery and Saftner 2019). Since the early 1980s, the American College of Nurse-Midwives, a professional association representing certified nurse-midwives and certified midwives, has established global outreach initiatives that support midwifery worldwide (http://midwife.org).

Certified Nurse Midwives in the USA are educated in the two disciplines of nursing and midwifery. They must earn a master's degree and pass a national certification exam. Ireland identifies the advanced nurse practitioner (ANP) and the advanced midwife practitioner (AMP) separately with two main titles. The titles are protected by law and must be registered with the Nursing and Midwifery Board of Ireland. A master's degree or higher is required (Lehwaldt and Lockwood 2023). The presence of nurse-midwives are context dependent roles that exist in some jurisdictions. Positive advances in nurse-midwifery and its relationship to the broader healthcare systems continue to evolve. The need for more midwives and nurse-midwives has been recognized internationally in the effort to continue to reduce maternal and neonatal mortality. Increasingly, nurse-midwives are engaged in collaborative policy efforts in order to shape the evolving nature of this field of practice (ACNM n.d.).

3.4 Nurse Practitioners

The nurse practitioner (NP) concept is usually associated with the idea of advanced practice nurses providing primary care services. NPs commonly provide care through diagnosis and treatment of healthcare concerns as well as a focus on disease prevention and health management (Sheer 2023; Lusk et al. 2019). As early as the late nineteenth century, during an era of rapid industrialization and social reform in the USA, public health nurses were providing aspects of what is today viewed as NP practice. In the UK, the NP concept was viewed as a role suitable for experienced nurses who could enhance patient care through the development of health assessment and diagnostic skills (Rogers and Gloster 2023). The early beginnings of advanced nursing in Canada date back to the 1890s, when outpost nurses worked in isolated areas and became more formalized in the 1960s. Even though the NP role was emerging at this time, initial legislation to enact the NP role did not occur until 1996 (Miller et al. 2023).

During the 1960s, the NP role was first described formally as a response to a shortage of primary care physicians in the USA In addition, there was a trend toward medical specialization with physicians moving away from clinical practice in primary care. At the same time, consumers were requesting accessible and affordable healthcare services (Sheer 2023; Lusk et al. 2019).

The identification of the origin of contemporary NP practice is often attributed to the description and formal implementation of the concept in outpatient pediatric clinics in the USA. The inception of the first pediatric NP (PNP) education program was launched by Loretta Ford, RN and Henry Silver, MD, at the University of Colorado in 1965 (Sheer 2023; Lusk et al. 2019). The program was designed to prepare professional nurses to provide comprehensive well-child care and manage common childhood health concerns.

NP clinical practice is viewed as integrating characteristics commonly associated with medicine, thus contributing to issues of interprofessional conflict as the role progressed. Although marked by early confrontations with medicine and other nurses when defining the role and level of practice, there was significant growth in the number of NPs. In addition, in the 1980s, new types of NPs emerged in fields of emergency, neonatal, and family practice. Even though the founders had envisioned NPs practicing in mainly outpatient or out-of-hospital settings, NPs with specialty preparation were increasingly present in tertiary settings such as neonatal intensive care units (Lusk et al. 2019).

In the decades following the launching of the first formal NP education program in 1965 in the USA, the number of NPs increased dramatically with clinical practice taking place in diverse settings in addition to pediatrics. Education progressed from achieving a diploma or certificate to the required completion of a master's degree, with increasing support to achieve a DNP (doctorate of nursing practice). The nature of NP practice with a focus on primary care led to a visible move to actively pursue regulations and legislation in support of increased autonomy that included prescriptive authority (Sheer 2023).

International interest in the NP concept began gaining momentum in the 1990s when a nurse from the UK attended an NP program in the USA, eventually resulting in the development of an NP program at the Royal College of Nursing in London. Following increased interest in the USA and UK a decision to hold international NP collaborative conferences followed in 1993 with an increased presence of additional nations. These collective efforts led to the launching of the ICN NP/APN Network in 2001 (Sheer 2023).

Over time, as these categories of advanced nursing practice have emerged and progressed, each area of expertise has had to deal with resistance from other nurses who saw these roles as developing outside of nursing. Each of the APN classifications faced intraprofessional struggles within the context of change. The respective levels of advanced practice challenged not only overlapping boundaries with medicine but the status quo of the nursing establishment and healthcare systems (Lusk et al. 2019). As these fields of advanced nursing practice continue to progress, the establishment of relevant health policy continues to be increasingly important.

4 Beginnings: Variations in Advanced Practice Nursing Evolution

Globally, the evolution of nursing and development of advanced practice nursing has notably been in response to population healthcare needs (Delamaire and LaFortune 2010; Maier et al. 2017; Woo et al. 2017). Even though there has been pride and enthusiasm over time for these accomplishments, there have been ongoing struggles to have the profession viewed in a positive light. In addition, key decision makers tend to underestimate the complexities of introducing a new nursing role and level of practice. Furthermore, the recognition and timeline of health policy supporting the advancement of these nursing categories originate from different sources.

Nurses who ventured into APN roles and advanced levels of practice in the years prior to formal credentialing and regulation deserve to have their stories told. These narratives provide continuity that offers guidance and connection to current practice and thinking. Identifying aspects of this history reveals the progress that has been made, while also reminding us of the need to continue to effect policy change supportive of the emerging dimensions of APN (Lusk et al. 2019). The trajectory of nurses who introduced APN roles and levels of practice prior to formal legislation and regulations set the stage for ongoing policy development.

Early APN concepts emerged in Canada as outpost nurses in the 1890s worked in isolated areas of the country (Miller et al. 2023). In the 1960s, the APN concept became more formalized with the development of an NP program preparing nurses to work in remote settings (Kaasalainen et al. 2010). This was followed by recommendations for legislative changes for advanced practice and university programs to educate NPs for urban and rural practice settings. However, by 1983, most programs were closed due to a lack of legislation, absence of compensation mechanisms, perceived oversupply of physicians in urban areas, limited awareness of the role by the public, and other healthcare professionals. Healthcare reform in the 1990s resulted in renewed interest in role development, along with a more robust approach to legislation and regulation (Miller et al. 2023). Canada today recognizes and identifies the CNS and NP with Advanced Practice Nursing: A Pan-Canadian Framework (CNA 2019).

In Jamaica, a response to the need for enhanced healthcare services included the introduction of NPs in 1977. There was no regulatory or legislative framework initially, and thus a lag in the presence of supportive health policies (McGrath 2023). In 2023, more than 40 years following the introduction of NP services, the Ministry of Health and Wellness for Jamaica announced amendments to the Nurses and Midwives Act and the Pharmacy Act to accommodate the registration and licensure of Advanced Practice Registered Nurses (Jamaica Ministry of Health and Wellness 2023).

In New Zealand (NZ), the Ministry of Health (MOH), looking at healthcare reform in the late 1990s, felt that the nursing workforce had more potential and was being underutilized. Central to the report was the priority to develop advanced clinical nursing roles, including nurse prescriber. It was determined that "nurse practitioner" would be a new scope of practice regulated by the Nursing Council of NZ. This was viewed as significant for protection of the NP role, allowing for regulation and legislation that resulted in revisions and updating over time. Even though this has been positive, there is a continued need for a national workforce policy to direct NP integration and improve healthcare equity for all populations of the country (Adams and Carryer 2023).

The Australian NP role began in the early 1990s with nursing leaders identifying the potential of nurses to address healthcare gaps, often in marginalized populations and contexts. Decades later, with substantial gains in the NP presence in the country, leaders and policymakers continue to work to synchronize legislation across all Australian jurisdictions. Strategic thinking and legislative reform continue to be essential as policy decision makers continue to address barriers to optimal NP practice (Helms and Boase 2023).

This section is intended to provide examples of how attention to APN policy occurs but does not include all nations that are engaged in development of health policy for APNs. Additional chapters in this book provide further in-depth coverage of national health policy initiatives and strategies. In addition, this section stresses that it is imperative to note that context often determines consideration of relevant policies and that active participation in the processes is ongoing.

4.1 Advanced Practice Nursing: From Inspiration to Reality

Despite increased international development comprehension of what advanced practice nursing represents varies from country to country, and even within countries. While there is impressive progress, the full potential of APN roles and level of practice have yet to be realized. APNs continue to be underutilized, despite clear evidence of their benefits to health systems worldwide (Delamaire and LaFortune 2010; Maier et al. 2017; Woo et al. 2017).

To ensure that populations worldwide have access to consistent, high-quality APN healthcare services, it is critical to enable effective workforce planning along with supportive health policy. Successful APN implementation and sustainability require:

- Increasing consistency and a consensus in role definition and level of clinical practice
- Informed development of educational curricula specific to APN practice
- Shaping government and organizational decisions supportive of optimal APN scope of practice
- Identifying and conducting ongoing research relevant to the APN concept

Exploring the historical perspective of APN development draws attention to the roots of insightful, responsive provision of caring healthcare, leading to a contemporary vision that continues to respond to societal needs. Evidence demonstrates that APNS provide safe, competent care (Delamaire and LaFortune 2010; Maier et al. 2017; Woo et al. 2017). In order to ensure public protection and the most advantageous APN healthcare services, it is essential to establish a health policy that includes definitive legislation, regulation, and a professional standard.

4.2 Strengthening Facilitators-Decreasing Barriers

Enthusiasm for the concept of advanced practice nursing roles and level of practice continues to grow worldwide. Nevertheless, there is a tendency for policy decision makers, healthcare administrators, and healthcare professionals themselves to underestimate the complexities of integrating APNs into the healthcare workforce.

Extensive literature demonstrates the value of the APN in diverse clinical settings, as well as identifying the facilitators and barriers that impact APN practice. However, there is a shortage of publications that pinpoint specific policies pivotal to successful and sustainable APN initiatives (Porat-Dahlerbruch et al. 2024). In addition, there is a need to recognize that individuals in positions of power and authority can facilitate or block interest in promoting APN roles and practice.

A core question emerges: What policy or policies can be implemented to maximize the effects of facilitators and minimize identified barriers?

Introducing APN roles alone does not directly translate to positive outcomes. Much of the existing literature focuses on identifying facilitators and barriers to effective integration of APNs (Porat-Dahlerbruch et al. 2024). This is useful, but successful integration requires identification and discussions of what specific policies can be implemented to maximize facilitators and minimize barriers. With increased attention and visibility worldwide, APNs no longer have the luxury of maintaining an invisible presence and contribution to the provision of healthcare services. There is a call to mobilize supporters, confront detractors and opposition, while also communicating and disseminating relatable information.

5 Conclusion

Early visionaries and pioneers of the APN concept envisioned a role and level of practice that promoted continuity of care for individuals and communities, while at the same time enhancing the professional status and career mobility for nursing. In the early years, informal and formal discussions seemed quite casual compared to the environment today. In the current healthcare milieu, there is increasing attention on health policy that contains regulations and legislation that officially codifies the APN concept, thus increasing professional credibility to the consumer, other healthcare professionals, and policymakers.

Over time, the concept of advanced practice nursing has progressed from a response to societal healthcare needs to an aspiration to achieve a global consensus on the dimensions of the role and this level of nursing practice. As the APN concept continues to evolve, there is an increasing need to continue to establish health policy that promotes clarity and credibility for this category of nursing but does not excessively restrict clinical practice. For the future sustainability of APN practice, a recognized professional standard based on a sound foundation of identifiable health policies that include legislation and regulation is essential. Lack of supportive health policy limits APN development and recognition.

Nations in the early stages of APN development are seeking guidance as they understand the necessity of health policies to guide APN implementation and future sustainability. It is imperative that APN leadership understand the contextual factors that influence health policy processes and contribute to policy decisions. To accomplish continued progress worldwide, APNs must actively participate in the decision-making based on an understanding of local, regional, and international standards, customs, and regulatory procedures that support or impede clinical practice. Consideration of strategic planning that includes use of a framework and a health policy toolkit could be instrumental in continuing to create incremental and positive change while shaping governmental and organizational decisions.

References

Adams S, Carryer J. The evolution and future of nurse practitioners in New Zealand. In: Thomas SL, Rowles JS, editors. Nurse practitioners and nurse anesthetists: the evolution of the global roles. Geneva: Springer Nature; 2023. p. 255–62.

American College of Nurse-Midwives (ACNM). ACNM's global outreach program: 2023 report. Author; n.d. https://annualreport.midwife.org/global-outreach/. Accessed 3 Aug 2025.

APRN Consensus Work Group, National Council of State Boards of Nursing APRN Advisory Committee. Consensus model for APRN regulation: licensure, accreditation, certification & education. Author; 2008. https://www.ncsbn.org>nursing-regulation>practice. Accessed 4 Jan 2024.

Avery MD, Saftner MA. The certified nurse-midwife. In: Tracy MS, O'Grady ET, editors. Hamric and Hanson's advanced practice nursing: an integrative approach. 6th ed. New York: Elsevier Inc.; 2019. p. 436–59.

Canadian Nurses Association (CNA). Advanced practice nursing: a Pan-Canadian framework. Author; 2019. https://hl-prod-ca-oc-download.s3-ca-central-1.amazonaws.com/CNA/2f975e7e-4a40-45ca-863c-5ebf0a138d5e/UploadedImages/documents/nursing/Advanced_Practice_Nursing_framework_e.pdf. Accessed 20 Jan 2023.

Chan GK, Holly VW. Global view of the clinical nurse specialist role. In: Fulton JS, Holly VW, editors. Clinical nurse specialist role and practice: an international perspective. Geneva: Springer Nature; 2021. p. 3–15.

Delamaire ML, LaFortune G. Nurses in advanced roles: a description and evaluation of experiences in 12 developed countries. OECD Health Working Papers No. 54. OECD Publishing; 2010. https://www.oecd.org/en/publications/nurses-in-advanced-roles_5kmbrcfms5g7-en.html. Accessed 3 Aug 2025.

Gray DC, Kgositau M, Lubinda-Sinombe G. The nurse practitioner role and practice in Botswana. In: Thomas SL, Rowles JS, editors. Nurse practitioners and nurse anesthetists: the evolution of the global roles. Geneva: Springer Nature; 2023. p. 225–34.

Helms C, Boase L. Transforming healthcare: the Australian nurse practitioner role. In: Thomas SL, Rowles JS, editors. Nurse practitioners and nurse anesthetists: the evolution of the global roles. Geneva: Springer Nature; 2023. p. 263–78.

International Council of Nurses (ICN). Guidelines on advanced practice nursing: nurse anesthetists. Author; 2021.

International Federation of Nurse Anesthetists (IFNA). In: Ouellette SM, Horton BJ, Rowles JS, editors. International Federation of Nurse Anesthetists (1989–2021): the global voice for nurse anesthetists. Author; 2021.

Jamaica Ministry of Health & Wellness. Parliamentary Statement of the Minister of Health & Wellness, Cabinet approval for amendments to the nurses and midwives act and the pharmacy act to accommodate the registration and licensure of advanced practice registered nurses. Press Release; 2023. https://www.moh.gov.jm/cabinet-gives-approval-for-prescriptive-rights-for-advanced-practice-registered-nurses/.

Kaasalainen S, Martin-Misener R, Kilpatrick K, Harbman P, Bryant-Lukosius D, Donald F, Carter N, DiCenso A. A historical overview of the development of advanced practice nursing roles in Canada. Nurs Leadersh (Tor Ont). 2010;23(Spec No 2010):35–60. https://doi.org/10.12927/cjnl.2010.22268. PMID: 21478686.

Lehwaldt D, Lockwood E. The nurse practitioner role in Ireland. In: Thomas SL, Rowles JS, editors. Nurse practitioners and nurse anesthetists: the evolution of the global roles. Geneva: Springer Nature; 2023. p. 197–206.

Lusk B, Cockerham AZ, Keeling AW. Highlights from the history of advanced practice nursing in the United States. In: Tracy MF, O'Grady MF, editors. Hamric and Hanson's advanced practice nursing: an integrative approach. 6th ed. Elsevier Inc.; 2019. p. 1–24.

Maier C, Aiken L, Busse R. Nurses in advanced roles in primary care: policy levers for implementation. OECD Health Working Papers No. 98. OECD Publishing; 2017. https://www.oecd.org/en/publications/nurses-in-advanced-roles-in-primary-care_a8756593-en.html. Accessed 3 Aug 2025.

McGrath H. The nurse practitioner role and practice in Jamaica. In: Thomas SL, Rowles JS, editors. Nurse practitioners and nurse anesthetists: The evolution of the global roles. Geneva: Springer Nature; 2023. p. 157–65.

Miller M, Prodan-Bhala N, Marchuk S. The NP role and practice in Canada. In: Thomas SL, Rowles JS, editors. Nurse practitioners and nurse anesthetists: the evolution of the global roles. Geneva: Springer Nature; 2023. p. 145–55.

Porat-Dahlerbruch J, Ratz S, Ellen M. Development of a taxonomy of policy interventions for integrating nurse practitioners into health systems. Int J Health Policy Manag. 2024;13:8194. https://doi.org/10.34172/ijhpm.2023.8194. Accessed 7 July 2024.

Reisen M, Hoekman J, Björkelund K. Global development of nurse anesthesia education from mid-nineteenth century into today's advanced nursing practice. In: Thomas SL, Rowles JS, editors. Nurse practitioners and nurse anesthetists: the evolution of the global roles. Geneva: Springer Nature; 2023. p. 343–65.

Rod P. The International Federation of Nurse Anesthetists: past, present, and future. In: Thomas SL, Rowles JS, editors. Nurse practitioners and nurse anesthetists: the evolution of the global roles. Geneva: Springer Nature; 2023. p. 331–42.

Rogers M, Gloster A. The evolution of the nurse practitioner role and practice in the United Kingdom. In: Thomas SL, Rowles JS, editors. Nurse practitioners and nurse anesthetists: the evolution of the global roles. Geneva: Springer Nature; 2023. p. 167–80.

Rothwell S. Advanced nursing practice in the Kingdom of Saudi Arabia. In: Thomas SL, Rowles JS, editors. Nurse practitioners and nurse anesthetists: the evolution of the global roles. Geneva: Springer Nature; 2023. p. 287–92.

Sheer B. Evolution in healthcare: the journey from a US demonstration project to an international concept. In: Thomas SL, Rowles JS, editors. Nurse practitioners and nurse anesthetists: the evolution of the global roles. Geneva: Springer Nature; 2023. p. 3–39.

Woo BFY, Lee JXY, Tam WS. The impact of the advanced practice nursing role on quality of care, clinical outcomes, patient satisfaction, and cost in the emergency and critical care settings: a systematic review. Hum Resour Health. 2017;15(1):63. https://doi.org/10.1186/s12960-017-0237-9. Accessed 3 Aug 2025.

Foundations for Health Policy Implementation and Improvement

Theoretical Foundations and Frameworks for Health Policy Implementation and Improvement

Kathy J. Wheeler and Garrett K. Chan

1 Introduction

Considerable policy implementation for advanced practice nurses (APNs) has occurred incrementally, often by circumstance and serendipity, sometimes bottom-up, sometimes top down, sometimes by intuition. However, policy implementation and improvement science does exist, and it can provide structure and guidance to those wanting more direction about the process for successful policy implementation. Eccles et al. (2005, p. 1) stated the application of research was often "an expensive version of trial and error." What seemed to be missing in the process was the application of theoretical foundations and structures. In a time when cost-effectiveness is an important metric of an evolving, improving healthcare system, any action that improves cost-effective implementation is worth study and consideration. These guiding structures consist of theories, models, frameworks, and guidelines (TMFGs). This chapter is devoted to simple presentations of several TMFGs that have or can be applied to policy implementation or improvement for APNs. This chapter can also serve as a springboard to the consideration, selection, and application of theoretical foundations that streamline policy implementation and improvement. As this is a limited list and discussion the reader is encouraged to adapt and explore as needed for the policy and research work they are undertaking, and also be open to exploring other theoretical foundations. The reader is encouraged to look at the Marmor and Wendt Policy Cycle in Healthcare in Chapter 1

K. J. Wheeler (✉)
University of Kentucky College of Nursing, Lexington, KY, USA
e-mail: kjwheeler623@gmail.com

G. K. Chan
University of California, San Francisco, Oakland, CA, USA

K. J. Wheeler, M. Acorn (eds.), *Health Policy for Advanced Practice Nursing: A Toolkit for Implementation and Improvement*, Advanced Practice in Nursing,
https://doi.org/10.1007/978-3-032-03667-4_4

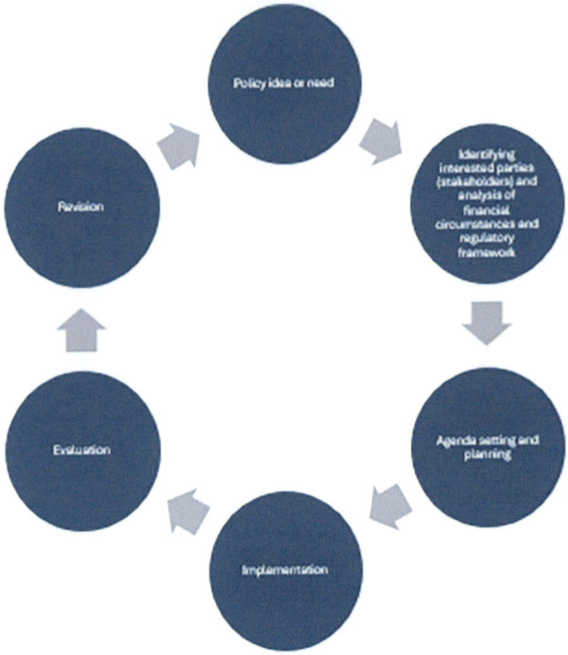
Policy idea or need
Identifying interested parties (stakeholders) and analysis of financial circumstances and regulatory framework
Agenda setting and planning
Implementation
Evaluation
Revision

Fig. 1 Policy cycle (Please note, the term interested parties will be used beside the term stakeholder in hopes of helping the transition to the more acceptable term. The term stakeholder carries a colonial or power differential connotation)

(Fig. 2), a healthcare cycle that aligns with common policy implementation/improvement cycles similar to the one above (Fig. 1). This cycle also aligns with the nursing process that all nurses know—SOAPIER (subjective data, objective data, assess, plan, implement, evaluate, revise) (Nurseslab.in 2025). Theoretical foundations can apply to the entire process or any piece of the process, according to what is needed for policy implementation and improvement.

2 Overview of Implementation Theories, Models, Frameworks, and Guidelines

Much of this overview is taken from Nilsen's 2015 article "Making Sense of Implementation Theories, Models and Frameworks," a seminal work dedicated to helping people understand theoretical foundations. A theory is a set of statements that represents what is seen or understood about the world (Nilsen 2015; Frankfort-Nachmias and Nachmias 1996; Wacker 1998; Carpiano and Daley 2006). A theory should provide an explanation for why and how things unfold and how variables lead to certain outcomes (Nilsen 2015; Frankfort-Nachmias and Nachmias 1996; Bluedorn and Evered 1980). Models are simple representations of an event or an occurrence. Theories and models are similar and often not easily distinguished.

Models are usually descriptive, while theories are both descriptive and explanatory. Theoretical frameworks are outlines or structural and relational representations of concepts or variables that explain an event or occurrence. APNs also rely on guidelines to define their professions. For APNs, these professional guidelines are detailed frameworks that address roles, populations, settings, and other broad details of the profession (as opposed to clinical guidelines that address specific conditions and provide evidence-based treatment options) (APA 2015). In nursing, these terms—theories, models, frameworks, and guidelines—are often used interchangeably, remaining as useful guides to shape, evaluate, and improve health policy for the APN profession.

These theoretical tools serve three purposes, specifically they: (1) explain and/or guide the process whereby research is translated into practice, (2) describe what affects the outcomes of implementation, or (3) assist in the evaluation of the implementation. These theoretical processes in policy implementation fall into five main categories: process models, determinant frameworks, classic theories, implementation theories, and evaluative frameworks (Nilsen 2015). Despite what seems like clear distinctions of application, those demarcations can be limiting to a new profession that is attempting to define itself globally, while on its path to deliver accessible, high-quality, cost-effective healthcare. Those attempting to structure change need to understand these foundations are meant to be adapted, adjusted, and blended according to context and need, revisited, and revamped repeatedly throughout the process.

3 General Implementation Theories, Models, Frameworks, and Guidelines

Table 1 provides descriptions and details of the five categories of implementation theories, models, and frameworks and some examples in common use among policy makers.

The United States National Institute of Health Fogarty International Center (n.d.) provides a list of policy implementation frameworks and models. Some are listed above, such as the PRECEDE PROCEED Model; the Dynamic Sustainability Model Framework for Reach, Effectiveness, Adoption, Implementation, and Maintenance (RE-AIM); and the Consolidated Framework for Implementation Research (CFIR). Strifler et al. cite a tool that identifies TMFGs, the Dissemination and Implementation Models Webtool. Developed through the work of Tabak et al. and Rabin et al. the tool is available at https://dissemination-implementation.org. Many of the above TMFGs have been used by nursing and APN policy makers and researchers. For example, the PRECEDE-PROCEED Model has been used so extensively and effectively that a systemic review and metanalysis was completed, with findings demonstrating strong evidence for effective use of the model (Kim et al. 2022).

Table 1 General implementation science theories, models, and frameworks

Process models	These models provide the steps in the process of translating research into practice. Action models are specific types of process models that offer more practical advice for the planning and implementation of projects. At times, the terms *model* or *framework* are used, but model is generally the term used most often	Exploration, Preparation, Implementation, Sustainment (EPIS) Framework Huberman Model Model by Landry et al. Model by Davis et al. Model by Majdzadeh et al. Canadian Institutes of Health Research Model of Knowledge Translation Knowledge-to-Action Framework Stetler Model Academic Center for Evidence Based Practice Star Model of Knowledge Transformation Knowledge-to-Action Model Iowa Model Ottawa Model Model by Grol and Wensing Model by Pronovost et al. Quality Improvement Framework
Determinant frameworks	These frameworks delineate types of determinants that act as enablers and barriers (variables) to implementation outcomes (dependent variables). The primary objective is to understand/ explain what influences implementation outcomes	Promoting Action on Research Implementation in Health Sciences (PARIHS) Active Implementation Frameworks Understanding-User-Content Framework Conceptual Models Framework by Grol. et al. Framework by Cochrane et al. Framework by Nutley et al. Ecological Framework by Durlak and DuPre Consolidated Framework for Implementation Research (CFIR) Framework by Gurses et al. Framework by Ferlie and Shortell Theoretical Domains Framework

(continued)

Table 1 (continued)

Classic theories	These are theories that have come from advanced practice nursing, nursing, sociology, psychology, and organizational theorists. They can be applied to implementation processes and provide strategies for change	Advanced practice nursing theories Nursing theories Social cognitive theories Social capital theories Cognitive processes and decision-making theories Social network theories Communities of practice Organizational theories Professional theories
Implementation theories	These theories have been created by implementation researchers to describe and/or explain implementation processes	Implementation climate Adsorptive capacity Organizational readiness Capacity-Opportunities-Motivation Behavior (COM-B) Normalization process theory
Evaluation models	These models identify aspects of implementation that lend themselves to evaluation of implementation success	Reach, Effectiveness, Adoption, Implementation, Maintenance (RE-AIM) PRECEDE-PROCEED Framework (predisposing, reinforcing, and enabling constructs in educational diagnosis and evaluation-policy, regulatory, and organizational constructs in educational and environmental development) Implementation Outcomes Taxonomy by Proctor et al.

Adapted from Nilsen (2015)

4 Implementation Theories, Models, and Frameworks Specific to Advanced Practice Nursing

Advanced practice nursing also has a number of TMFGs that provide guidance on the many complicated aspects of advanced practice nursing, particularly role distinctions. As has been shared throughout the text, the variations in APN titling, recognition, regulation, research, education, credentialing, and practice around the world make these documents extremely helpful in policy work. Table 2 provides a partial list, presented in no particular order. The most recent or updated version of the link to the framework is presented whenever possible. Theoretical foundations of curriculum and education are presented in their respective chapters.

Table 2 Implementation theories, models, frameworks, and guidelines specific to advanced practice nursing

Theory, model, framework, guideline Developers Year of publication or update Target countries	Important elements	Source or link
ICN Guidelines on Advanced Practice Nursing 2020 International Council of Nurses 2020 International	Updated definition for APN (new recommendation for master's degree) Primarily discussed nurse practitioners (NPs) and clinical nurse specialists (CNSs) Differentiated specialized nurse and CNS Discussed educational preparation, nature of practice, and regulatory issues for NPs and CNSs	https://www.icn.ch/system/files/documents/2020-04/ICN_APN%20Report_EN_WEB.pdf
ICN Guidelines on Advanced Practice Nursing Nurse Anesthetists 2021 International Council of Nurses and International Federation of Nurse Anesthetists 2021 International	Updated definition for APN (new recommendation for master's degree) Discussed educational preparation, nature of practice, and regulatory issues for NAs	https://www.icn.ch/system/files/documents/2021-05/ICN_Nurse-Anaesthetist-Report_EN_WEB.pdf
ICM Professional Framework for Midwifery 2021 International Confederation of Midwives 2021 International	Replaces 2009 ICM professional framework (three pillars: education, regulation, association) 2021 framework elements Midwifery philosophy Essential competencies for midwifery Education Regulation Association Research Midwife-led continuity of care model of practice Leadership Enabling environment Commitment to gender equality and justice, equity, diversity, and inclusion	https://www.internationalmidwives.org/assets/files/general-files/2022/05/professional-framework-2022.pdf

Consensus model for APRN regulation: Licensure, accreditation, Certification & Education APRN Consensus Work Group & the National Council of State Boards of Nursing APRN Advisory Committee 2008 US	Endorsed by 48 US nursing organizations Recognized four roles under the title Advanced Practice Registered Nurse (APRN): certified registered nurse anesthetist (CRNA), certified nurse-midwife (CNM), clinical nurse specialist (CNS), and certified nurse practitioner (CNP) Specified APRN education was to be broad-based and to include graduate-level courses in advanced physiology/pathophysiology, health assessment, and pharmacology Education programs to be housed in nationally accredited graduate programs and prepare graduates for national certification and state licensure Program graduates will sit for certification exams to assess national competencies of the APRN core, role, and at least one population focus Certification programs will be accredited by a national certification accrediting body, and will require a continued competency mechanism Education, certification, and licensure will be congruent in terms of role and population foci APRN may specialize but cannot be licensed solely within a specialty	https://www.aacnnursing.org/Portals/0/PDFs/Teaching-Resources/APRNReport.pdf
Hamric integrative model of APN Various iterations by Ann B. Hamric, as well as Charlene M. Hanson and/or Judith A. Spross 2023 Originally United States but used by multiple other countries	Most recent version: Primary criteria Graduate education Certification Practice focused on patient/family Central competency Direct clinical practice Core competencies Guidance and coaching Consultation Evidence-based practice Leadership Collaboration Ethical decision-making skills Critical environmental elements affecting advanced practice nursing Regulatory and credentialing requirements Business aspects Health policy Payment mechanisms Outcome evaluation and performance improvement Marketing and contracting Organizational structure and culture	Available in Hamric & Hanson's advanced practice nursing: An integrative approach, seventh edition

(continued)

Table 2 (continued)

Theory, model, framework, guideline Developers Year of publication or update Target countries	Important elements	Source or link
Advanced nursing practice framework Department of Health, Northern Ireland 2016 Northern Ireland	Based on national and international work, particularly Hamric et al. (2009) Emphasis on direct clinical care, supported by leadership and collaborative practice, education and learning, and research and evidence-based practice	https://www.health-ni.gov.uk/sites/default/files/publications/health/advanced-nursing-practice-framework.pdf
Multi-professional framework for advanced practice in England National health service England 2025 England	New definition for advanced practice Four pillars of practice Clinical practice Leadership and management Education Research Competence and capability based on work-based assessment, professional portfolios, and other considerations Accredited programs listed on website	https://yhtraininghubs.co.uk/wp-content/uploads/2025/05/Multi-professional-framework-for-advanced-practice-in-England-Edition-2025.pdf
Caring advanced practice nursing model/Nordic model of APN Lisbeth Fagerström 2011 Finland/Norway	Similar to Hamric model and ICN APN definitions, but added case management and emphasized theoretical premises such as holism, health, and caring	Fagerstrom L. Definition of advanced € practice nursing in a nordic perspective. In Advanced practice nurse in theory and praxis (Fagerstrom L ed.), € 2011, Studentlitteratur, Lund, 69–77 (in Swedish). 34 Jennings BM, staggers N

Participatory evidence-informed, patient-centered process framework (PEPPA) and PEPPA plus Developed by researchers from Cancer Care Ontario, McMaster University, Laurentian University, and regional cancer centers in Ontario, Canada 2004 Originally Canada, now international	Framework defines nine steps to assess the need for APNs in a practice and guide implementation and evaluation (Bryant-Lukosius and Dicenso 2004, p. 532) (1) Define the patient population and describe the current model of care (2) Identify interested parties (stakeholders) and recruit participants (3) Determine the need for a new model of care (4) Identify priority problems and goals to improve the model of care (5) Define the new model of care and the APN role (interested party [stakeholder] consensus about alignment of goals, new care model, and APN roles) (6) Plan implementation strategies (outcomes, evaluation plan, collection of baseline data; identify role facilitator and barriers) (7) Initiate APN role implementation plan (provide education, resources, and support; develop APN policies and protocols; begin role development and implementation) (8) Evaluate the role's effectiveness and the new model of care in the short term (9) Provide long-term monitoring of the APN role and new model of care	Bryant-Lukosius and Dicenso (2004)
Schober conceptual policy framework for advanced practice nursing Developed by Madrean Schober, Kate Gerrish, and Ann McDonnell 2017 Originally Singapore, now international	Critical points for policy development (Schober et al. 2016, p. 1322): Assess the need and motivation for APNs Establish the legitimacy and feasibility of the APN concept Identify pivotal decision makers and their spheres of influence Establish title protection, and define the role, anticipated scope of practice, and position within the healthcare workforce Identify measures needed to accomplish the action for policy development and implementation Verify broad-based support from those in positions of authority, as well as managers, healthcare professionals, and staff on the ground Critical point for policy/role implementation (Schober et al. 2016, p. 1322): Include managers, medical directors, consultants, other nurses, and ancillary staff in discussions Develop clear role/job descriptions and scope of practice prior to implementation Define reporting mechanisms for evaluation and performance review Identify who the advanced practice nurse will report to in the clinical setting: nursing, medicine, or both Establish infrastructure for collegial communication: APN councils, journal club, continuing education workshops Define a specific plan for dissemination of information to healthcare professionals and the public, offering opportunities for questions and discussion Institute processes to evaluate the APN in actual clinical practice, aligned with a reporting mechanism for composite and future role development	Schober et al. (2016)

5 Other Useful Implementation Theories, Models, Frameworks, and Guidelines

There are additional theoretical foundations that apply to advanced practice nursing policy work. These range from general nursing theories to other commonly used theories, some for somewhat limited but specific uses.

5.1 General Nursing Theories

General nursing theories also apply to advanced practice nursing and policy work—what applies to nursing applies to advanced practice nursing. From Florence Nightingale's "Environmental Theory" to Patricia Benner's "Novice to Expert Theory" to Lillian Wald's "Theory of Public Health Nursing," and many in between, the list is extensive, and they all can apply to advanced practice nursing. Because the sweep is so wide-ranging a full discussion is beyond the scope of this toolkit. Readers and policy makers are encouraged to recognize the value of these theoretical foundations to APN policy work and access information from the many general nursing theory resources as needed. Multiple texts are available as are numerous websites.

- Mayo Clinic Libraries: Provides a list of nursing theories/theorists as well as a listing of texts dedicated to theory/theorists (https://libraryguides.mayo.edu/c.php?g=280182&p=186710).
- American Nurses Association: Provides a discussion of nursing theory classifications and applications, links to lists of theories/theorists (https://www.nursingworld.org/content-hub/resources/becoming-a-nurse/nursing-theory/).
- Nurselabs: Provides a discussion of history, classification, and application of nursing theories, links to multiple theories/theorists (https://nurseslabs.com/nursing-theories/).

5.2 Logic Models and Change/Action Models

A significant body of tools useful to policy and program development, implementation, and evaluation are logic models and change/action models. These terms are often used interchangeably but are different, serving different but complementary functions. A logic model defines a logical sequence of interventions—the what—that leads to results. A theory of change defines the causal relationship—the how and why—between interventions and certain outcomes. A logic model is descriptive, and a change/action model is explanatory. Administrations and funders often expect one or both, so they can understand what change is to be anticipated and how

Inputs	Activities	Outputs	Outcomes		
			Short Term Outcomes	Intermediate Term Outcomes	Long Term Outcomes

Fig. 2 Logic model

to plan financially. Evaluators rely on them to anticipate what to expect as they evaluate the level of success and return on investment. Logic models tend to be linear representations, but theories of change may be very complex, with multiple components at play at various times (Sharp 2021; Clark and Anderson 2004).

One of the best examples of a logic model is the one developed and extensively used by the United Way in the late 1990s. Figure 2 is a visual representation of that model.

To clarify (United Way 2015):

Inputs refers to the needed resources to carry out a desired activity. These could include such things as money, staff/volunteers, equipment, organizational resources, community resources, and research.

Activities refers to all the services or what might need to be done to bring about desired results, namely the tools, processes, actions, and events. These could include workshops, training, counseling, and assessments.

Outputs refers to the direct results of the activities—the products, the participation. These are usually listed in number format, so may include sessions completed, clients served, and number of referrals.

Outcomes are the anticipated changes in the served population and fall into short-term outcomes, intermediate-term outcomes, and long-term outcomes. Hopefully, what starts as changes in knowledge, skills, and attitudes will result in changed behavior and long-term improvements.

Once an issue is identified and goals (outcomes) are set, the policymaker/s can use forward logic and process through the model (if-then), or reverse logic and process backward through the model (but how?). Logic models can be adapted specifically for advocacy and policy change, such as the one developed by Coffman et al. (2007)—the Composite Logic Model (CLM). Important process questions and evaluation questions, a visual representation, and glossary are available at the following link: https://kq.freepressunlimited.org/wp-content/uploads/2020/11/Advocacy-and-Policy-Change-Composite-Logic-Model.pdf. Among the development guidance questions are those related to consideration of the opposition or competition, how to develop contingency plans, and how to prioritize given time and resource constraints.

5.3 Kingdon's Multiple Streams Framework

Kingdon (2010) developed the Multiple Streams Framework (MSF) in 1984, with a major revision in 2010. The MSF is a well-respected framework to analyze public policymaking and the opportunities for policymaking to take place. It has particular importance in the policy agenda-setting phase of policymaking. There are three streams: the policy problem stream, the policy solutions stream, and the political stream. The three streams must converge in order for a policy window to open and for successful public or health policy to be enacted, commonly understood as: (1) getting official approval; (2) making something into law, regulation, or policy; and (3) implementing the change.

The policy problems stream is a bad situation in which affected groups or populations could greatly benefit from a governmental solution. According to Hoefer (2022), "the problem is put on the government agenda for action. It may be seen to be a problem in search of a solution" (p. 3). The policy solutions stream consists of potential policy solutions that can be created by academia, experts, think tanks, or entrepreneurs. While these potential policy solutions might be good solutions to the problem, not all will have equal chances of being accepted since some solutions may lack feasibility, are too expensive, or are beyond the limits of acceptable policy solutions at the time of proposal (Hoefer 2022). The third stream is the political stream. This is the most difficult to understand because it involves all of the forces and nuances that affect the political stream. Some factors that can affect the political stream include, but are not limited to, the national discourse on a particular topic (e.g., affordable healthcare, access to a specific type of care such as reproductive freedom or gender-affirming care), elected or appointed officials active in decision-making, and then special interest groups who have political capital and can influence governmental officials. These ever-changing variables in the political stream make it clear that the process is not always a rational process where clear goals are achieved through evidence-based solutions, but rather the process is "random and depends on skilled framing and coupling of both identified and defined problems and general solutions to appeal to a majority of decision-makers during a brief time when action is possible" (Hoefer 2022, pp. 3–4). The MSF is particularly useful as the analysis structure to look for windows of opportunity for policymaking.

5.4 Rogers' Diffusion of Innovation

Another useful theory is Everett Roger's "Diffusion of Innovation" (DOI) theory, first created in 1962 and now in its fifth edition (Rogers 2003). This theory is particularly important in understanding the rate of adoption after a policy has been enacted. In a broad overview of DOI, the theory describes how, why, and at what rate new ideas diffuse or spread through any given population. There are five players in the theory—innovators, early adopters, early majority, late majority, and laggards or resistors, and a five-stage process in the innovation-decision process—knowledge, persuasion, decision, implementation, confirmation. The DOI theory posits that any given population exists in a bell curve. At one tail end of the bell curve, innovators, either individuals or a unit made up of individuals, make up approximately 2.5% of the population. Innovators, as they disseminate their innovation, influence the early adopters, who make up approximately 13.5% of the population, have high social status, are socially more forward, have a high degree of opinion leadership, and can help diffuse the innovation to the next group—the early majority, which make up approximately 34% of the population. The early majority adopt an innovation after a time that is longer than innovators and early adopters. They are open to the innovation and want to understand how the innovation works with the early adopters. The fourth type of players are the late majority, making up approximately 34% of the population. People in this category adopt the innovation after the average participant. They have a higher degree of skepticism and only adopt the innovation after the majority of the society or intended population has adopted the innovation. Lastly, the laggards, approximately 16% of the population, are the last to adopt the innovation, if they ever fully adopt the innovation. It is important for the innovators and early adopters to listen to the laggards as they have some good insights to consider modifying the innovation as it is being diffused across the population.

5.5 Centers for Disease Control and Prevention's Polaris Policy Process

The Centers for Disease Control and Prevention's (CDC) Polaris Policy Process (2024) provides an additional framework to develop and implement policies to address public health problems. The policy process involves five domains: problem identification, policy analysis, strategy and policy development, policy enactment, and policy implementation. In all domains, interested party (stakeholder) engagement and education are essential for policy work to be successful. Additionally, continuous evaluation in each domain according to four standards, utility, feasibility, propriety, and accuracy, when engaging interested parties (stakeholders), describing the program, focusing on evaluation design, gathering credible evidence, justifying conclusions, and ensuring use and sharing lessons learned (CDC 1999). The CDC Polaris Policy Process website has many great resources and examples to help develop and implement public health policy.

5.6 SWOT Analysis

The SWOT (strengths, weaknesses, opportunities, threats) analysis is such a broadly useful process in policy implementation and improvement that it deserves a separate discussion. Though more procedural than conceptual, this technique is commonly used early in policy work. Attributed to Albert Humphrey from the United States, the procedure was used initially in business in the 1960s and later applied to healthcare. It has been found to be effective for individuals, organizations, and

	STRENGTHS	WEAKNESSES
INTERNAL		
	OPPORTUNITES	THREATS
EXTERNAL		

Fig. 3 SWOT (strengths, weaknesses, opportunities, threats) template

jurisdictions (Teoli et al. 2023). Since every policy initiative requires a comprehensive assessment of the landscape surrounding an issue—need, applications, supporters, barriers—a thorough analysis provides an opportunity to understand the complexity of the situation in order to plan appropriately.

A visual representation is presented in Fig. 3. Strengths are internal characteristics that reflect things being done well or advantages that help achieve goals. Weaknesses are internal characteristics that reflect things being done poorly or that undermine the achievement of goals. Opportunities are external characteristics that can be used to improve things or accomplish initiatives, and threats are external characteristics that limit abilities to achieve objectives (Schober 2016).

As simple as this process seems, there have been limitations. Some have found the tool to be simplistic and superficial, leading to poor information. To counter these concerns, users recommend thorough and careful discussions by multiple informed individuals or groups, and the recognition that the data provided is only a snapshot of one point in time against an ever-changing landscape that exists in healthcare (Teoli et al. 2023). Gandolf (2024), Chief Executive Officer of Healthcare Success, recommends doing the following when performing a SWOT analysis (para 16):

1. Be specific—avoid vagueness
2. Be objective—ask for input from multiple, well-informed individuals and interested parties (stakeholders)
3. Be realistic—apply a practical, pragmatic perspective to the evaluation
4. Apply context—consider setting in the analysis, and recognize context applies to now and in the future

5. Contrast and compare—make comparisons along the way
6. Keep it short and simple—avoid over analysis and getting bogged down in minutiae
7. Update goals—identify concerns then develop a plan and set priorities

The last step offered by Gandolf is critical to the process. Some feel the work is done once the SWOT information is collected. But the real work is just beginning. This is the time for policymakers to prioritize and create plans, either through a business plan, a project plan, or an implementation or improvement plan (Raeburn 2023).

6 Moving from Theory to Implementation/Improvement

As useful as a list of TMFGs are at some point policy makers and interested parties (stakeholders) must start to make some decisions about the process and implementation science frameworks that might be needed, understanding some TMFGs are all inclusive while others are aimed at specific goals, such as assessment of the policy landscape (e.g., SWOT Analysis), assessment of background and rate of adoption (e.g., Roger's DOI Theory), or the timing for windows of opportunity (e.g., Kingdon's Multiple Streams Framework). A limitation in scope often leads to the need to apply and blend multiple TMFGs to policy implementation/improvement. The following implementation authorities offer the following to guide some of the decisions:

1. Lynch et al. (2018, p. 10) recommend considering the following questions, adapted below:
   (a) Who is involved—individuals, groups, or is the setting wider?
   (b) When in the process is a TMFG needed?
   (c) Why is the TMFG needed (what is the aim and what is needed to understand)?
   (d) How will data be collected or made available?
   (e) What resources are available to support the change?
2. Fernandez et al. (2021, para 4) recommend implementation mapping, a process involving five steps:
   (a) Conduct a needs and asset assessment. Identify adopters and implementers.
   (b) Identify adoption and implementation outcomes, performance objectives and determinants, and create matrices of change.
   (c) Choose theoretical methods; select or create implementation strategies.
   (d) Produce implementation protocols and materials.
   (e) Plan evaluation of implementation outcome.
3. Moullin et al. (2020, pp. 3–11) recommend the following steps, acknowledging they only follow an approximation of stages in the process, the order of which might change based on the needs and context of the project:
   (a) Select suitable framework(s) (see #4 or #5 below).
   (b) Establish and maintain community interested party (stakeholder) engagement and partnerships.

(c) Define issue and develop research or evaluation questions and hypotheses.
(d) Develop an implementation logic model.
(e) Select research and evaluation methods.
(f) Determine implementation factors/determinants.
(g) Select and tailor, or develop, implementation strategy(s).
(h) Specify implementation outcomes and evaluate implementation.
(i) Use framework(s) at micro level to conduct and tailor implementation.
(j) Write the proposal and report.

4. To select a framework, Birken et al. (2018, p. 8) offer the following checklist, called the Theory Comparison and Selection Tool (T-CaST). It consists of sixteen criteria in four categories, adapted as follows:

Usability	1. The TMFG includes relevant constructs (e.g., self-efficacy, climate) 2. Key interested parties (stakeholders; e.g., researchers, clinicians, funders) are able to understand, apply, and operationalize the TMFG 3. The TMFG has a clear and useful figure depicting included constructs and relationships among them 4. The TMFG provides a step-by-step approach for applying it 5. The TMFG provides methods for promoting implementation in practice 6. The TMFG provides an explanation of how included constructs influence implementation and/or each other
Testability	1. The TMFG proposes testable hypotheses 2. The TMFG includes meaningful, face-valid explanations of proposed relationships 3. The TMFG contributes to an evidence base and/or TMFG development because it has been used in empirical studies
Applicability	1. The TMFG focuses on a relevant implementation outcome (e.g., fidelity; acceptability) 2. A particular method (e.g., interview, survey, focus groups, chart review) can be used with the TMFG 3. The TMFG addresses a relevant analytical level (e.g., individual, organizational, community) 4. The TMFG has been used in a relevant population (e.g., children, adults with mental illness) and/or conditions (e.g., attention deficit hyperactivity disorder, cancer) 5. The TMFG is generalizable to other disciplines (e.g., education, health services, social work), settings (e.g., schools, hospitals, community-based organizations), and/or populations (e.g., children, adults with mental illness)
Acceptability	1. The TMFG is familiar to interested parties (stakeholders; e.g., researchers, scholars, clinicians, funders) 2. The TMFG comes from a particular discipline (e.g., education, health services, social work)

5. Reviewing and simplifying the work of Lynch et al. and Moullin et al. (above), Strifler et al. (2024, p. 8) developed the following decision tool regarding TMFG choice:
   (a) What is the purpose or goal of the implementation process?
   (b) What guidance is needed?
      (i) Develop or guide the implementation process (i.e., a process model)
      (ii) Understand or explain determinants of implementation or sustainability (i.e., a determinant framework)
      (iii) Understand or explain implementation outcomes and/or sustainability (i.e., an evaluation framework)
   (c) For what stage/s are guidance needed?
      (i) Select and/or adapt evidence
      (ii) Identify barriers and facilitators and/or select, tailor, and implement strategies
      (iii) Monitor evidence use and/or evaluate outcomes
      (iv) Sustain use of evidence
   (d) What is the target level for the change?
      (i) Individual
      (ii) Organizational
      (iii) Broad policy level

As helpful as these decision tools are, implementation/improvement scientists note there are times when the selection may not be as helpful as hoped, so the policy maker or the APN needs to be flexible, patient, willing to communicate with interested parties (stakeholders), and willing to add or substitute other theoretical foundations, where appropriate.

7 Policy Exemplar: Enteral Feeding Tube Connectors and Patient Safety

The following exemplar was previously written for the American Association of Colleges of Nursing's Health Policy Toolkit (AACN 2022). AACN has given permission to reproduce this exemplar for this chapter. This exemplar focuses on the policy implementation after the enactment of the law. The work of individuals, the healthcare system writ large, and manufacturing took over 6 years to implement the policy, highlighting the sustained efforts needed for implementation.

Historically, when an error occurred, the user was the first to be blamed. However, patient safety experts recognized that humans worked in organizations and systems that could make mistakes more prone to happen. Therefore, a major policy initiative in the United States was focused on improving the safety of healthcare delivery. A landmark report by the Institute of Medicine (2000), titled "To Err Is Human," called on the health professions to reduce healthcare professional errors, reduce patient injuries, and improve the use of evidence-based medicine.

In California, there were a few deaths and medical errors related to enteral feeding tube feedings. The enteral tubes were connected via the substitution of intravenous lines and epidural lines because enteral feeding tubes were manufactured with Luer Lock connections, then only compatible with intravenous and epidural lines. As a result, the California Hospital Association, nursing organizations, and patient advocacy groups collaborated and discussed the need to incorporate human factors engineering (also known as human factors design or human factors ergonomics) to advance health safety policy through legislation. Human factors engineering considers many elements in eliminating hazards, such as patient and healthcare professional factors, task factors, technology and tool factors, environmental factors, and organizational factors (Karsh et al. 2006; Pelayo et al. 2021). To avoid blaming the nurse (who knew tube feedings connected via these methods could cause severe morbidity and mortality but who had no alternative) and to focus on human factors engineering to help improve patient safety, the coalition partnered with California State Senator Dean Florez to introduce Senate Bill 158 (SB 158) in 2008. SB 158 prohibited health facilities from using an intravenous connection, epidural connection, or enteral feeding connection that would fit into a connection port other than the type it was intended for. The bill was successfully signed into law by the Governor of California on September 25, 2008, and was codified in California Health and Safety Code Section 1279.7. Senator Florez and the healthcare community knew that enteral-specific connectors did not already exist—all enteral feeding tube connectors on the market were Luer Lock connections. Therefore, the bill allowed the law to be delayed until January 1, 2011. The passage of SB 158 was a major impetus for the device manufacturing companies to develop an alternative connector for enteral feeding tubes and syringes. In 2009, AdvaMed, the manufacturers' trade association, successfully pushed legislation to delay the bill's effects to 2017 or until an international standards group reached a decision on appropriate standards for enteral feeding tube connection design (U Deliver Medical 2018).

Subsequently, the deadline had to be extended to allow manufacturers to design and manufacture appropriate tubing and syringes. A *New York Times* article published in 2010 written by Harris (2010) profiled multiple people who died as a result of tubing misconnections and identified opportunities within the manufacturer trade associations and the Food and Drug Administration bureaucracy that caused delays in improving patient safety.

A research study published by Simmons and colleagues (2011) reviewed 116 published cases of nutrition tubing misconnections with inappropriate tubing and devices. Of the 116 cases, 21 patients died and 95 survived. Out of the 95 survivors, 84 had at least one diagnosis reported. Diagnoses included respiratory conditions, including cardiopulmonary arrest ($n = 37$, 44%), sepsis ($n = 16$, 19%), neurological harm ($n = 11$, 13%), and renal impairment ($n = 8$, 9.5%). Additionally, ECRI, an independent nonprofit organization dedicated to improving the safety, quality, and cost-effectiveness of healthcare and the only organization worldwide that conducts independent medical device evaluations, identified enteral feeding tube misconnections as one of the top ten technology hazards in 2012 (ECRI 2012).

In 2015, the new international design standard for enteral feeding tube devices was released. The initiative by the Global Enteral Device Supplier Association (GEDSA™), titled "Stay Connected," unveiled ENFit®, the enteral feeding tube connection (GEDSA™ 2025; Harding 2025). The healthcare industry was then able to order appropriate supplies, train staff, and improve safety in patient care.

This exemplar illustrates the complexity and extended amount of time it took for policy implementation. As may commonly happen, unforeseen issues had an impact—the healthcare manufacturing industry was unprepared for the impact of the policy and legislative action to advance patient safety.

8 Conclusion

Implementing or improving any policy in any APN setting, whether related to practice, education, or regulation, is extremely complex. The process is multifaceted, challenging, and unpredictable. This chapter can only offer a beginning for what an APN or policy maker might consider when applying theoretical foundations to policies that affect people, populations, and professions. Readers and policy makers are encouraged to use this chapter as a springboard to the study and planning that may be required to provide the scaffolding necessary to implement effective, meaningful healthcare policy and to know when and how improvement might be necessary.

References

American Association of Colleges of Nursing (AACN). Health policy concept: why, who, what, when, where, and how. AACN; 2022. https://www.aacnnursing.org/essentials/database/kit/i/c_health_policy_doc. Accessed 4 Mar 2025.

American Psychological Association (APA). Professional practice guidelines. APA; 2015. https://www.apa.org/about/policy/professional-practice.pdf. Accessed 4 Mar 2025.

Birken SA, Rohweder CL, Powell BJ, Shea CM, Scott J, Leeman J, Grewe ME, Alexis Kirk M, Damschroder L, Aldridge WA II, Haines ER, Straus S, Presseau J. T-CaST: an implementation theory comparison and selection tool. Implement Sci. 2018;13(1):143. https://doi.org/10.1186/s13012-018-0836-4. PMID: 30466450; PMCID: PMC6251099.

Bluedorn AC, Evered RD. Middle range theory and the strategies of theory construction. In: Pinder CC, Moore LF, editors. Middle range theory and the study of organizations. Boston: Martinus Nijhoff; 1980. p. 19–32.

Bryant-Lukosius D, Dicenso A. A framework for the introduction and evaluation of advanced practice nursing roles. J Adv Nurs. 2004;48(5):530–40. https://doi.org/10.1111/j.1365-2648.2004.03235.x. PMID: 15533091.

Carpiano RM, Daley DM. A guide and glossary on post-positivist theory building for population health. J Epidemiol Community Health. 2006;60(7):564–70. https://doi.org/10.1136/jech.2004.031534. PMID: 16790824; PMCID: PMC2566228.

Centers for Disease Control and Prevention (CDC). Framework for program evaluation in public health. Morbidity and Mortality Weekly Report: MMWR. 48 (No. RR-11). U.S. Dept. of Health, Education, and Welfare, Public Health Service, Center for Disease Control; 1999. https://www.cdc.gov/mmwr/PDF/rr/rr4811.pdf. Accessed 5 Mar 2025.

Centers for Disease Control and Prevention (CDC). CDC policy process. CDC; 2024. https://www.cdc.gov/polaris/php/cdc-policy-process/index.html. Accessed 5 Mar 2025.

Clark H, Anderson AA. Theories of change and logic models: telling them apart. [Presentation at American Evaluation Association Atlanta Georgia]. 2004. https://www.theoryofchange.org/wp-content/uploads/toco_library/pdf/TOCs_and_Logic_Models_forAEA.pdf. Accessed 4 Mar 2025.

Coffman J, Hendricks A, Kaye J, Kelly T, Masters B. Advocacy and policy change composite logic model. 2007. https://kq.freepressunlimited.org/wp-content/uploads/2020/11/Advocacy-and-Policy-Change-Composite-Logic-Model.pdf. Accessed 4 Mar 2025.

Eccles M, Grimshaw J, Walker A, Johnston M, Pitts N. Changing the behavior of healthcare professionals: the use of theory in promoting the uptake of research findings. J Clin Epidemiol. 2005;58:107–12.

Emergency Care Research Institute (ECRI). ECRI's top 10 health technology hazards for 2012. Biomed Saf Stand. 2012;42(2):9–10. https://doi.org/10.1097/01.BMSAS.0000411011.94193.b8. Accessed 5 Mar 2025.

Fernandez M, Walker TJ, Rome A. Featured framework: Implementation mapping. 2021. https://thecenterforimplementation.com/toolbox/implementation-mapping. Accessed 4 Jan 2025.

Fogarty International Center. Toolkit: overcoming barriers to implementation in global health. Part 1. Implementation science methodologies and frameworks. n.d. https://www.fic.nih.gov/About/center-global-health-studies/neuroscience-implementation-toolkit/Pages/methodologies-frameworks.aspx. Accessed 4 Sept 2025.

Frankfort-Nachmias C, Nachmias D. Research methods in the social sciences. London: Arnold; 1996.

Gandolf S. SWOT: the high-level self exam that boosts your bottom line. 2024. https://healthcare-success.com/blog/case-studies-best-practices/swot.html. Accessed 2 Jan 2024.

Global Engineered Device Supplier Association (GEDSA™). ENFit®. 2025. https://stayconnected.org/enteral-enfit/. Accessed 4 Mar 2025.

Hamric A, Spross J, Hanson C. Advanced practice nursing—an integrative approach. 4th ed. Missouri: Saunders Elsevier; 2009.

Harding J. ENFit transition for enteral management in an acute care setting. Patient Saf. 2025;7(2). https://doi.org/10.33940/001c.129694.

Harris G. U.S. inaction lets look-alike tubes kill patients. New York Times, 20 Aug 2010. https://www.nytimes.com/2010/08/21/health/policy/21tubes.html. Accessed 6 Mar 2025.

Hoefer R. The multiple streams framework: understanding and applying the problems, policies, and politics approach. J Pol Prac Res. 2022;3(1):1–5. https://doi.org/10.1007/s42972-022-00049-2.

Institute of Medicine (IOM). To err is human: building a safer health system. Washington, DC: National Academy Press; 2000.

Karsh BT, Holden RJ, Alper SJ, Or CK. A human factors engineering paradigm for patient safety: designing to support the performance of the healthcare professional. Qual Saf Health Care. 2006;15(Suppl 1):i59–65. https://doi.org/10.1136/qshc.2005.015974. PMID: 17142611; PMCID: PMC2464866.

Kim J, Jang J, Kim B, Lee KH. Effect of the PRECEDE-PROCEED model on health programs: a systematic review and meta-analysis. Syst Rev. 2022;11(1):213. https://doi.org/10.1186/s13643-022-02092-2. PMID: 36210473; PMCID: PMC9549687.

Kingdon J. Agendas, alternatives and public policy. 2nd ed. New York: Pearson; 2010.

Lynch EA, Mudge A, Knowles S, Kitson AL, Hunter SC, Harvey G. There is nothing so practical as a good theory: a pragmatic guide for selecting theoretical approaches for implementation projects. BMC Health Serv Res. 2018;18:857.

Moullin JC, Dickson KS, Stadnick NA, Albers B, Nilsen P, Broder-Fingert S, Mukasa B, Aarons GA. Ten recommendations for using implementation frameworks in research and practice. Implement Sci Commun. 2020;1:42. https://doi.org/10.1186/s43058-020-00023-7. PMID: 32885199; PMCID: PMC7427911.

Nilsen P. Making sense of implementation theories, models and frameworks. Implement Sci. 2015;10:53. https://doi.org/10.1186/s13012-015-0242-0. PMID: 25895742; PMCID: PMC4406164.

Nurseslab.in. SOAPIER nursing documentation: structured approach to patient care. Author; 2025. https://nurseslab.in/nursing-blog/nursing-education/soapier-nursing-documentation-structured-approach-to-patient-care/. Accessed 15 Sept 2025.

Pelayo S, Marcilly R, Bellandi T. Human factors engineering for medical devices: European regulation and current issues. Int J Qual Health Care. 2021;33(Supplement_1):31–6. https://doi.org/10.1093/intqhc/mzaa103. PMID: 32991690.

Raeburn A. SWOT analysis. 2023. https://asana.com/resources/swot-analysis. Accessed 2 Jan 2025.

Rogers EM. Diffusion of innovation. 5th ed. New York: Free Press; 2003.

Schober M. In: Schober M, editor. Role and practice development: environmental scanning and SWOT analysis. Switzerland: Springer; 2016. p. 98–9.

Schober MM, Gerrish K, McDonnell A. Development of a conceptual policy framework for advanced practice nursing: an ethnographic study. J Adv Nurs. 2016;72(6):1313–24. https://doi.org/10.1111/jan.12915. Epub 2016 Feb 9. PMID: 26858010.

Sharp S. Logic models vs theories of change. Center for Research Evaluation. https://sites.olemiss.edu/cere/blog/logic-models-vs-theories-change. 2021. https://sites.olemiss.edu/cere/blog/logic-models-vs-theories-change. Accessed 4 Mar 2025.

Simmons D, Symes L, Guenter P, Graves K. Tubing misconnections: normalization of deviance. Nutr Clin Pract. 2011;26(3):286–93. https://doi.org/10.1177/0884533611406134. PMID: 21586413.

Strifler L, Fahim C, Hillmer MP, Barnsley JM, Straus SE. Development and usability testing of an online support tool to identify models and frameworks to inform implementation. BMC Med Inform Decis Mak. 2024;24(1):182. https://doi.org/10.1186/s12911-024-02580-6. PMID: 38937692; PMCID: PMC11209996.

Teoli D, Sanvictores T, An J. SWOT analysis. 2023. https://www.ncbi.nlm.nih.gov/books/NBK537302/#:~:text=SWOT%20Analysis%20(short%20for%20strengths,but%20this%20attribution%20remains%20debatable. Accessed 2 Jan 2024.

U Deliver Medical. What is ENFit? Easier tube feeding—no more messy syringes. 2018. https://www.udelivermedical.com/what-is-enfit. Accessed 28 Feb 2025.

United Way. A guide to developing an outcome logic model and measurement plan. 2015. https://www.yourunitedway.org/wp-content/uploads/2015/12/UWGRP-Guide-to-Outcomes-and-Logic-Models-6-8-15.pdf. Accessed 20 Sept 2025.

Wacker JG. A definition of theory: research guidelines for different theory-building research methods in operations management. J Oper Manag. 1998;16:361–85.

The Language of Health Policy

Kathy J. Wheeler

1 Introduction

Word choice matters. In health policy, word choice and the understanding of terms are critical. For that reason, most policy documents include a list of definitions or a glossary of terms, organizations involved in policy work publish extensive lists of policy terms, and those leading policy discussions devote time to agreeing on terms. Nurses and advanced practice nurses (APNs) are great communicators when it comes to patient care. A significant amount of their schooling is devoted to principles of patient-centered communication, and how to help patients deal with difficult situations. However, the amount of time educating these same clinicians to communicate with policymakers and speak the language of policy may not be as extensive as what is needed. Nurses tend to devote their time to learning about patient care, not seeing themselves as potential policymakers of their profession. And yet, a defining characteristic of being a profession is that practitioners regulate and control their own practice (Larson 1978). That requires not only an understanding of policy implementation and improvement but a command of policy language. Doing so allows APNs to communicate effectively when making policy and ensures credibility as they do so. This chapter is a brief introduction to the language of health policy, why valuing it is important, and what language issues may be particularly important to APNs.

K. J. Wheeler (✉)
University of Kentucky College of Nursing, Lexington, KY, USA
e-mail: kjwheeler623@gmail.com

K. J. Wheeler, M. Acorn (eds.), *Health Policy for Advanced Practice Nursing: A Toolkit for Implementation and Improvement*, Advanced Practice in Nursing,
https://doi.org/10.1007/978-3-032-03667-4_5

2 Policy Words and Glossaries

Addressing this topic is particularly challenging since policy language is complicated, many-layered, and affected by context and location. For APNs, policy implementation and improvement primarily takes place in the three policy domains of governance, clinical practice, and education, but also in leadership and certainly in research. Each domain is composed of dozens of subdomains, with some terms shared between domains and some terms quite unique. This text could not possibly provide an exhaustive list, but Table 1 represents several glossaries and websites

Table 1 Examples of common healthcare glossaries and websites devoted to terms to use

Glossary/website name	Organization/ author	Details	Link
Governance example: I.C.E. Basic Guide to Credentialing Terminology (ICE 2021)	Institute for Credentialing Excellence	"Designed to serve as a definitive reference to credentialing terms and their definitions for the credentialing community." (ICE 2020, para 1)	https://www.credentialinginsights.org/Article/back-to-basics-ice-releases-updated-terminology-guide-1
Clinical example: W.H.O. Health Promotion Glossary of Terms (WHO 2021)	World Health Organization	"The list of terms is not intended to be either exhaustive or exclusive, and draws upon the wide range of disciplines in which health promotion has its roots." (WHO 2021, para 1)	https://www.who.int/publications/i/item/9789240038349
Education example: Education Terms Glossary (ProctorFree n.d.)	ProctorFree	"Education related terms can seem like a unique language, on this page you will find some commonly used education terms, along with friendly definitions we could find or create." (ProctorFree n.d., para 1)	https://www.proctorfree.com/education-terms-glossary/
Leadership example: Leadership Glossary and Concepts (ALL 2018)	Arceil Leadership Limited	"Here is a compendium of terms we use in *Fundamentals of Leadership*, *The Art of Leadership*, *Master Class in Leadership*, and *The Serving Leader*." (ALL 2018, para 1)	https://www.arceil.com/resources/glossary-of-terms
Research example: Glossary of Research Terms (USC 2025)	University of Southern California	"This glossary is intended to assist you in understanding commonly used terms and concepts when reading, interpreting, and evaluating scholarly research." (USC 2025, para 1)	https://libguides.usc.edu/writingguide/researchglossary

Table 2 Examples of common healthcare glossaries and websites devoted to terms to avoid and terms to use that improve inclusivity and clarity

Glossary/ website name	Organization/ author	Details	Link
Inclusive and Empathetic Language Use Guidelines (AHC n.d.)	Canada-Alliance for Healthier Communities	"Language is a powerful tool. The way we talk about people and communities facing barriers has a tremendous impact on the way they are viewed in our society. Words can either empower people and affirm the value of diversity and difference, or demean them and perpetuate the stigma they already face." (AHC n.d., para 1)	https://www.cityofboise.org/media/12897/optional-readings-week-1.pdf
Plain Language and Word Choice (Australian Government 2024)	Australian Government Style Manual	"People can relate to content when it uses inclusive language. Choose words that respect all people, including their rights and their heritage." (Australian Government 2024, para 1)	https://www.stylemanual.gov.au/writing-and-designing-content/clear-language-and-writing-style/plain-language-and-word-choice
Avoid Emotive Words, Jargon, and Policy Speak (PCO n.d.)	New Zealand Parliamentary Counsel Office	"The theory is simple: use plain, clear words and satisfy readers. Do the opposite and risk confusing and annoying readers." (PCO n.d., para 2)	https://www.pco.govt.nz/making-secondary-legislation/plain-language/supporting-documents/5-1
Words and Phrases You May Want to Think Twice About Using (Hwang 2021)	CBC Radio-Canada	"…it's a tricky question, but it's less about being politically correct and more about listening to the lived experiences of others." (Hwang 2021, para 7)	https://www.cbc.ca/news/canada/ottawa/words-and-phrases-commonly-used-offensive-english-language-1.6252274

useful to someone involved in shaping health policy. Some are global in application and some more regional or jurisdictional. Their presentation is more to show the types and categories of glossaries that someone active in health policy might need to understand in order to be prepared for policy discussions and planning.

Then there are words that either need to be avoided or used preferentially. Careful word choice assures inclusiveness, minimizes offensiveness, and provides clarity. Some words commonly used in policy have fallen into disfavor. For example, the terms grandfather or grandfathered are considered insensitive or inappropriate to use. Employed to describe policies or processes exempt from updated rules, there are better alternatives, such as excused, preapproved, or legacied (Okeh 2021). The list of outdated terms is extensive. It is important for policymakers to understand the basis for the offense and seek out alternative terms to use. Table 2 provides a limited list of glossaries and websites devoted to terms to avoid or terms to use to improve inclusivity and clarity.

3 Importance of Health Policy Language to Advanced Practice Nursing

The importance of understanding and using a shared, inoffensive language in policy discussions cannot be diminished. As the Institute for Credentialing Excellence stated, "After all, if professionals don't agree on a shared language, it can become difficult to achieve…complicated tasks" (ICE 2021, para 1). When policy vocabulary is agreed on and known, the discussions are more efficient and less confusing. Publications are understandable, and policies are more transferable and adaptable. Research and data collection are more reliable because comparisons are made between comparable items via a more correct apples-to-apples comparison. As more and more attention is directed at achieving universal health coverage in a global, interconnected world, the need for agreement on policy terms is even more imperative. So, if APNs are going to participate in policy discussions and shape policy, they need to not only be familiar with appropriate policy terms, they also need to drive consensus on policy terminology whenever and wherever possible.

4 Specific Language Issues for Advanced Practice Nursing

The most obvious language problem for APNs around the world pertains to the titles used by the various advanced roles, with titles varying from country to country or even institution to institution. Multiple studies have documented the immense variation in titles used for APNs (Wheeler et al. 2022; Maier and Aiken 2016a; Heale and Buckley 2015; Pulcini et al. 2010), and the resulting problems from these variations. Lack of standardization affects professional credibility and branding and also limits the ability of APNs to meet unmet health needs of their communities, to participate in scholarly exchanges, to lead and participate in reliable research, and to collaborate across borders (Wheeler et al. 2022; Scanlon et al. 2019; Maier and Aiken 2016b; Kooienga and Carryer 2015). There are four commonly accepted APN roles, with the International Council of Nurses codifying the terms *nurse practitioner* (ICN 2020), *clinical nurse specialist* (ICN 2020), and *nurse anesthetist* (ICN 2021), and the International Confederation of Midwives (ICM 2023) recognizing a category of midwifery that follows education as a nurse (e.g., nurse midwife). Additionally, the ICN recently added the requirement of a master's degree as the educational credential needed for APNs (ICN 2020). Jurisdictions and institutions will follow respective laws/regulations that are in operation, and there are some where various titles are allowed and perhaps not well regulated; nonetheless, there is a general movement toward title consistency (Wheeler et al. 2022). Additionally, in some countries, there are many serving as nurse practitioners (NPs), nurse specialists (NSs), nurse anesthetists (NAs), and nurse midwives (NMs) who do not have master's or doctoral degrees (Wheeler et al. 2022). Over time, with intent, resources, and planning, the means will be provided to allow APNs to meet those higher education standards when deemed helpful and necessary. In the meantime, the critical message, when involved in policy discussions, is to use correct local terms as decided by the profession and not be drawn into the use of terms that do not fairly represent the profession.

Other examples of terms that have plagued the APN profession are *midlevel provider* and *physician extender*. The term midlevel provider is thought to have originated with the Department of Justice's Drug Enforcement Administration (DEA) of the United States (Bishop 2012), where the DEA used the term midlevel practitioner to distinguish nurse practitioners, nurse midwives, nurse anesthetists, clinical nurse specialists, and physician assistants from physicians, dentists, veterinarians, or podiatrists (USDEA n.d.). As early as 2009, the American Association of Nurse Practitioners (AANP) called for the disuse of these terms in reference to NPs, either individually or in aggregate (AANP 2024). The position paper for this stance was revised as recently as 2022, demonstrating that the terms have continued to be used despite the efforts of AANP. Schools and organizations in the United States and around the world are urged to educate nursing and APN students, APNs, and policymakers to avoid the use of these terms and refer to the respective APN group under discussion (e.g., nurse practitioner, nurse midwife, clinical nurse specialist, or nurse anesthetist).

5 Conclusion

A working knowledge of the language of health policy is valuable to any APN who hopes to influence health policy or who is the recipient of policies they hope to better understand. To improve the understanding, development, and utilization of optimal policy terms, APNs and APN interested parties (stakeholders) may want to consider the following:

1. Look for applicable policy glossaries when developing policies that apply to education, practice, governance, leadership, and research.
2. When policy work is being done, devote time at the beginning to language consensus, defining pertinent terms as needed.
3. Watch for offensive, culturally insensitive terms, and agree to use inclusive, culturally sensitive terms.
4. Include content on health policy terminology in policy courses and policy education.

References

Alliance for Healthier Communities (AHC). Inclusive and empathetic language use guidelines. n.d.. https://www.cityofboise.org/media/12897/optional-readings-week-1.pdf. Accessed 2 July 2024.

American Association of Nurse Practitioners (AANP). Use of terms such as mid-level provider and physician extender. 2024. https://www.aanp.org/advocacy/advocacy-resource/position-statements/use-of-terms-such-as-mid-level-provider-and-physician-extender. Accessed 2 May 2025.

Arceil Leadership Limited (ALL). Leadership glossary and concepts. 2018. https://www.arceil.com/resources/glossary-of-terms. Accessed 1 May 2025.

Australian Government. Australian government style manual. 2024. https://www.stylemanual.gov.au/writing-and-designing-content/clear-language-and-writing-style/plain-language-and-word-choice. Accessed 2 July 2024.

Bishop CS. Advanced practitioners are not mid-level providers. J Adv Pract Oncol. 2012;3(5):287–8.

Heale R, Buckley R. An international perspective of advanced practice nursing regulation. Int Nurs Rev. 2015;62(3):421–9. https://doi.org/10.1111/inr.12193.

Hwang PKS. Words and phrases you may want to think twice about using. 2021. https://www.cbc.ca/news/canada/ottawa/words-and-phrases-commonly-used-offensive-english-language-1.6252274. Accessed 1 July 2024.

Institute for Credentialing Excellence (ICE). Back to basics: I.C.E. releases updated terminology guide. 2020. https://www.credentialinginsights.org/Article/back-to-basics-ice-releases-updated-terminology-guide-1. Accessed 1 June 2024.

Institute for Credentialing Excellence (ICE). I.C.E. basic guide to credentialing terminology, 2nd ed. 2021. https://www.credentialinginsights.org/Article/back-to-basics-ice-releases-updated-terminology-guide-1. Accessed 1 June 2024.

International Confederation of Midwives (ICM). Post-nursing midwifery programme guide. 2023. https://www.internationalmidwives.org/assets/files/education-files/2023/05/en-tc_30112022-icm-post-nursing-programme-guide_v0.8-jan-15.pdf. Accessed 1 July 2024.

International Council of Nurses (ICN). Guidelines on advanced practice nursing 2020. 2020. https://www.icn.ch/system/files/documents/2020-04/ICN_APN%20Report_EN_WEB.pdf. Accessed 1 July 2024.

International Council of Nurses (ICN). Guidelines on advanced practice nursing nurse anesthetists 2021. 2021. https://www.icn.ch/system/files/documents/2021-05/ICN_Nurse-Anaesthetist-Report_EN_WEB.pdf. Accessed 1 July 2024.

Kooienga SA, Carryer JB. Globalization and advancing primary health care nurse practitioner practice. J Nurse Pract. 2015;11(8):804–11. https://doi.org/10.1016/j.nurpra.2015.06.012.

Larson MS. The rise of professionalism: a sociological analysis. Berkeley: University of California Press; 1978.

Maier C, Aiken L. Task shifting from physicians to nurses in primary care in 39 countries: a cross-country comparative study. Eur J Publ Health. 2016a;26(6):927–34. https://doi.org/10.1093/eurpub/ckw098.

Maier C, Aiken L. Expanding clinical roles for nurses to realign the global health workforce with population needs: a commentary. Isr J Health Policy Res. 2016b;5:1–5. https://doi.org/10.1186/s13584-016-0079-2.

Okeh N. Say this instead: grandfathering. 2021. https://practicalesg.com/2021/07/say-this-instead-grandfathering/. Accessed 2 July 2024.

Parliamentary Counsel Office (PCO). Avoid emotive words, jargon, and policy speak. n.d.. https://www.pco.govt.nz/5.1/. Accessed 2 July 2024.

ProctorFree. Education terms glossary. n.d.. https://www.proctorfree.com/education-terms-glossary/. Accessed 2 June 2024.

Pulcini J, Jelic M, Gul R, Loke AY. An international survey on advanced practice nursing education, practice and regulation. J Nurs Scholarsh. 2010;43(1):31–9. https://doi.org/10.1111/j.1547-5069.2009.01322.x.

Scanlon A, Bryant-Lukosius D, Lehwaldt D, Wilkinson J, Honig J. International transferability of nurse practitioner credentials in five countries. J Nurse Pract. 2019;15(7):487–93. https://doi.org/10.1016/j.nurpra.2019.02.007.

United States Department of Justice Drug Enforcement Administration (USDEA). Mid-level practitioners authorization by state. n.d.. https://www.deadiversion.usdoj.gov/drugreg/practioners.html. Accessed 2 May 2025.

University of Southern California (USC). Glossary of research terms. 2025. https://libguides.usc.edu/writingguide/researchglossary. Accessed 1 May 2025.

Wheeler KJ, Miller M, Pulcini J, Gray D, Ladd E, Rayens MK. Advanced practice nursing roles, regulation, education, and practice: a global study. Ann Glob Health. 2022;88(1):42. https://doi.org/10.5334/aogh.3698.

World Health Organization (WHO). Health promotion glossary of terms. 2021. https://www.who.int/publications/i/item/9789240038349. Accessed 2 June.

Critical Building Blocks for Health Policy Implementation and Improvement

Andrea Brassard and Sarah J. Locke

1 Assessing the Need for Change

Advanced practice nurses (APNs) caring for patients in every healthcare setting can identify the need to change health policy. When considering policy changes, the APN needs to identify what exactly needs to be changed. Is there a written policy or guideline, or are APNs constrained by unwritten cultural norms? If there is an actual policy, what is the policy level—departmental, institutional, jurisdictional, or other? Is the policy or guideline part of an institution's policy book? Is the policy or guideline from a jurisdiction or national professional governing body or from a professional organization? Consulting with APN leaders for clarification is critical. Is APN practice restricted by laws or regulations? In the United States, for example, the most difficult way to change policy is through a state regulation or an act of Congress. Before going the legislative route, consider if there are alternative paths to policy change.

When there is a barrier to APN practice and care, frame the issue from the patient's perspective. How does this barrier limit patients' access to APN care? What evidence is there? Is the evidence anecdotal? Is patient care delayed? Do delays have negative consequences? How would changing the current policy benefit patients and their families?

Again, talking to APN colleagues in the institution or geographical area is essential. APN colleagues may be able to provide some background information on the policy issue or can provide an exemplar or template on which to model a proposed policy change. If the need for a regulatory or legislative change is identified, the

A. Brassard (✉)
New Jersey State Nurses Association, Newfoundland, NJ, USA
e-mail: andreabelanusbrassard@gmail.com

S. J. Locke
University of Arizona College of Nursing, Tucson, AZ, USA
e-mail: slocke@arizona.edu

K. J. Wheeler, M. Acorn (eds.), *Health Policy for Advanced Practice Nursing: A Toolkit for Implementation and Improvement*, Advanced Practice in Nursing,
https://doi.org/10.1007/978-3-032-03667-4_6

next step is to go to the source and carefully study the current policy language and the specific laws or regulations that govern APN practice. This analysis includes researching the history of the issue and how the laws or regulations changed to get where they are presently and any previous attempts at policy changes that did not pass. Has there been a specific stance of opposition? Have any other laws or regulations recently changed that impact the identified policy issue and now support the need to update it?

How large a change is needed? Is it incremental—a small change or a gradual phase in, or something more significant? Incremental changes are small adjustments to the status quo. Incremental changes are limited and manageable, building on each other over time. Radical change transforms the healthcare system. Removing barriers to APN practice and care affects APNs and their patients, physicians and other providers, healthcare institutions, and government entities. Because of this, radical change requires more resources and engenders more resistance. Thus, most healthcare policy changes are incremental.

It is important to continue to gather evidence. Published research is ideal, but case reports, expert opinions, quality improvement studies, position statements, or clinical guidelines are also evidence of the need for change. Evidence from other institutions, geographical areas, or other countries can be powerful to demonstrate workable solutions. Reports of cost savings are strong evidence and can gain the support of interested parties (stakeholders) at the organizational and healthcare system levels. Patient stories or testimonials can also be used to support a health policy change, but to be a positive influence, they should be rooted in evidence and potential challenges and pitfalls need to be considered (Fadlallah et al. 2019).

2 Identifying Interested Parties (Stakeholders) and Influencing Decision-Makers

Identifying interested parties (stakeholders) is the first step in assessing the policy environment. *Interested parties (stakeholders)* are defined as individuals or groups who are responsible for, or affected by, health- and healthcare-related decisions. In a healthcare setting, interested parties (stakeholders) always include nurses, APNs, physicians, patients, and their family caregivers. However, to change healthcare policy, it is important to identify the interested parties (stakeholders) who are the decision-makers. Who has the power to write or revise an organizational policy? Key decision-makers within an organization are primarily the administration, but it depends on the culture of the organization. Many healthcare organizations have unit- or department-level committees, taskforces, or shared governance models that allow front-line staff direct input into ideas and direction for organizational change. Following the current processes or change of command is vital to getting a proposed change to the appropriate decision-makers. Similarly, if regulatory or legislative changes are needed, identify the process and the decision-makers. Can meetings be arranged to meet directly with legislators? Does the Board of Nursing or Nursing Council hold open meetings for community or interested parties (stakeholders) input? Is there a professional organization with APN advocates or lobbyists for representation? To affect policy change, it is necessary to not only identify key interested parties (stakeholders) but also the various approaches that can be taken to reach the decision-makers.

The next step is to determine target audiences. The primary targets of health policy change may include the minister of health, the head of a health committee, or members of the legislature. These primary targets may not be easily accessible to APNs, so it is important to identify secondary targets, those persons or institutions that can influence the primary targets.

A visual way to identify primary and secondary targets is by drawing a Power Map. In the United States, the National Organization of Nurse Practitioner Faculties (NONPF) developed a policy toolkit, Integration of Health Policy Education throughout DNP Nurse Practitioner Curricula (2022), that includes a power mapping exercise. Developed by nurse practitioner faculty for nurse practitioner students, the power mapping steps can be applied by any APN to situations needing change. Power mapping creates a visual representation of decision-makers and their personal and professional connections (Klein et al. 2022).

2.1 Steps in Power Mapping

1. Identify the critical decision-maker needing to be influenced. The entity could be a person or an institution.
2. Identify the decision-maker's critical personal and professional relationships that could influence the decision-maker in supporting or opposing the policy issue. When considering relationships, think of family members, campaign donors, constituency groups, employment affiliations, religious affiliations, neighborhood and community groups, and organizations in the community that employ a large number of people. In this step, think broadly and brainstorm. Make a list of at least ten people or institutions that influence the decision-maker. Keep track of sources that can be used when creating the list.
3. Next, consider the connections, also called the relational power lines. Think about how the decision-maker targets are related to the people and institutions that have been identified, and also note how the people and institutions connect to each other.
4. Diagram software can be used to draw a chart similar to the one in Fig. 1. Using the list created in step 2, write the person or institution's name in the chart in the area that best describes the relationship to the decision-maker. The chart in Fig. 2 can be used to determine where to place the person or institution on the Power Map. Draw lines to connect them to the decision-maker in the center of the map.

   Think about the questions:

   - Are they with us/do they agree with us, and are they influential? Place near the upper left.
   - Are they with us/do they agree with us, and have little influence? Place near the upper right.

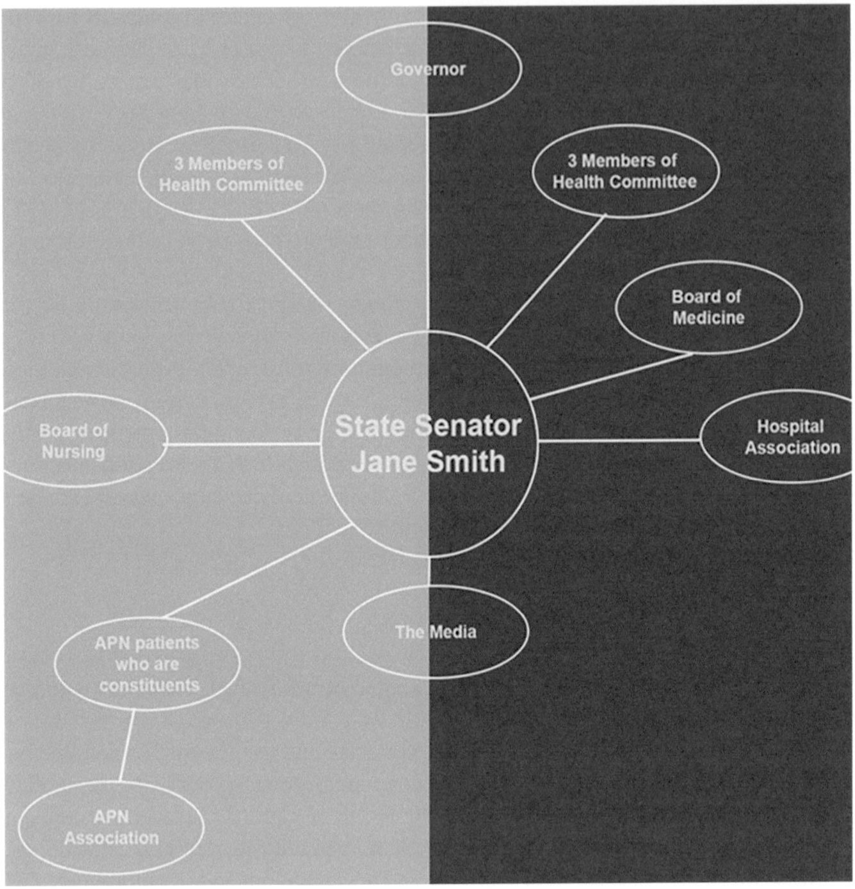

Fig. 1 Power mapping example

With Us a lot of influence	Against Us a lot of influence
With Us a little influence	Against Us a little influence

Fig. 2 Diagram support or opposition and influence

- Are they against us/do they disagree with us, and are they influential? Place near the lower left.
- Are they against us/do they disagree with us, and have little influence? Place near the lower right.
- If unsure of their influence or if they agree/disagree, place them closer to the center.

5. Next, consider how the individuals and institutions connect to the other decision-makers on the Power Map. Draw a line to indicate a connection between the individuals/institutions with commonalities.
6. Consider identified connections to determine priority relationships. Notice which individuals/institutions have the most lines drawn to them.
7. Identify which relationships need to be cultivated or developed, and which overlapping concerns are shared among the entities.
8. Create a plan for influencing the targeted decision-maker.
   - Decide how and where action can be taken, strategies that can be used, and what resources are available that will amplify the likelihood that support for the health policy issue is increased.
   - Decide how and where you can be taken, strategies that can be used, and what resources are available to diminish opposition to the health policy issue. Describe how to address or debunk the opposition's statements used to influence the legislators.

3 Assessing the Policy Environment

A common framework for assessing the policy environment is the Kingdon model (Hoefer 2022). John Kingdon is an American political scientist who developed the multiple streams framework in 1984 (updated in 2010). The multiple streams framework has been cited in numerous English-language publications. The three streams in this framework are delineating the policy problem, proposing a policy solution, and assessing the political will to do something about the issue (Hoefer 2022). Do the policymakers identified and analyzed through power mapping have the political will to implement the health policy change? If so, a window of opportunity opens for policy change (Fig. 3).

APNs and policy interested parties (stakeholders) must be alert to the opening of a window of opportunity, recognizing the window may close without action being taken, leaving the current policy in place. The Kingdon framework can be helpful as APNs advocating for legislative change are reminded that the process of health policy change can seem random, perhaps irrational (Hoefer 2022). In *America the Unusual*, Kingdon (1999) explains the American system of government as being different from other Western democracies. Nonetheless, much APN policy work in the United States has progressed during some window of opportunity and may be useful as a guide for potential APN policy change.

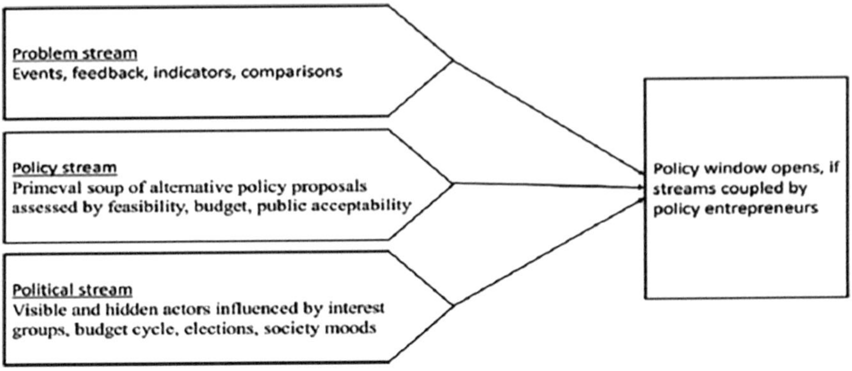

Fig. 3 John Kingdon multiple streams framework. (Reprinted with permission from "Why Digitalization is NOT on the Local Political Agenda: Findings from Danish Local Governments," by K. Kristensen, 2023, *Scandinavian Journal of Public Administration*, *27*(4), 52–68. https://doi.org/10.58235/sjpa.2023.10663). Reprinted with permission from the School of Public Administration, University of Gothenburg. Framework material based on *Agendas, Alternatives, and Public Policies*, by J.W. Kingdon, 2011, Pearson)

An example of a window of opportunity that resulted in a major policy change was the COVID-19 epidemic. Since patients could not get to their providers' offices, state and federal policymakers greatly expanded telehealth in the United States (Giese 2022). This expansion of telehealth required a reimbursement change by the Center for Medicare and Medicaid Services (CMS), the federal insurance system in the US Language in the 2016 Coronavirus Aid, Relief, and Economic Security Act, also known as the CARES Act, had to be changed (Shaver 2022). In the aftermath of the COVID-19 pandemic, there has been an influx of proposed state and federal-level bills in the United States to continue or permanently enact many of the loosened regulations, particularly around telehealth and removing barriers to APN practice and care.

At the organizational level, it is vital to have a strong grasp of the organizational culture: How things work, who has formal and informal power, and internal communication networks. Does the organizational culture have a spirit of inquiry or excellence where process improvement is the norm? Or is there toxicity, and everyone tries to keep their head down and maintain the status quo? Understanding the inner workings of an organization, such as committee structure and governing bylaws, will help to anticipate whether a policy change will be embraced or not, as well as the best way to approach it. Any type of proposed policy change should align with an organization's mission, vision, values, and strategic plan. Keep in mind the overall political, legislative, and regulatory environments, and the potential impact on the organization in relation to issues being explored for policy change or implementation.

4 Working with Lobbyists

In the United States, for example, most state and federal APN organizations have a legislative committee and hire lobbyists to champion legislation that benefits APNs and their patients. APNs rely on lobbyists to draft and monitor legislation, maintain relationships with decision-makers, and advise the APN organization on legislative strategies and tactics. In the United States, lobbying is federally regulated. Activities and monies received and spent on the organization's behalf must be reported. Lobbyists typically have backgrounds in health policy, political science, or law. Through their direct work with legislators, lobbyists can offer valuable insight into how potential policy changes may be perceived by individual politicians, as well as possible issues with the proposed change. Changing legislation is a time-consuming process, marked by stops and starts and pitfalls. Professional lobbyists are expensive, so local APN groups enlist APN volunteers for advocacy. Similar to lobbyists, APN advocates form relationships with their elected officials. Legislators respond more readily to their constituents. Nursing organizations and their lobbyists can provide strategies and talking points for APNs wanting to get more engaged and active in health policy and advocacy.

One communication strategy used by APN advocacy volunteers and paid lobbyists is the elevator speech. An elevator speech is a tool used to promote an issue, idea, oneself, or one's profession. The term elevator is used because it is a short 60-second speech, which is enough time to share the information on an elevator ride with an intended targeted audience member. APNs use elevator speeches in advocating for the advanced practice nursing role, as well as policy changes, be it organizational or legislative. Sometimes referred to as an elevator pitch, the 60-second speech begins by introducing oneself, describing the problem, proposing the solution, and ending with a pitch or ask (Yonkaitis 2020). A three-minute version of an elevator speech is described in the NONPF Health Policy toolkit (DeClerk et al. 2022).

A short speech or encounter with a decision-maker should ideally be accompanied by a takeaway or handout. Similar to the elevator speech, the takeaway document or "leave behind" should include information about the APN organization, the problem, the solution, and an ask. A one-page fact sheet is described in the NONPF Health Policy toolkit (Brassard 2022). It is important that the fact sheet be easy to read and written without medical or nursing jargon.

5 Working with Media

In today's era, access to a variety of media sources is widely available, such as print, online news sources, television, and social media. However, the regulation of media can vary greatly between countries. The use of media is a powerful tool to support, promote, and advocate for, or against, a policy issue or change. At the organizational level, it is imperative to be aware of any policies about employee use of social media. Finding the right approach to reach decision-makers is important; going about it the right way is even more important. It is also important to consider any potential criticism, or even repercussions, from addressing the policy issue in the media. The media is also a major source of biased information or misinformation. To use media to support an intended policy change, it is important to research various media outlets and focus on one that is trusted and is either objective in nature or is in line with the side of the policy issue of the intended policy change. It is important to remember that legislators and interested parties (stakeholders) outside of healthcare receive the same misinformation as the public. As an APN working for policy change, it is vital to be aware of the current news to dispel any associated false information or myths, as well as keeping current with positive and negative evidence to support the policy change. Social media, especially, has driven increased awareness of healthcare issues, which can benefit proposed policy change, particularly if organizational, state, or federal decision-makers deem the issue a priority. Aligning with the discussion from Sect. 3, media can be a major influencer in providing the window of opportunity for policy change, and often timing is the pivotal factor deciding if action will be taken to advance a policy change. Awareness of current news also guides lobbyists in their approach to conversations with legislators.

Two common ways that health policy issues are presented to the media are social media campaigns and opinion editorials (more commonly called OpEds). In the NONPF policy toolkit, cited above, a plan is outlined for social media communications strategy (Swint 2022a). Having a communications strategy for social media provides a detailed blueprint that takes the what, when, how, and why into consideration for the content posted (Swint and Miller 2022).

The social media communications strategy plan should include:

- Target audience: Identify the specific audience the campaign will be geared toward.
- Objectives: What is the goal trying to be achieved through a social media campaign?
  - Write objectives in SMART format (specific, measurable, attainable, realistic, and timely).
  - Use market research or community data to support and describe the communication needs of targeted audiences.
  - Align the objectives with the organization's mission, as indicated.
- Content, message, and tools:
  - Create just two to three well-designed key messages. These should align with the objectives and intended audience.
  - Identify an individual or team to create the content and oversee the online campaign.
  - Consider using more than one social media tool to connect with the target audience.
  - Detail logistics of how long the information will be posted and how long the viewer will interact with the content.
- Partners: Consider up to three key partners to support the campaign and define their roles and responsibilities.

- Evaluation: Create a plan to determine if the social media campaign was successful, using at least two processes and two outcome evaluation measures.
- Reflection: Was the campaign successful? Is another campaign needed? What could be improved for future campaigns? (Swint 2022a)

Historically located in the editorial section of the newspaper, OpEds (opinion editorials) are the writer's opinion on a given topic or issue, geared toward a targeted audience, presented with a strong voice, and supported by valid information or evidence. For the OpEd to be effective, the chosen media format and outlet need to reach the intended target audience. OpEds are less formal than academic writing, but still need to be well written and evidence based. The APN writer demonstrates their credibility on the issue by highlighting their professional role and credentials. Including an unnamed patient story strengthens the emotional value of communicating the message to the target audience of interested parties (stakeholders) and decision-makers. In the past, OpEds were published in print media, but OpEds can also be a part of the social media communication plan.

The NONPF policy toolkit includes more thorough instructions on how to write an OpEd (Swint 2022b), but an OpEd should be about 600–800 words in length and include these main points:

- Lead: Grab the reader's attention with a bold statement to set the scene.
- Thesis: Clearly state the argument being specific and precise, and include fact, not opinion.
- Argument: Provide three points to support position or opinion on the topic. With each point, provide two statements of evidence (fact) and a conclusion statement. This is the substance of the OpEd to sway the reader into caring about the issue or supporting the proposed position or opinion.
- "To be sure" paragraph: This is where any flaws or limitations to the discussion are addressed.
- Conclusion: Wrap-up with a strong ending tied to the lead, and end with a call to action for the reader using an active verb tense (Swint 2022b).

6 Initiating, Monitoring, and Evaluating the Policy Project

Ideas must include action to drive change, and initiating a policy project is the first part of the process. As discussed so far in this chapter, assessing the need for change, identifying interested parties (stakeholders) and decision-makers, and assessing the policy environment lay the groundwork for starting a policy project.

Steps in initiating, monitoring, and evaluating a policy project:

1. *Determine the type of policy change*: What change is needed? An amendment to an existing policy? An idea for a new bill to introduce into legislation? Revision of organizational procedure? Minor verbiage changes to policy or bylaws?

2. *Review the evidence*: Compile and organize the information, research, and documents from assessing the need for change. Identify themes, gaps, or redundancies. Is there enough background to support the need for policy change?
3. *Preliminarily consult with interested parties (stakeholders)*: Discuss the identified need for change and thoughts on the solution. Listen to the stance and feedback of interested parties (stakeholders). This is an important step needed to build consensus. Early discussions with interested parties (stakeholders) could be APN colleagues, mid-level organizational leadership, community members, patients, and local professional organizations. Discussions with decision-making interested parties (stakeholders) will come later in the process.
4. *Put together a team*: Policy projects can be grassroots efforts by one determined individual, but compiling a team brings support, expertise, and power in numbers. The team members can include interested parties (stakeholders) that were preliminarily consulted, but further expertise from varied perspectives may also be needed based on the type and breadth of policy change. Determining the type of policy change needed will help determine who needs to be on the team to reach the target audience. One organization that is a good resource for advice and support is seeds for change, available at seedsforchange.org.uk.
5. *Create a delivery plan*: There are many types of formats for this, but a delivery plan should include goals, objectives, deliverables, a timeline, and the team members involved or accountable. Goals are the results intended to be achieved. Objectives are the desired outcomes to be achieved by the project. Deliverables are the items produced to meet objectives. The timeline outlines each task and due dates to keep everyone on track. Finally, it is important to assign team members to specific tasks to create ownership and accountability. If money is needed for certain activities, identifying a plan to secure funding or who will cover the costs needs to be planned.
6. *Develop a solution*: Determining the type of policy change is part of the solution, but before a policy change is presented to higher-level decision-makers, a potential solution needs to be thought through. What specific aspects of the issue need to be addressed? Does the solution align with organizational mission, vision, values, and strategic plan? Will this solution lead to the expected outcomes? When developing a solution, it is important to consider the perspective of the interested parties (stakeholders), as well as any other people, departments, programs, and funding that could be directly or indirectly impacted. From a systems perspective, everything is connected, and one change can trigger a chain reaction. More foresight in addressing or mitigating potential impact can strengthen the proposed solution. Depending on the nature of the solution, a cost-benefit or cost-effectiveness analysis may be needed to demonstrate cost savings or improved outcome potential above and beyond cost. Finally, is the solution sustainable? Expert consultation and/or collaboration may need to be pursued, as needed.
7. *Draft a proposal*: This can be done in several formats, depending on the nature of the policy change and the targeted audience, such as a slide presentation, a policy brief, a health policy memo, or an executive summary. Sometimes an

organization may have a proposal template or online process to follow. A slide presentation can be appropriate in smaller, less formal settings for lower-stakes changes. The table here introduces three types of proposals. The terms are often used interchangeably, but policy briefs focus on an argument with specific policy recommendations, whereas a health policy memo presents a broader perspective addressing an issue from both sides and ends with a call to action. The shortest format, the executive summary, typically includes an introduction, objective, methodology, findings, recommendations, and conclusion. Policy briefs and health policy memos often include an executive summary, but more so as an abstract or brief overview.

Policy brief (Swint and Miller 2022)	Health policy memo (UC n.d.)	Executive summary (Harvard n.d.)
Title Executive summary Context or scope of the problem Identify interested parties (stakeholders) Policy alternatives Policy recommendation/call to action Appendices References	Heading in memo format Executive summary Background and methodology Key findings Opinions/alternative options Recommendations Conclusion References	Introduction Objective/policy issue Methodology Findings Recommendations Conclusion References

8. *Map a course of action*: The course of action can be added to the delivery plan, but once the policy proposal is ready to go, it is time to bring it to the decision-makers' attention. The key is to get on a committee's agenda. In an organization, there may be a policy council, a shared governance committee, or a policy and procedure committee. Reach out to the committee's chair, an executive assistant, or follow the organizational chain of command. Proposing legislation needs the support of a legislative sponsor. This is where the lobbyists can liaise with legislative aides and meet with them or be able to set up a meeting with a legislator. If an elected official is a nurse, they may or may not be the ideal sponsor, but a lobbyist and/or the state's nurses association should be able to provide guidance on which legislators may sponsor and/or support a bill. The legislative aide will arrange the appointment with the legislator. Mapping a course of action is also where the media communications plan will be integrated to start promoting the chosen policy change, but the media communications plan can be implemented sooner or later in the process, as necessary.
9. *Action time*: Meeting with a legislator or legislative committee can seem intimidating, but it is important to not let nerves take over. Getting organized and taking the time to be well prepared is essential (Whited et al. 2022). Also review the legislative committee or legislator's webpage, recent actions or votes, and decide which team members will attend (Whited et al. 2022). Mapping logistics of weather, the commute, and parking ahead of time reduces stress the day of the meeting, as does arriving early and being dressed professionally. Conversations with policy- or decision-makers should include the provision of a fact sheet, so

they can refer to it during the discussion and have it available to reference or disseminate after the meeting. The conversation on the issue should be clear and concise on what is being asked (Whited et al. 2022). If they are being asked to sponsor or support a legislative change, they should know why it is important for them to do so. Providing a list of talking points and a synopsis of the collective evidence and background information supporting the policy change helps them understand why change is necessary. Be sure to describe the proposed solution, incorporate discussion from the perspective of various interested parties (stakeholders), and explain why other potential solutions would not work as well. Incorporate information on the financial component, as this aspect can significantly sway support or opposition. Policymakers should be thanked for their time, provided contact information, and informed of what follow-up might happen—a call, email, or future meeting—depending on the outcome of what was discussed (Whited et al. 2022). After the meeting, notes should be written about what transpired, shared with others working on the issue if appropriate, and plans made to meet with the team on the next steps.

It is not uncommon to be turned away, hear "no," or not hear back. Perseverance is needed, as there will be many speed bumps and hurdles to overcome. Lots of work is needed to develop a draft for an institutional policy or legislative bill. Organizational committee members, leadership team, lobbyists, or legislative administration can instruct on specifics about the process. Bills are often reintroduced several times before they get traction. As discussed earlier, timing in the right political environment can make all the difference. Getting to the monitoring phase of a policy is a huge feat! Keeping the momentum going with the social media communication plan, social and professional networking, and word-of-mouth is ongoing work. Local news media outlets and professional organizations can provide further exposure if they are updated periodically. Attendance at any open meetings within the organization or open legislative sessions where the proposal or new bill is on the agenda is recommended. The team must be continuously updated and meet on a regular basis to discuss ways to mitigate threats and roadblocks, and look for opportunities for improvement, especially if the proposal or bill gets turned down. Communication on progress must be maintained with relevant interested parties (stakeholders), such as legislative aides or project sponsors. If the policy change gets implemented or enacted, congratulations! Given how many steps, stakeholders, and barriers there are to change policy, getting to the end of the policy process is a major accomplishment. Even if the policy project was successful, it is important to discuss and celebrate what went well and what could be improved for next time. As mentioned earlier, once a change occurs, there are often other changes that are needed because of the given change, or to keep the process going incrementally to achieve greater change. If the policy proposal was stopped at any part in the process, it is important to determine why and what needs to change to be successful. Did the proposal not have enough supporting evidence? Was there not enough buy-in and support? Was it the right solution, timing, or approach? Make sure to capture any feedback received and use that as fuel to revise and reattempt. As economic and societal needs change, the proposed solution may need to be updated. Revisit the initiation steps each time and make appropriate adjustments as needed.

References

Brassard A. Fact sheet. In: Swint C, DeClerk L, NONPF's Health Policy Education Special Interest Group, editors. A tool kit: integration of health policy education throughout DNP nurse practitioner curricula. NONPF; 2022. p. 69–71. https://cdn.ymaws.com/www.nonpf.org/resource/resmgr/faculty_resources/NONPF_Health_Policy_Educatio.pdf. Accessed 1 Aug 2025.

DeClerk L, Clement D, Hopla D, Sanford M. Elevator speech/elevator pitch. In: Swint C, DeClerk L, NONPF's Health Policy Education Special Interest Group, editors. A tool kit: integration of health policy education throughout DNP nurse practitioner curricula. NONPF; 2022. p. 47–9. https://cdn.ymaws.com/www.nonpf.org/resource/resmgr/faculty_resources/NONPF_Health_Policy_Educatio.pdf. Accessed 1 Aug 2025.

Fadlallah R, El-Jardali F, Nomier M, Hemadi N, Arif K, Langlois EV, et al. Using narratives to impact health policy-making: a systematic review. Health Res Policy Syst. 2019;17:26. https://doi.org/10.1186/s12961-019-0423-4.

Giese K. Coronavirus disease 2019's shake-up of telehealth policy: application of Kingdon's multiple streams framework. J. Nurse Pract. 2022;16(10):768–70.

Harvard University, Kennedy School Communications Programs. How to write an executive summary. Harvard Kennedy School Communications Program, Harvard University; n.d.. https://projects.iq.harvard.edu/files/hks-communications-program/files/how_to_write_an_exex_summ_to_use_4_18_18.pdf. Accessed 1 Aug 2025

Hoefer R. The multiple streams framework: understanding and applying the problems, policies, and politics approach. J Policy Pract Re. 2022;3:1–5.

Kingdon JW. America the unusual. New York: Worth Publishers; 1999.

Klein T, Kaplan L, Swint C. In: Swint C, DeClerk L, NONPF's Health Policy Education Special Interest Group, editors. A tool kit: integration of health policy education throughout DNP nurse practitioner curricula. Washington, DC: NONPF; 2022. p. 29–33. https://cdn.ymaws.com/www.nonpf.org/resource/resmgr/faculty_resources/NONPF_Health_Policy_Educatio.pdf. Accessed 1 Aug 2025.

National Organization of Nurse Practitioner Faculties (NONPF). A tool kit: integration of health policy education throughout DNP nurse practitioner curricula. 2022. https//cdn.ymaws.com/www.nonpf.org/resource/resmgr/faculty_resources/NONPF_Health_Policy_Educatio.pdf. Accessed 1 Aug 2025.

Shaver J. The state of telehealth before and after the COVID-19 pandemic. Prim Care Clin Office Pract. 2022;49:517–30.

Swint C. Social media communications strategy plan. In: Swint C, DeClerk L, NONPF's Health Policy Education Special Interest Group, editors. A tool kit: integration of health policy education throughout DNP nurse practitioner curricula. Washington, DC: NONPF; 2022a. p. 86–9. https://cdn.ymaws.com/www.nonpf.org/resource/resmgr/faculty_resources/NONPF_Health_Policy_Educatio.pdf. Accessed 1 Aug 2025.

Swint C. Op-ed. In: Swint C, DeClerk L, NONPF's Health Policy Education Special Interest Group, editors. A tool kit: integration of health policy education throughout DNP nurse practitioner curricula. Washington, DC: NONPF; 2022b. p. 63–5. https://cdn.ymaws.com/www.nonpf.org/resource/resmgr/faculty_resources/NONPF_Health_Policy_Educatio.pdf. Accessed 1 Aug 2025.

Swint C, Miller J. Policy brief. In: Swint C, DeClerk L, NONPF's Health Policy Education Special Interest Group, editors. A tool kit: integration of health policy education throughout DNP nurse practitioner curricula. Washington, DC: NONPF; 2022. p. 34–7. https://cdn.ymaws.com/.www.nonpf.org/resource/resmgr/faculty_resources/NONPF_Health_Policy_Educatio.pdf.

University of Chicago (UC), Harris Public Policy Leadership Programs. How to write a policy memo that matters. Author; n.d.. https://harris.uchicago.edu/files/how_to_write_a_policy_memo_that_matters_0.pdf. Accessed 1 Aug 2025

Whited T, DeClerk L, Hopla D. Planning a face-to-face interaction with policymakers. In: Swint C, DeClerk L, NONPF's Health Policy Education Special Interest Group, editors. A tool kit: integration of health policy education throughout DNP nurse practitioner curricula. Washington, DC: NONPF; 2022. p. 50–4. https://cdn.ymaws.com/www.nonpf.org/resource/resmgr/faculty_resources/NONPF_Health_Policy_Educatio.pdf. Accessed 1 Aug 2025.

Yonkaitis CF. The elevator pitch: a 60-second advocacy tool for nurses. ANJ. 2020;16:54–6.

Building a Culture of Leadership and Advocacy

Diana J. Mason and Richard Ricciardi

1 Introduction

Patient care is a highly political endeavor, whether we want to recognize it as such or not. Politics shapes the allocation of scarce resources, whether in a health care organization, government, or nursing organizations. Politics determines the policies that all of these entities adopt—or choose not to adopt. It determines who gets what kind of care when and from whom through policies that, for example, define who is authorized and paid for giving care. Increasingly, the standards for care are set in national policy through payment mechanisms and scorecards that require clinicians to document and health systems to report on certain aspects of care and outcomes.

The importance of advanced practice nurses (APNs) engaging in health policy should be readily apparent, particularly for those who have long advocated for the authority and resources needed to improve access to high-quality, person-centered care and advance health equity. In the United States, the nurse practitioner (NP) role emerged in the 1960s as a certificate program designed to improve access to care for children in underserved communities and to expand the role of nurses in primary care settings (Silver et al. 1985).

As the role of the NPs took hold, the preparation of NPs moved into the universities at the master's level, preparing an APN who could practice independently in underserved communities where access to care was limited or nonexistent. Over the

D. J. Mason
Hunter College, Center for Health Policy and Media Engagement, George Washington University School of Nursing, Washington, DC, USA
e-mail: djmasonrn@gmail.com

R. Ricciardi (✉)
Center for Health Policy and Media Engagement, George Washington University School of Nursing, Washington, DC, USA
e-mail: ricricciardi@gwu.edu

K. J. Wheeler, M. Acorn (eds.), *Health Policy for Advanced Practice Nursing: A Toolkit for Implementation and Improvement*, Advanced Practice in Nursing,
https://doi.org/10.1007/978-3-032-03667-4_7

years, APNs in 28 states, the District of Columbia, and two territories in the United States have laws or regulations that define their role as full practice authority (FPA). FPA is defined as the authorization of APNs to evaluate patients, diagnose, order, and interpret diagnostic tests and initiate and manage treatments, including prescribing medications under the exclusive licensure authority of the state board of nursing. Evidence supporting the safety and quality of APN care has accumulated (McMenamin et al. 2023; Newhouse et al. 2011).

The success of the APN role in the United States has led to its spread globally, but many countries still lack the legal authorization and regulation of the role. But the evidence is clear on the value of the APN role, and the stage has been set to advance the role globally. In 2021, the US National Academies of Science, Engineering, and Medicine issued a report titled "Implementing High Quality Primary Care" with the aim of promoting health and reducing the marked disparities that exist in the country (National Academies of Sciences, Engineering, and Medicine 2021). The report called for rethinking primary care, calling for team--based care, including the essential role of APNs. This message of reducing health disparities through the expanded role of nurses was further articulated in the International Council of Nurses (ICN) report on the 76th World Health Assembly and its role in that international body's deliberations, including prioritizing universal health coverage (ICN 2023).

2 The Mandate for APNs to Be Leaders in Policy

So what is keeping APNs from being leaders in policy development, implementation, and evaluation? Perhaps the greatest barrier is the longstanding socialization of nurses that fails to encourage them and equip them to be leaders in policy work that promotes the health of people. This socialization arises in societies that fail to embrace women's roles in the public sphere, normalizing their confinement to the private sphere of family and home or as followers who follow orders (Reverby 1987). The Women's Movement and focus on gender equity are changing how society sees women, as well as men who are nurses; however, until all levels of nursing education fully integrate competencies on leadership, politics, policy, and advocacy, change will be slow.

In a seminal article describing the stages of nurses' political development, Cohen et al. (1996) describe four stages of the profession's involvement in policy and politics.

- *Buy-in:* This stage involves helping nurses to understand the importance of policy work and learn the language and processes of policy development and political strategy. One of the purposes of this book is to help APNs understand both the importance of policy and equip them with some tools for beginning to think about policy and equip them with basic tools for influencing policy. The focus is a reactive one, and mostly on nursing issues. A few nurses garner political appointments but usually because of the individual's own achievements as leaders in nursing and health care.

- *Self-interest:* The second stage moves nurses to using more sophisticated tools (e.g., coalition-building, though largely confined to nursing groups) to advance a policy agenda focused on the interests of nursing. For example, higher payment or reimbursement of APNs is advocated as an end in itself, rather than positioning and framing the aim as a key factor in improving the health of people. While the focus remains on nursing, the efforts are coordinated by nursing organizations that advocate for nurses to be appointed to political positions that focus on nursing.
- *Political sophistication:* Stage 3 sees nurses being proactive on both nursing and broader health care issues. Nurses and their organizations become integral to health care coalitions and are sought for their support of broader health care issues. The associations advocate for nursing to be appointed to nursing--designated policy positions, such as a seat on the health payment reform commission.
- *Leading the way:* This last aspirational stage is exemplified by nurses and their associations leading efforts to improve the health of people through health and social policies that go beyond the self-interests of the profession. Coalition--building is with nonnursing organizations that are critical interested parties (stakeholders) and leaders in health care reforms. Nurses are appointed or elected to key policy positions because of their expertise and focus on advancing the health of people.

Although APNs in most countries continue to focus on advocating laws and regulations that establish or advance practice authority and payment, framing these issues in terms of the public's health, societal costs, and benefits to the economic prosperity of the nation will garner support from multiple interested parties (stakeholders) who care about the broader issues affecting the health of people. But we must move beyond nursing's self-interests. Stage 4, leading the way, is what we should be striving for. In some places, on some issues, at some times, nurses and their organizations demonstrate behaviors that reflect this stage. Gaining a critical mass of APN leaders who are leading the way in policy development requires that nurses broaden their focus beyond self-interest and recognize the interconnections among important determinants of health and the health and well-being of the population.

3 But What Are We Leading? Social Determinants of Health and the SDGs

Sir Michael Marmot's foundational work on the social determinants of health spurred changes in world views of where and how health is promoted and supported (Marmot 2005). He led the development of a framework that organized what nurses such as Lillian Wald in the early 1900s understood as they cared for people in communities: factors such as housing, access to nutritious food, education, a safe environment, and socioeconomic security shape the health and well-being of individuals, families, communities, and societies. A 2014 review of the factors that account for variability in health found that only 25% of this variability was due to health care (McGovern 2014). Consider the implications of this for a country's health: The United States spends more on health care than other high-income countries and half as much as these countries on social services (Butler 2016; Schneider et al. 2021); and yet, it lags behind these other countries on leading health indicators, such as maternal mortality and longevity.

In 2015, the 191 member countries of the United Nations committed to action on 17 UN Sustainable Development Goals, or SDGs. These include: no poverty, zero hunger, quality education, gender equity, clean water and sanitation, affordable and clean energy, decent work and economic growth, reduced inequalities, climate action, life below water, life on land, and partnerships for the goals. All of the SDGs can be related to health and well-being, but Goal 3 specifically addresses "good health and well-being." These countries agreed to develop policies that address these SDGs, and their progress toward reaching the SDGs is ranked and available publicly (https://dashboards.sdgindex.org/rankings).

Nurses see the impact of social determinants of health and the failure of nations to accomplish the SDGs every day, whether from poor access to care, limited nutritious foods, inadequate housing, contaminated water, unaffordable education, or violence. Clearly, APNs need to be an enduring voice in calling for policies that will have a real and meaningful impact on the health of people. APNs can lead the development of policies at local, national, regional, and global levels to promote health and well-being. The SDGs have specific targets that can guide action by APNs and others, particularly when the actions are aligned with the priorities of the Minister of Health, who reports to the UN on their nation's progress. APNs can also advocate for health-promoting policies in other ways, including ensuring that reporting of research findings or practice improvement initiatives include policy recommendations or implications, speaking out about the conditions that undermine health, educating the public and policymakers about the potential policy solutions, lobbying for the right solution, leading efforts to implement a policy, and ensuring that the policy's impact is evaluated and sustainable, if effective.

Success in progressing on the SDGs requires a team effort, including other health professionals, community-based organizations (CBOs), establishing public–private partnerships, and engaging other key interested parties (stakeholders). It also requires an understanding of the economic implications of policies and building into position papers and policy briefs the cost and human impact of a course of action or inaction.

4 Economics of Policy Development

Advancing policies requires attention to the costs and benefits of policy options. Cost-benefit analyses (CBA) can provide policymakers with the comparative value of any particular policy option to a society (Edge 2021). It is only one consideration in setting public policy, but it has an important place in a world of competing interests and limited resources.

Consider the economic value of nursing to a country. A healthy labor force contributes directly to a country's Gross Domestic Product (GDP). Labor productivity is a direct determinant of the economic growth of a country, and health is a major predictor of labor productivity (Ozyilmaz et al. 2022). In addition, studies have found APNs to be cost-effective providers, including when compared with physicians (Abraham et al. 2019; AANP 2013).

This evidence bolsters arguments in favor of establishing the APN role, authorizing APNs to practice to the top of their education and training, ensuring that regulations governing APN practice support full practice authority, and advocating for adequate pay to retain highly qualified APNs and a diverse nursing and APN workforce.

Increasingly, economic perspectives are being incorporated into arguments for building and using the nursing workforce globally, noting that investing in the nursing workforce will have economic payoffs for nations (PAHO 2022). In fact, there is evidence of a stimulus effect of nurses on GDP growth in OECD (Organization for Economic Co-operation and Development) countries (Amiri and Solankallio-Vahteri 2019). The evidence suggests that a 1.0% increase in the number of practicing nurses per 1000 population is associated with a 0.4% increase in a country's GDP.

Unfortunately, most nurses, even APNs, are not equipped to provide CBAs; however, nurses can collaborate on interprofessional teams to conduct such analyses. It is another example of the value of a team-based approach and partnerships to provide an evidence-informed approach to policymaking, policy implementation, and evaluation.

5 APN Advocacy and Leadership in Policy: From Barriers to Solutions

The model of nursing's stages of political development suggests that individual nurses' leadership role in policy may reflect the profession's nascent engagement in leading policy. In some countries, even discussing political strategies to influence national policy can be dangerous. And in countries where political discourse is the norm, seeing oneself as a leader in policy may be lagging because of nursing's roots in societies that marginalized women. Policy and politics receive some attention in the curricula of Western nursing education programs, but are rarely threaded throughout courses or taught as an integral part of what nurses do. But this is changing, as gender equity gains attention on the global stage (including being one of the 17 SDGs), and as both individual nurses and the societies in which they live and work are more open to women and nurses as leaders. Chapter 18 offers curricula and a discussion of how to introduce leadership into APN programs.

Nonetheless, it is incumbent upon APNs to examine their own feelings about being policy leaders, their readiness to serve in this capacity, and the opportunities for building their policy leadership skills. It is essential for APNs to be strategic about gaining seats at policy tables, whether governments, medical societies, and other interested parties (stakeholders) want them there or not. APNs must claim their space as policy leaders—and not just on APN practice authority and payment—and build the partnerships and coalitions that are needed for most policy work. Good leaders are visionaries. When we frame our issues within the context of promoting the health of people and speak out about the broader health and social issues of our times, we are no longer viewed as being focused solely on our own self-interests.

Fortunately, there are roadmaps and tools available to assist APNs to conduct policy analysis and lead advocacy efforts. For example, using the framework of the eightfold path to conduct policy analysis developed by Bardach and Patashnik (2023). The following eight steps provide a roadmap and an evidence-informed approach to the policy analysis: define the problem, assemble the evidence, construct the alternatives, select the criteria, project the outcomes, confront the trade-offs, decide, and tell your story. Further, to support advocacy efforts, there are a number of resources available to APNs, such as the ICN publication *Nurses: A Voice to Lead* (2021) and the Association of Public Health Nurses advocacy guidebook and toolkit (APHN 2021). Sigma has also developed a Global Nursing Leadership Competency Framework, accessible at https://www.sigmanursing.org/global-nursing-leadership-competency-framework.

These resources and those cited in Table 1 provide a springboard for APNs to build knowledge and skills and lead advocacy efforts in support of public policy. Kidner (2022) also published a useful text on the subject, *Successful Advanced Practice Nursing Role Transition*, available at https://www.link.springer.com/book/10.1007/978-3-030-53002-0. Additionally, many master's and DNP programs around the world offer leadership programs in a variety of formats, many specifically focusing on leadership.

The APN movement globally provides an opportunity for collaboration in leading policy change that will improve the health of people and communities. The challenge is for APNs to recognize and seize this opportunity.

Table 1 Leadership programs around the world

Program	Access Link
American Association of Colleges of Nursing's Leadership Programs	https://www.aacnnursing.org/leads
American Association of Colleges of Nursing--Wharton Executive Leadership Program	https://www.aacnnursing.org/conferences-webinars/leadership--development/senior-academic-leaders-program
American Association of Critical-Care Nurses Nurse Leaders Resource and Tool Center Nurse Leader Development	https://www.aacn.org/nurse-leader-resources

(continued)

Table 1 (continued)

Program	Access Link
American Association of Nurse Practitioners Executive Leadership Program	https://www.aanp.org/practice/professional-development/leadership-program
American Organization for Nursing Leadership Certification for Nurse Leaders	https://www.aonl.org/initiatives/certification
Duke Advanced Practice Provider Leadership Institute	https://sites.duke.edu/appli/
Harvard Comprehensive Leadership Programs (Four Programs Available: Owner/President Management, General Management, Advanced Management, Program for Leadership Development)	https://www.exed.hbs.edu/comprehensive-leadership-programs
Harvard Global Nursing Leadership Program	https://hsph.harvard.edu/fellowship-special-program/global-nursing/
Harvard Strategy Execution for Public Leadership (Individual Course)	https://www.harvardonline.harvard.edu/course/strategy-execution--public-leadership?&utm_source=google&utm_medium=cpc&utm_campaign=fy25_all_us&utm_content=brand&keyword=harvard%20kennedy%20plc&matchtype=e&keyword=harvard%20kennedy%20plc&matchtype=e&gad_source=1&gclid=CjwKCAjw0aS3BhA3EiwAKaD2ZTls9XySeOlX-kXtOC-AMAfZm--Vx50iUAka6kFedDT9Ype8Y3YJOoxoCW-gQAvD_BwE
Harvard Women Leaders: Advancing Together, A Multi-Week Leadership Program	https://professional.dce.harvard.edu/prgrams/women-leaders-advancing-together/
International Council of Nurses Global Nursing Leadership Institute™	https://www.icn.ch/how-we-do-it/nna-development-leadership--programmes/global-nursing-leadership-institutetm-gnli
International Council of Nurses Leadership for Change Programme	https://www.icn.ch/how-we-do-it/nna-development-leadership-programmes/leadership-changetm-lfc
Robert Wood Johnson Foundation Health Policy Fellowship	https://healthpolicyfellows.org/
Sigma Healthcare Leadership Program	https://www.sigmamarketplace.org/healthcare-leadership-program-online-course
University of Global Health Equity (Rwanda), Master's in Global Nursing Leadership Program	https://ughe.org/admissions-masters-in-global-nursing-leadership-program-mgln/

The list is presented in alphabetical order, some degree-granting, some certificate-granting, many short-term and/or providing continuing education units

References

Abraham CM, Norful AA, Stone PW, Poghosyan L. Cost-effectiveness of advanced practice nurses compared to physician-led care for chronic diseases: a systematic review. Nurs Econ. 2019;37:293–305. PMID: 34616101; PMCID: PMC8491992.

American Association of Nurse Practitioners (AANP). Nurse practitioner cost effectiveness. 2013. https://www.aanp.org/advocacy/advocacy-resource/position-statements/nurse-practitioner--cost-effectiveness. Accessed 1 Aug 2025.

Amiri A, Solankallio-Vahteri T. Analyzing economic feasibility for investing in nursing care: evidence from panel data analysis in 35 OECD countries. Int J Nurs Sci. 2019;7:13–20. https://doi.org/10.1016/j.ijnss.2019.06.009. PMID: 32099854; PMCID: PMC7031164.

Association of Public Health Nurses (APHN). Public health policy advocacy guide book and tool kit. 2021. https:// www.phnurse.org/assets/docs/APHN%20Public%20Health%20Policy%20Advocacy%20Guidebook%20and%20Toolkit%20_May%202021.pdf. Accessed 1 Aug 2025.

Bardach E, Patashnik EM. A practical guide for policy analysis: the eightfold path to more effective problem solving. 7th ed. Washington, DC: CQ Press; 2023.

Butler S. Social spending, not medical spending, is key to health. Brookings; 2016. https://www.brookings.edu/articles/social-spending-not-medical-spending-is-key-to-health/. Accessed 1 Aug 2015.

Cohen S, Mason DJ, Kovner C, Leavitt J, Pulcini J, Sochalski J. The stages of nursing's political development: where we've been and where we ought to go. Nurs Outlook. 1996;44:259–66.

Edge D. The role of cost-benefit analysis in public policy decision-making. Berkeley Public Policy J. 2021. https://bppj.berkeley.edu/2021/12/14/the-role-of-cost-benefit-analysis-in-public--policy-decision-making/.

International Council of Nurses (ICN). 76th World Health Assembly ICN report: nursing advocacy and influence in global health policy. Geneva: ICN; 2023. https://www.icn.ch/sites/default/files/2023-11/WHA76_ICN_Report.pdf. Accessed 1 Aug 2025.

International Council of Nurses (ICN). Nurses: a voice to lead—a vision for future healthcare. Author; 2021. https://www.icn.ch/resources/publications-and-reports/nurses-voice-lead--vision-future-healthcare. Accessed 1 Aug 2025.

Kidner M. Successful advanced practice nursing role transition. Cham: Springer Nature; 2022. https://www.link.springer.com/book/10.1007/978-3-030-53002-0.

Marmot M. Social determinants of health inequalities. Lancet. 2005;365:1099–104. https://doi.org/10.1016/S0140-6736(05)71146-6. PMID: 15781105.

McGovern L. The relative contributions of multiple determinants to health (Health Policy Brief). Health Aff. 21 Aug 2014. https://www.healthaffairs.org/do/10.1377/hpb20140821.404487.

McMenamin A, Turi E, Schlak A, Poghosyan L. A systematic review of outcomes related to nurse practitioner-delivered primary care for multiple chronic conditions. Med Care Res Rev. 2023;80(6):563–81. https://doi.org/10.1177/10775587231186720. Epub 2023 Jul 12. PMID: 37438917.

National Academies of sciences, engineering, and medicine. Implementing high-quality primary care: rebuilding the foundation of health care. Washington, DC: The National Academies Press; 2021. https://doi.org/10.17226/25983.

Newhouse RP, Stanik-Hutt J, White KM, Johantgen M, Bass EB, Zangaro G, Wilson RF, Fountain L, Steinwachs DM, Heindel L, Weiner JP. Advanced practice nurse outcomes 1990-2008: a systematic review. Nurs Econ. 2011;29(5):230–50; quiz 251. PMID: 22372080.

Ozyilmaz A, Bayraktar Y, Isik E, Toprak M, Er MB, Besel F, Aydin S, Olgun MF, Collins S. The relationship between health expenditures and economic growth in EU countries: empirical evidence using panel Fourier Toda-Yamamoto causality test and regression models. Int J Environ Res Public Health. 2022;19:15091. https://doi.org/10.3390/ijerph192215091. PMID: 36429808; PMCID: PMC9690520.

Pan American Health Organization (PAHO). The strategic importance of national investment in nursing professionals in the region of the Americas. Washington, DC: PAHO; 2022. https://iris.paho.org/bitstream/handle/10665.2/55957/PAHOHSSHR220012_eng.pdf?sequence=5&isAllowed=y.

Reverby S. Ordered to care: the dilemma of American nursing. New York: Cambridge Press; 1987.

Schneider EC, Shah A, Doty M, Tikkanen R, Fields K, Williams R II. Mirror, mirror 2021: reflecting poorly: health care in the U.S. compared to other high-income countries. The Commonwealth Fund; 2021. https://www.commonwealthfund.org/sites/default/files/2021-08/Schneider_Mirror_Mirror_2021.pdf. Accessed 1 Aug 2025.

Silver HK, Ford LC, Ripley SS, Igoe J. Perspectives 20 years later. From the pioneers of the nurse practitioner movement. Nurse Pract. 1985;10(1):15–8. PMID: 3881.

Creating and Sustaining an Advanced Practice Nursing Professional Organization

Kathy J. Wheeler, Beth Partin, and Jackie Rowles

1 Introduction

Nursing and advanced practice nursing organizations play a critical role in policy advocacy for APNs as well as services and social structure for the profession. According to Benton et al. (2017), there are three types of organizations devoted to nursing and advanced practice nursing: trade unions, regulatory bodies, and professional organizations. Trade or labor unions are dedicated to the financial and working conditions of nurses. Regulatory bodies are devoted to regulatory oversight of nurses, specifically for the benefit and protection of the public. Professional associations or organizations are devoted to advancing the interests of the profession, including policy advocacy. These distinctions are not absolute; in a few countries or some situations, organization functions do crossover. However, for the most part, organizations identify and function as what has been described. This chapter is devoted to professional organizations as defined above. These organizations can be powerful advocates for role-specific issues, with their impact strengthened when aligned and supported by a country's national nurses association, their local chapters, and other members of the broad nursing community.

K. J. Wheeler (✉)
University of Kentucky College of Nursing, Lexington, KY, USA
e-mail: kjwheeler623@gmail.com

B. Partin
Kentucky Association of Nurse Practitioners and Nurse Midwives; Taylor Regional Health Clinic, Campbellsville, KY, USA
e-mail: epartinfnp@gmail.com

J. Rowles
Texas Christian University School of Nurse Anesthesia, Fort Worth, TX, USA

K. J. Wheeler, M. Acorn (eds.), *Health Policy for Advanced Practice Nursing: A Toolkit for Implementation and Improvement*, Advanced Practice in Nursing,
https://doi.org/10.1007/978-3-032-03667-4_8

Professional organizations operate at a variety of levels, from institutional to international. This chapter presents three levels of professional organizations, providing successful exemplars from subnational, national, and international levels. Each discussion highlights several important aspects of professional organizations, including organization structure, common membership services, and policy advocacy efforts. Despite multiple differences, common threads for these extraordinarily successful organizations include the following:

- Demonstrated need
- Thoughtful planning and prework
- Sound, transparent organizational structure that evolves as needed
- Meaningful, dynamic goals
- Representative membership
- Financial structure that sustains the organization to accomplish stated goals

1.1 Benefits of Organization Membership

Whatever the level of professional organization, there must customarily be recognized benefits for members to participate, particularly if dues are a part of membership. Time and money are significant considerations as to whether individuals choose to participate in organizations (Walsh and Daddario 2015). That hundreds of nursing organizations have overcome those hurdles are testaments to the benefits they provide to members and to the public.

A 2007 study of nurses found a lengthy list of reasons members join professional organizations: education, opportunities for self-improvement, programs, support, professionalism, social events, fun, travel, friendship, group benefit plans, and networking with peers (Alotaibi 2007). Cline lists two other benefits, the first being the opportunity to broaden professional perspectives when professional organizations include members from outside a specific profession (e.g., professional organizations directed at a specific clinical issue or organizations that include patients) or organizations that cross jurisdictions or borders (e.g., regional, national, or international). And the second added benefit to membership is the potential to impact policy. Cline et al. stated, "Membership is one way to engage and potentially serve on boards or committees to ensure a nursing perspective informs practice-leading policy and guidelines" (2019, p. 544). Though some may not see the connection, it should be clear; when the professional is well supported, the result is better care delivery and better patient outcomes.

Another professional organization is a subgroup of a professional organization, one that honors its members through a fellows program. This type of program is one that identifies and supports members recognized for their expertise and leadership. They are often sponsored by academic institutions, non-profit organizations, private companies, or governmental agencies. Membership is usually very selective, with members benefitting from networking, special programs, mentoring opportunities, research, and leadership training (Inspire Pearls 2026). Though professional recognition of this sort is often reward enough, most fellows programs provide community service as well as contributions to policy work, research, and scholarly dissemination.

2 Exemplar 1: A Subnational Advanced Practice Nursing Organization: The Kentucky Association of Nurse Practitioners and Nurse Midwives

The landscape of health care is evolving rapidly, and the role of advanced practice nurses (APNs) has become increasingly crucial in providing high-quality patient care. As the demand for advanced practice nursing grows, there is a need for an organized structure that supports and empowers APNs. APNs are leaders and should take ownership of their profession by seizing every opportunity to increase their visibility and promote positive changes in health care systems. Working through a professional organization can help achieve these goals.

Establishing and sustaining an APN organization is a complex, but rewarding endeavor that requires careful planning, collaboration, and dedication. Many existing state organizations were developed years ago to meet specific needs and have evolved over time, while others have been formed more recently as the need for representation of the profession was recognized. However, all organizations require certain components to succeed. The process is the same regardless of the size of the organization.

2.1 Conduct Needs Assessment

The first step in forming an APN organization is to identify the needs and challenges faced by APNs, who are the intended recipients of the organization's offerings, in a target area. The target area may be an institution, a local community, or a state or other jurisdiction. Therefore, understanding the needs of APNs in the target area is key to decoding the organization's purpose. Assessing and identifying the needs and challenges faced by APNs in the target area will also help in defining the scope of the organization.

A group of APNs, or the founding team, may come together to conduct a needs assessment to help establish the organization's goals and objectives. The team may examine some common problems faced by APNs to determine if any of the issues are those the newly created organization can incorporate as part of its purpose. Some common issues faced by APNs are:

- Antiquated laws and policies hindering APNs from practicing to the full extent of their education and training
- Confusion regarding the role of the APN
- Lack of local opportunities for continuing education
- Need for strong advocacy and lobbying for role clarity and policy and statutory changes
- A lack of a community of peers to whom APNs may look to for support and advice

The assessment helps identify the needs of APNs and the services that may be offered by the organization. The assessment should help to describe the goals the organization aims to achieve. Whether short-term milestones or long-term visions, understanding these goals provides clarity on the purpose and the strategic path the organization is pursuing.

The Kentucky Association of Nurse Practitioners and Nurse Midwives (KANPNM) is an example of how APN needs, a target area, and a founding team came together in the 1980s to form an organization. At that time, there were some local nurse practitioner (NP) and nurse midwife (CNM) groups that were meeting in Louisville and Lexington, Kentucky. These groups saw a need for APN representation and a common voice. In the 1980s, Kentucky advanced practice registered nurses did not have prescriptive authority; were not recognized as primary care providers; could not easily access meaningful continuing education; and did not have cohesive, consistent professional advocacy.

The igniting factor that brought these two groups together was the failure of Kentucky HB 807, a prescriptive authority bill put forth in 1988. Despite 100 nurse practitioners and nurse midwives appearing and testifying before the Kentucky House Health and Welfare Committee, the bill did not make it out of committee.

In a letter to Kentucky APNs, founding President Michael Sheets announced a plan to form a new organization dedicated to addressing the issues of APNs. The letter listed the following goals, all of which are still pertinent today (Wheeler and Partin 2023):

- Work toward improvement of access to care for everyone in the state
- Provide a yearly continuing education conference
- Update mailing lists of nurse practitioners and nurse midwives
- Assist with coordination of APNs and employers
- Improve visibility of APNs in the state
- Ensure APN input in any state policy changes pertinent to APNs

The KANPNM remains a strong and vital professional organization today. Over the years it has grown and now provides an annual regional educational conference and online continuing education offerings, has successfully led the way to passage of key APN legislation, has raised the visibility and recognition of NPs and CNMs, and is called upon by state policymakers for opinions related to health care. Other states have sought advice from the organization as they have established their own organizations.

2.2 Define Purpose, Scope, Mission, and Values

Understanding the core identity, scope, and purpose of an organization is fundamental to its success and provides valuable insights into its mission and strategic direction. Identifying and articulating objectives based on the needs assessment helps define the organization's purpose, scope, goals, and values and directs the founding team in developing the mission statement.

Defining a clear mission and vision is the foundation of any successful organization. A well-crafted mission statement reinforces organizational values and culture, creates loyalty, and clarifies strategic priorities. It is the first impression of the organization (Palaniapan 2025). The mission should articulate the purpose of the APN organization, while the vision outlines the desired future state (Wright 2024). Crafting compelling and concise statements will guide decision-making and strategy development.

A mission statement should be concise, describe the purpose of the organization, and be consistent with the organization's values (Palaniapan 2025). Therefore, a clear understanding of the organization's purpose, identity, and goals is imperative. It is also important to consider what sets the organization apart and its long-term aspirations. Here are the steps to creating a well-crafted mission statement:

- Gather input from leadership and organization members to ensure a comprehensive perspective.
- Keep the statement to the point. Aim for clarity and brevity to ensure the essence of the message is easily understood.
- Identify the principles that guide decision-making and behavior within the organization. Ensure that these values are reflected in the mission statement.
- Clearly state the reason for the organization's existence. What does it aim to achieve and for whom? This is a fundamental component of the mission statement.
- Keep in mind the audience for the mission statement. It should resonate with both APNs, external interested parties (stakeholders), and the broader community.
- Use inspirational language that inspires and motivates. It should evoke a positive and meaningful response.
- Avoid overly technical language. The mission statement should be easily understood by a diverse audience.
- Be specific about what the organization does, while maintaining some flexibility. This allows for adaptability as the organization evolves.
- Aim for a mission statement that remains relevant over time.
- Review and revise the mission statement, seeking input, to ensure that it accurately reflects the organization's identity.

The mission statement of the Kentucky Association of Nurse Practitioners and Nurse-Midwives was developed to align with the organization's purpose and values. "To empower Kentucky Advanced Practice Registered Nurses in providing quality, accessible and compassionate healthcare through education, leadership, and advocacy" (KANPNM n.d., para 1).

A vision statement outlines an organization's long-term aspirations and the impact it hopes to make in the future. It serves as a guiding beacon that inspires and aligns interested parties (stakeholders) toward a common future. "The bottom line is that a vision statement isn't just a nice-to-have. It should be included in every business plan and strategy discussion, especially during the strategic planning process, to ensure the organization and its departments stay aligned with its vision and don't get sidetracked" (Kati 2022, para 2). Unlike a mission statement, a vision statement should not be overly specific or tied to specific strategies. It should capture the overarching direction without getting into detailed tactics. Here are steps and guidelines to help write an effective vision statement:

- A vision statement is about the future. It should articulate the organization's long-term goals and the desired impact it wants to achieve.
- A vision statement should convey a sense of purpose about the future.
- Ensure the vision statement aligns with the organization's core values.
- Keep the vision statement concise and memorable. Avoid overly complex language or lengthy descriptions.
- The vision statement should not be tied to strategies but should capture the overreaching direction of the organization.
- Aim for a vision statement that remains relevant over time. While strategies and tactics may change, the vision should stand the test of time.

The vision statement of the Kentucky Association of Nurse Practitioners and Nurse-Midwives was developed years ago but remains relevant today. "Kentucky APRNs will be recognized as full partners and leaders in the development of health policy, provision of quality health care, and advocacy for the people of the Commonwealth" (KANPNM n.d., para 2).

2.3 Legal and Regulatory Considerations

Professional associations, like other organizations, can adopt different legal structures based on the legal requirements and preferences of their members. The legal structure chosen often influences the association's governance, liability, and tax status. Below are common legal structures for professional associations in the United States. Though specific to the United States, they demonstrate the types of legal structuring organizations might consider:

- Unincorporated association: It is the simplest form of an organization. It is a group of individuals who come together for a common purpose without formally incorporating. While it offers simplicity, it may lack legal and financial recognition and protection (Penman 2023).
- 501(c)(3) Tax-exempt status: These nonprofit corporations can apply for tax-exempt status from the US Internal Revenue Service (IRS). The status allows the association to receive tax-deductible donations and grants. To qualify, the association must operate exclusively for charitable, educational, or scientific purposes. These corporations are restricted in how much political and lobbying activities they may conduct, and they may not participate in any campaign activity for or against political candidates (IRS 2025a).
- 501(c)(6) Tax-exempt status: Some professional associations may qualify for 501(c) (American Association of Nurse Practitioners 2026e) status, which is specific to business leagues, chambers of commerce, and professional associations.

This status allows for tax-exempt income, but contributions are not tax deductible. Professional associations often fall into this category (IRS 2025b).

At its start, the KANPNM was registered as a 501(c)(3) corporation. This suited the organization's needs, as the thrust of its activities involved continuing education for NPs and CNMs through its annual conference, educating the public about nurse practitioners and nurse-midwives, and advocating for improving the health of Kentuckians. Professional advocacy and lobbying efforts, while important, consumed a small portion of the organization's income. Much of the legislative lobbying in the early years of the organization was done through grassroots efforts and volunteer APNs. However, as the organization grew, the needs of the organization and its members changed. The need to have a greater impact and influence on policymaking and legislation supportive of APNs became apparent. This transformation required a larger financial investment toward advocacy and more sophisticated lobbying efforts. Therefore, the organization was required to change its tax status to a 501(c)(6) corporation. While the mission and the vision of the organization did not change, the means of accomplishing its goals did shift.

The choice of legal structure depends on various factors, including the association's size, mission, activities, and the preferences of members. It is advisable for professional associations to seek legal counsel to determine the most suitable legal structure based on their specific needs and goals. Additionally, legal and tax regulations may vary by jurisdiction, so associations should comply with the laws applicable to their location.

2.4 Founding Team, Leadership, and Governance

Developing a robust governance structure is essential for effective organizational functioning. This involves establishing officers, a board of directors, defining roles and responsibilities, and creating bylaws that govern the organization's operations. A transparent and accountable governance structure ensures sound decision-making and organizational integrity.

Recruiting experienced APNs to serve on the founding team is crucial in ensuring the success and sustainability of the organization. A strong founding team brings diverse skills, perspectives, and expertise to the table. This team will determine the leadership roles, such as president, vice president, secretary, treasurer, and board of directors, needed for governance of the organization. Important considerations for these roles include clinical expertise, leadership skills, financial acumen, legal knowledge, and organizational management skills.

The founding team will also develop a plan for organizational structure. This should include bylaws that outline the rules, decision-making processes, responsibilities, and committees within the organization. There are many online tutorials with instructions on writing bylaws. One example of an easy-to-understand article, written by Sonia Urlando (2023), describing how to write bylaws for an association, is available online. A copy of KANPNM bylaws is available at https://cdn.ymaws.com/www.kcnpnm.org/resource/resmgr/by-laws/association_bylaws_finalappr.pdf.

2.5 Membership

Building membership in a professional organization requires a strategic and inclusive approach. Here are some steps to build and grow membership in an APN organization:

- Clearly articulate the benefits of joining the organization. Highlight professional development opportunities, networking events, access to resources, and any other advantages.
- Identify the specific needs and preferences of potential APN members. Different segments of APNs may have unique interests and priorities. Tailor membership offerings to address the diverse needs of APNs.
- Establish a website that provides information about the organization's mission, benefits of membership, and upcoming events. Utilize social media platforms to engage potential members and create a sense of community.
- Offer and promote educational programs, workshops, and conferences. Highlight how participation in these offerings can contribute to continuing education requirements and career growth.
- Host networking events to provide members with opportunities to connect with peers, mentors, and leaders.
- Establish connections with educational institutions, health care organizations, and other interested parties (stakeholders) in the nursing community.
- Advocate for issues relevant to APNs. Engage in legislative initiatives, policy discussions, and public awareness campaigns. Position the organization as a voice for APNs and advocate for policies that positively impact the profession.
- Solicit feedback from existing members to continuously improve offerings and address evolving needs. Encourage member involvement in committees, leadership roles, or special projects to foster a sense of belonging.

Building membership is an ongoing effort that requires adaptability and a focus on delivering value to members. Regularly assess strategies and adjust to ensure sustained growth and member satisfaction.

Looking back at history again, the Kentucky Coalition of Nurse Practitioners and Nurse Midwives (KCNPNM) followed the same path for establishing a professional organization. The first meeting of the KCNPNM took place on May 21, 1988. Work included bylaws preparation, plans for fundraising, newsletter publication, planning the first educational conference for the following year, and surveying the policy landscape (Wheeler and Partin 2023). Later, the organization name was changed to the Kentucky Association of Nurse Practitioners and Nurse-Midwives to accommodate the aforementioned change to a 501(c)(6) corporation. Membership was small at the beginning, but leadership that was goal oriented, newsletters to keep members informed, educational offerings, and opportunities for networking grew membership and filled a void for Kentucky APNs.

2.6 Financial Management

Establishing sound financial management for the organization is critical for its success and sustainability. Effective management ensures that the organization can meet its goals, allocate resources efficiently, and maintain long-term viability. Here are the steps to establish sound financial management:

- Establish a dedicated bank account for the organization.
- Create a comprehensive budget that outlines income, expenses, and financial projections.
- Develop clear financial policies and procedures to guide the organization's activities.
- Establish internal controls to safeguard financial assets and prevent mismanagement.
- Hire an accountant who has a clear understanding of nonprofit accounting principles.
- Generate regular financial reports that provide an overview of the organization's financial health. Share reports with officers and the board of directors to ensure transparency and accountability.
- Engage in financial planning to anticipate future financial needs.
- Conduct regular financial audits by outside auditors to ensure accuracy and compliance with regulations.
- Stay informed about best practices in financial management and adapt strategies accordingly.

2.7 Advocacy and Public Awareness

Advocating for APNs and raising public awareness about the organization's contributions are essential for sustainability. Engaging in policymaking, participating in community outreach programs, and collaborating with interested parties (stakeholders) enhances the organization's visibility and impact.

KANPNM provides a long list of policy information and tools for its members, posted on its website, useful since policy work is ongoing and might be needed at any time. A guide to meeting with legislators, entitled *Meeting with Legislators: Dos and Don'ts*, is available at https://cdn.ymaws.com/www.kcnpnm.org/resource/resmgr/legislative/do_s_don_tswithlegislators.pdf. Each year, KANPNM updates talking points for association priority bills and makes the document available to members.

To improve public awareness, the organization publishes an informational flyer, entitled *Who Are Nurse Practitioners (NPs) and Nurse-Midwives (CNMs)?*, available at https://cdn.ymaws.com/www.kcnpnm.org/resource/resmgr/legislative/legislative2021/who_are_aprns_2021.pdf. The flyer is used to educate the public, but also legislators and interested parties (stakeholders).

2.8 Kentucky Association of Nurse Practitioners and Nurse-Midwives Summary

Creating and sustaining an APN organization is a multifaceted journey that demands strategic planning, collaboration, and a commitment to excellence. By understanding the evolving health care landscape, addressing specific needs, and building a strong organizational foundation, APN organizations can play a pivotal role in advancing patient care and shaping the future of health care delivery.

The KANPNM began as a small group of dedicated nurse practitioners and nurse midwives who were determined to change the face of health care in Kentucky. In 1988, membership in the organization was less than 50; APNs could not prescribe medication, were not considered primary care providers, and could not bill directly for the services they provided. Today, the organization has grown to over 2000 members; APNs prescribe medication autonomously, bill directly, and are considered primary care providers. Professional APN organizations provide an avenue for APNs to flourish. The labor to create and sustain an organization is well worth the effort.

3 Exemplar 2: A National Advanced Practice Nursing Organization: The American Association of Nurse Practitioners

The American Association of Nurse Practitioners (AANP) is a national member service and nurse practitioner (NP) advocacy organization formed in 2013, when the American Academy of Nurse Practitioners (founded in 1985; often referred to as the Academy) merged with the American College of Nurse Practitioners (founded in 1995; often referred to as the College). The American Academy of Nurse Practitioners was the first organization formed to represent all the nurse practitioner (NP) specialties in the United States (AANP 2026a). The association has grown to be the largest NP organization in the world, and recently added international membership. As of 2026, the AANP website states the organization represents the interests of more than 461,000 NPs in the United States (AANP 2026b).

3.1 The American Association of Nurse Practitioners Mission

According to the mission statement, AANP "empowers all nurse practitioners (NPs) to advance accessible, person-centered, equitable, high-quality health care for diverse communities through practice, education, advocacy, research and leadership" (AANP 2026c, para 1). Intent on providing services to the NP profession, the organization has adopted the P.E.A.R.L acronym to represent the categories of service—*P*ractice, *E*ducation, *A*dvocacy, *R*esearch, and *L*eadership (AANP 2026c, para 8).

3.1.1 Practice

As a clinical practice profession, it was appropriate for an organization devoted to practicing NPs to be created. At the time, there were few organizations at any level dedicated specifically to NPs in clinical practice. The National Organization of Nurse Practitioner Faculties (NONPF) was created in 1980 but was devoted to United States NP faculty and their unique needs (Pulcini et al. 2019). Across the country, many practice issues were not well defined in law or regulation—scopes of practice, title protection, prescriptive authority, reimbursement, and many others. AANP took the lead on these issues, primarily at the national level but also at the state and local levels when appropriate. Through the policy work of AANP, many practice barriers have been identified and eliminated. Specific materials and programs devoted to practice issues have included clinical resources for use with patient care and patient education, practice management info, state-specific practice fact sheets, two journals, the NP Career Center full of resources, the NP Job Center for employers and job seekers, and NP Finder so patients can find a local NP for care (AANP 2026d).

3.1.2 Education

AANP has been a steadfast provider of continuing education for NPs via an annual national conference, an annual fall conference, an annual policy conference, annual regional meetings, continuing education sessions available at conferences and online, and continuing education credits available within the two journals AANP publishes. In addition to the two journals, the Journal of the American Association of Nurse Practitioners (JAANP) and Journal for Nurse Practitioners (JNP), AANP has provided education materials for students, interested parties (stakeholders), and patients (AANP 2026e). An ongoing media campaign was initiated via the *Did You Know?* video, about the NP role. The video was aired to international, national, and state media markets multiple times (AANP 2026a). Media work has continued, with a recent offering of podcasts.

3.1.3 Advocacy

From the beginning, both the Academy and the College focused on NP advocacy. Over the years, many of the materials published by AANP referred to the organization as the voice of the nurse practitioner, so much so the term was trademarked and used for the title of the podcast, *NP Pulse: The Voice of the Nurse Practitioner.*

Advocacy has been the hallmark of everything AANP has done, advocating for NPs and their ability to provide "accessible, person-centered, equitable, high-quality health care for diverse communities" (AANP 2026c, para 1). Aside from policy work at the federal and state levels, with dedicated staff and devoted resources at both levels, AANP has provided multiple advocacy initiatives and materials. A partial list includes the following: NP fact sheet, NP infographic, position statements, position papers, discussion papers, and policy-related clinical practice briefs. Each is periodically reviewed and updated. The Advocacy Center highlights critical legislation and policy issues, allowing NPs (member and nonmember) to generate letters to respective legislators (AANP 2026f).

3.1.4 Research

One of the first actions the Academy took related to research was the creation of the NP database, started the year the Academy was founded. As an ongoing initiative, the database is the most comprehensive repository of NP information in the United States Through the delivery of quality surveys to NP members and nonmembers, AANP has provided extensive data on NP roles, practice, practice settings, compensation, and demographics. The studies have all met ethical study standards, attentive to informed consent, privacy, confidentiality, and thoughtful data protection. AANP has published the data in research briefs, infographics, and fact sheets, affecting policy throughout the United States. AANP also has provided research funds through annual grants and research guidance through the AANP Network for Research (AANP 2026g).

3.1.5 Leadership

AANP has been the NP policy leader in the U.S., sharing expertise with thousands of NPs and interested parties (stakeholders) across the United States. Few APN policy initiatives in the United States have not been shaped in some way by the foundational and ongoing policy work of AANP. AANP has concentrated on *doing the work*, providing the leadership that changed the practice climate and regulatory foundations of advanced practice. But it has also devoted extensive resources to recognizing and developing policy and practice leaders.

> A prime example of recognizing NP leaders is the Fellows of the Association of Nurse Practitioners (FAANP) program. Established in 2000, the "FAANP program is dedicated to the advancement of nurse practitioners and the high quality healthcare NPs deliver. By engaging recognized NP leaders who have made outstanding contributions to NP education, policy, clinical practice or research, and developing leaders of the future, FAANP is furthering the NP role while enhancing AANP's mission". (AANP 2026h, para 1). Members are selected annually, meet twice a year, and are assessed annual dues. At this writing there were close to 1000 Fellows, several from outside the U.S. (AANP 2026h).

AANP also offers an impactful leadership program, called The Loretta Ford Visionary Leadership Program. The program combines multiweek in-person and virtual experiences culminating in a capstone workshop and pinning ceremony at the AANP Annual Conference. AANP members can apply and are competitively selected only after completing the Jan Towers Foundational Leadership Program (continuing modules delivered virtually) (AANP 2026i).

3.2 Organization Funding, Structure, and Operations

Much of the success of AANP has been because of the strength of its funding, structure, and operations. Each deserves a brief discussion.

3.2.1 Funding

Both the Academy and the College recognized each needed funding to do the important work they planned and did so primarily via membership fees and the provision of numerous financially successful conferences. This allowed them to gradually add staff so the NP leaders could not only practice unhindered but also allow time for meaningful, direct policy work best done by NPs.

3.2.2 Structure

Although the Academy was incorporated in Texas and the College was incorporated in Virginia AANP incorporated in Austin, Texas, breaking ground for the AANP National Headquarters building in January, 2018. The AANP Office of Government Affairs is housed in Washington, D.C. Staff are split between the two offices according to duties.

AANP has a complete administrative and leadership structure. Executive staff consists of the following: chief executive officer, vice president of accreditation, conference and education; vice president of association governance, associate vice president of building operations, vice president of communications and marketing, vice president of finance, vice president of human resources, vice president of information technology, vice president of legal affairs, vice president of membership, vice president of professional practice, vice president of research, vice president of federal government affairs, DC office and external alliances, and vice president of state government affairs (AANP 2026j).

The AANP board of directors (BOD) is composed of the following: president, president elect or immediate past president, treasurer, recording secretary, and 11 regional directors (representing various combinations of various states and territories). The BOD is elected by annual membership elections, though terms are staggered to assure continuity. Members of the BOD also serve as liaisons to standing and ad hoc committees, composed of a mix of AANP members. Each US state and territory is represented by a state liaison, also elected by the members of the respective states and/or territories (AANP 2026j).

Aside from individual membership, AANP offers international membership and international student membership. International membership rates are significantly reduced, informed by the World Bank Classification of Income Economies, accessible via https://www.aanp.org/membership/international-membership. Businesses, organizations, and state associations also have the opportunity to connect via organization membership. Aside from networking opportunities, this type of membership includes special membership benefits, such as access to AANP publications and mailing lists (AANP 2026k). AANP also offers numerous member-only community groups for members to join according to their specific clinical and professional interests. AANP Communities are available as follows: acute care; cardiology; dermatology and aesthetics; emergency and convenient/urgent care; endocrine; entrepreneur, functional and lifestyle medicine; gastroenterology; gerontology; health equity, diversity and inclusion; healthcare technology; hospice and palliative care; industry and executive NP; infectious disease/HIV and immunology/rheumatology; interagency government; international; men's health, urology and nephrology; neonatal; neurology; obesity; occupational and environmental health; oncology; ophthalmology and otolaryngology; orthopedics; pain management; pediatrics; primary care; psych and mental health; pulmonary and sleep; women's health; and wound care. (AANP 2026l).

3.2.3 Operations

Association operations are based on organization bylaws and a strategic plan. The strategic plan is updated periodically by the AANP BOD and is used as a metric for organizational success. As a not-for-profit organization, AANP directs all money earned or contributed toward organization objectives (Kenton 2023). As an organization devoted to investing all earned money back into the association, it has allowed AANP to support NP members in multiple ways, such as scholarships, grants, funding to attend conferences if presenting, and funding to attend some meetings if attending.

The BOD meets multiple times a year in face-to-face meetings and virtually. All BOD members receive training on governance standards and fiduciary responsibility, and new BOD members receive specific orientation training. Similar to any organization of this structure and size, committees and staff make reports, and the directors make decisions about the internal processes of the company, the strategic plan, and finances at these meetings.

3.3 Historical Policy Initiatives

Many of the policy initiatives accomplished by AANP were pivotal to the profession in the United States. Policy efforts have been directed at two levels, national and state. It is noteworthy that two critical staff positions reflect this two-tiered effort, with both a Vice President of Federal Government Affairs, DC Office & External Alliances and a Vice President of State Government Affairs. Table 1 highlights many policy accomplishments achieved over the years. Two particular policy programs were foundational to the success of many of the policy initiatives, one primarily directed at national policy issues and the other directed primarily at state policy issues. Both are described below.

The first was an annual program of policy meetings held in Washington, D.C. By invitation, AANP would select NPs who were active or interested in policy issues. Coordinated to occur when US legislators were in Washington, Dr. Jan Towers

Table 1 Organization timeline and significant policy initiatives

Year		Initiative	Policy significance
1984	Academy[a]	Steering committee met to discuss need for a national NP organization	Provided groundwork for needed national NP organization
1985	Academy[a]	American Academy of Nurse Practitioners formed	Established first national NP organization for NPs of all specialties
1985	Academy[a]	National NP database created	Initiated process of collecting national NP data
1986	Academy[a]	Formal efforts taken to affect legislation at national level	Addressed need for NP voice at national level
1987	Academy[a]	US federal government invests $100 million on education of NPs	Provided critical funding to launch NP programs across US
1987	Academy[a]	Member survey regarding malpractice liability insurance conducted	Resulted in affordable malpractice insurance made available
1989	Academy[a]	Journal of the American Academy of Nurse Practitioners (JAANP) began publication	Launched first association connected NP journal
1989	Academy[a]	First national conference held in Philadelphia, Pennsylvania	Resulted in first national NP conference
1989	Academy[a]	NP preparation and practice survey published	Provided national info on NP education and practice
1992	Academy[a]	Met with Royal College of Nursing (UK) to develop role internationally	Began process for initiation of role internationally
1993	Academy[a]	American Academy of Nurse Practitioners Certification Program formed	Provided quality national certification
1995	College[b]	American College of Nurse Practitioners formed	Provided additional NP organization at national level
1995	Academy[a]	Corporate Advisory Council formed	Enhanced communication with health care industries
1999	Academy[a]	National NP survey conducted	Compared 1999 survey data to 1989 survey data
1999	Academy[a]	American Academy of Nurse Practitioners Certification Program incorporated separately from American Academy of Nurse Practitioners	Eliminated conflict of interest and maintained exam integrity
2000	Academy[a]	Fellows Program created	Created organization to recognize exemplary NPs
2000	Academy[a]	First international NP conference started in the United States	Encouraged international development and reflected international leadership
2002	Academy[a]	American Academy of Nurse Practitioners Network for Research (AANPNR) created	Created first national practice-based research network for NPs
2002	Academy[a]	Practice Site Survey conducted	Provided national info on NP practice
2003	Academy[a]	SmartBrief made available to members	Provided daily electronic newsletter of health-related news
2003	Academy[a]	Membership survey conducted	Provided national info on NPs

(continued)

Table 1 (continued)

Year		Initiative	Policy significance
2004	Academy[a]	National NP Week recognized as a proclamation by US Congress	Created national NP recognition system
2004	Academy[a]	National NP Sample Survey conducted	Provided national info on NPs
2005	College[b]	Journal for Nurse Practitioners (JNP), publication of the American College of Nurse Practitioners began publication	Established an additional association connected NP journal
2005	Academy[a]	Practice Site Survey conducted	Provided national info on NP practice
2006	Academy[a]	Membership Survey conducted	Provided national info on NPs
2006	Academy[a]	Education Needs Survey conducted	Provided national info on NP education
2006	Academy[a]	Fellows launched Mentorship Program	Provided high-level mentoring program
2007	Academy[a]	National NP Income Survey conducted	Provided national info on NP income
2007	Academy[a]	NP Finder launched	Provided web-based site to list NP practices so patients could locate NPs in their community
2007	Academy[a]	NP Compensation Survey conducted	Provided national info on NP compensation
2007	Academy[a]	Online CE Center made available for CE learning and credits	Made online CEs available
2008	Academy[a]	Developed program to track online CE learning	Provided easy tracking of CE learning and credits
2008	Academy[a]	Practice Site Survey, Compensation Survey, and Educational Needs Assessment Survey conducted	Provided national info on NP practice, compensation, and education needs
2008	Academy[a]	Pharmaceutical companies and other health care product suppliers petitioned to use provider-neutral language	Clarity provided regarding NP ability to prescribe and recommend via neutral language
2009	Academy[a]	"Did You Know?" video, about NP role, created and distributed. Video distributed to international, national, and state media markets	Aired hundreds of times to 200 US markets in all 50 states. Voice of America aired daily to international market of 96 million viewers in 200 cities and 127 countries
2009	Academy[a]	Membership Survey, National NP Sample Survey, and Educational Needs Assessment Survey conducted	Provided national info on NPs and NP education
2009	Academy[a]	E-Bulletin launched	Provided weekly email communication to members
2009	Academy[a]	Webnp.org launched	Created social networking site for members

(continued)

Table 1 (continued)

Year		Initiative	Policy significance
2010	Academy[a]	Policy activities concentrated on Health Care Reform, CMS regulations, Medicare payment, Appropriations, Medical Home, and multiple other issues of importance to NPs and their patients	Targeted critical national policy issues targeted
2010	Academy[a]	Participated in White House meeting on health reform. Later attends President Obama's White House briefing on Health Care Reform legislation	Reflected participation and recognition at a national level on policy issues
2013	Association[c]	Academy and College merge. Members receive both JAANP and JNP journals	Unified national NP organizations
2020	Association[c]	National NP Sample Survey on Practice conducted	Provided national info on NP practice
2021	Association[c]	Membership Survey conducted	Provided national info on NPs
2022	Association[c]	National NP Workforce Survey conducted	Provided national info on NP workforce

Adapted from AANP Historical Timeline (2026a), available at https://www.aanp.org/about/about-the-american-association-of-nurse-practitioners-aanp/historical-timeline

[a]Academy refers to American Academy of Nurse Practitioners

[b]College refers to American College of Nurse Practitioners

[c]Association refers to American Association of Nurse Practitioners

(AANP founder) would educate and dialogue with participants on issues related to NP practice, education, and funding. The last day of the meeting was devoted to nonpartisan visits with respective US senators and representatives, educating them on NP roles and education, asking for legislators to act on one or several policies impacting NP practice. At the end of those visits, the NPs would provide feedback to AANP policy staff, summarizing the visits. The program has now been replaced by the Health Policy Conference, which occurs once a year and is open to all AANP members. The program is much larger, involving many more NPs, but retains the same format, including visits with legislators and legislative aides.

A second pivotal policy program refers to regional policy and membership meetings, held throughout the year and according to region membership, as described previously. Those meetings were largely dialogue based, allowing members to discuss and brainstorm on local policy issues with AANP policy staff and BOD members. These meetings continue via virtual meeting format.

3.4 American Association of Nurse Practitioners Summary

AANP continues to grow in membership and influence but is faithful to its initially stated goals as well as updated strategic objectives. The organization has shown remarkable flexibility, adapting to changes in health care issues, changing political

Table 2 (continued)

International Council of Nurses Nurse Practitioner/Advanced Practice Nurse Network (ICN NP/APNN) (professional association) Referred to as the Network https://icnnpapnnetwork.wildapricot.org (for access and for details about information provided here)	Membership/representation: Network affiliation with the ICN, direct membership representing APNs from 121 countries, membership in NNAs recognized Key goals (ICN NP/APNN n.d., para 3): Making relevant and timely information about practice, education, role development, research, policy and regulatory developments, and appropriate events widely available Providing a forum for sharing and exchange of knowledge expertise and experience Supporting nurses and countries who are in the process of introducing or developing NP or ANP roles and practice Accessing international resources that are pertinent to this field Organization structure: Aside from the Core Steering Group, there are six subgroups (practice, education, health policy, communications, research, students). An alumni group is also available for those who have made significant contributions to the network Activities: Holds biennial conference that rotates globally, publishes a network bulletin
Sigma Theta Tau International Honor Society of Nursing (professional association for qualifying members) Referred to as Sigma https://www.sigmanursing.org (for access and details about information provided here)	Membership/representation: membership offered to students and nursing leaders who meet specific nursing achievements, currently 100,000 from over 100 countries, divided among global regions Key goals: Sigma is an international community of nurses, dedicated to the advancement of knowledge, teaching, learning, and service through the cultivation of communities of practice, education, and research (Sigma 2026, para 3). Organization structure: Aside from a Board of Directors, there are 600 chapters, housed primarily at institutions of higher learning Activities: Holds annual Research Congress that rotates globally and a biennial conference held in United States; publishes the *Journal of Nursing Scholarship*, the *Worldviews on Evidenced-Based Nursing*, and multiple books; offers webinars, online programs, scholarships, and research grants; and, along with the Johnson and Johnson Foundation, provides the Global Nursing Leadership Competency Framework

(continued)

Table 2 (continued)

International Confederation of Midwives (professional association for member associations) Referred to as "… the global voice of midwives (ICM n.d., para 2)" https://internationalmidwives.org (for access and for details about information provided)	Membership/representation: Represents over 131 midwives' associations in 116 countries Key goals: The "mission is to strengthen midwives' associations and to advance the profession of midwifery globally by promoting autonomous midwives as the most appropriate caregivers for childbearing women and in keeping birth normal, to enhance the reproductive health of women, their newborns and their families" (ICM n.d., para 4) Organization structure: A governing council composed of two delegates per member organization and the members of the governing board, the chief executive executes the strategic plan Activities: Holds triennial Congress that rotates globally; known for multiple documents related to midwifery practice, standards, and education
Royal College of Nursing (RCN) (professional association and trade union) Referred to as "the voice of nursing (RCN 2026, para 1) https://www.rcn.org.uk (for access and details about information provided here)	Membership/representation: Described as largest nursing organization in the world, representing over a half million nurses, midwives, and nursing support workers (NSWs) Key goals (ICN 2026, para 3): To promote the science and art of nursing and education and training in the profession of nursing To promote the advancement of nursing as a profession in all or any of its branches To promote the professional standing and interests of members To assist members who, by reason of adversity, ill-health, or otherwise, are in need of assistance of any nature To promote all of these objects in other countries, with the help of international agencies Organization structure: RCN Council is advised by a Trade Union Committee and a Professional Nursing Committee, as well as boards representing each region and country. Activities: Holds annual Research Congress with the United Kingdom; works on policy initiatives to raise the profile of the nursing community and improve working conditions for nurses, midwives, and NSWs; publishes documents defining workforce standards, nursing, and principle of nursing; offers nursing education scholarships; provides access to extensive library services; elects fellows and honorary fellows

6 Conclusion

Although this chapter presented three examples of extremely successful, profession-centered organizations, as well as a listing of other nursing organizations, the main purpose of this chapter is to encourage APNs to recognize the critical impact organizations play in the success of the profession, a profession devoted to improving the lives and health of patients and systems of care everywhere in the world. While individuals may not be *joiners*, for a variety of reasons, APNs and nurses would do well to engage with organizations relevant to their professional lives, at institutional, subnational, national, and international levels. When considering an organization for membership, Cline et al. (2019, p. 544) recommend asking the following questions:

1. Does the organization offer continuing education materials that can support my professional growth or license renewal?
2. Does the organization offer peer-reviewed journals or other materials to support my practice?
3. Does membership offer discounts toward certification or conference registration?
4. Does the organization offer the opportunity for engagement on policy or guideline development?
5. How have other nurses been engaged with the organization?
6. How does the organization advocate for my profession or professional interests?
7. Does the organization have a formal mentoring opportunity?
8. Is there an opportunity for me to actively participate at the local or national level?
9. Does the organization have a local chapter?

Where organizations do not exist, APNs and nurses should create needed professional organizations. The provided exemplars demonstrate some of the steps to organization creation. As professionals, APNs should invest in the work of building and sustaining professional organizations at all levels. It is an important step toward self-regulation, a defining step of being a profession.

References

Alotaibi M. Factors affecting nurses' decisions to join their professional association. Int Nurs Rev. 2007;54(2):160–5. https://doi.org/10.1111/j.1466-7657.2007.00555.x. PMID: 17492989.

American Association of Nurse Practitioners (AANP). Historical timeline. 2026a. https://www.aanp.org/about/about-the-american-association-of-nurse-practitioners-aanp/historical-timeline. Accessed 10 Mar 2026.

American Association of Nurse Practitioners (AANP). About the American Association of Nurse Practitioners. 2026b. https://www.aanp.org/about/about-the-american-association-of-nurse-practitioners-aanp. Accessed 10 Mar 2026.

American Association of Nurse Practitioners (AANP). Strategic focus. 2026c. https://www.aanp.org/about/about-the-american-association-of-nurse-practitioners-aanp/strategic-focus. Accessed 10 Mar 2026.

American Association of Nurse Practitioners (AANP). Practice. 2026d. https://www.aanp.org/practice. Accessed 10 Mar 2026.

American Association of Nurse Practitioners (AANP). Education. 2026e. https://www.aanp.org/education. Accessed 10 Mar 2026.
American Association of Nurse Practitioners (AANP). Advocacy. 2026f. https://www.aanp.org/advocacy. Accessed 10 Mar 2026.
American Association of Nurse Practitioners (AANP). Practice-related research. 2026g. https://www.aanp.org/practice/practice-related-research. Accessed 10 Mar 2026.
American Association of Nurse Practitioners (AANP). The Fellows of the American Association of Nurse Practitioners. 2026h. https://www.aanp.org/membership/fellows-program. Accessed 10 Mar 2026.
American Association of Nurse Practitioners (AANP). The Loretta Ford visionary leadership program. 2026i. https://www.aanp.org/practice/professional-development/leadership-program. Accessed 10 Mar 2026.
American Association of Nurse Practitioners (AANP). AANP leadership. 2026j. https://www.aanp.org/about/about-the-american-association-of-nurse-practitioners-aanp#:~:text=Your%20association%20is. Accessed 10 Mar 2026.
American Association of Nurse Practitioners (AANP). Membership for organizations. 2026k. https://www.aanp.org/membership/memberships-for-organizationss. Accessed 10 Mar 2026.
American Association of Nurse Practitioners (AANP). AANP communities. 2026l. https://www.aanp.org/membership/aanp-communities. Accessed 15 May 2026.
Benton DC, Thomas K, Damgaard G, Masek SM, Brekken SA. Exploring the differences between regulatory bodies, professional associations, and trade unions: an integrative review. J Nurs Regul. 2017;8(3):4–11. https://doi.org/10.1016/S2155-8256(17)30154-0.
Cline D, Curtin K, Johnston PA. Professional organization membership: the benefits of increasing nursing participation. Clin J Oncol Nurs. 2019;23(5):543–6. https://doi.org/10.1188/19.CJON.543-546. PMID: 31538979.
Inspire Pearls. What is a fellows program? 2026. https://inspirepearls.com/blogs/words/what-is-a-fellows-program-1. Accessed 14 Mar 2026.
Internal Revenue Service (IRS) (U.S.). Exemption requirements—501(c)(3) organizations. Author; 2025a. https://www.irs.gov/charities-non-profits/charitable-organizations/exemption-requirements-501c3-organizations. Accessed 8 Sept 2025.
Internal Revenue Service (IRS) (U.S.). 2025b. https://www.irs.gov/charities-non-profits/other-non-profits/business-leagues. Accessed 8 Sept 2025.
International Confederation of Midwives (ICM). We are the global voice of midwives. n.d. https://nternationalmidwives.org. Accessed 14 Mar 2026.
International Council of Nurses (ICN). The global voice of nursing. n.d.-a. https://www.icn.ch. Accessed 14 Mar 2026.
International Council of Nurses (ICN). Mission, vision and strategic plan. n.d.-b. https://www.icn.ch/who-we-are/mission-vision-constitution-and-strategic-plan. Accessed 14 Mar 2026.
International Council of Nurses Nurse Practitioner Advanced Practice Nurse Network (ICN NP/APNN). n.d. https://icnnpapnnetwork.wildapricot.org. Accessed 14 Mar 2026.
Kati G. How to write a vision statement. LinkedIn. 2022. https://www.linkedin.com/pulse/how-write-vision-statement-gideon-kati/. Accessed 2 Sept 2025.
Kenton W. Not for profit: definitions and what it means for taxes. Investopedia; 2023. https://www.investopedia.com/terms/n/not-for-profit.asp. Accessed 5 Mar 2025.
Kentucky Association of Nurse Practitioners and Nurse Midwives (KANPNM). Who we are and what we do. n.d. https://www.kcnpnm.org/page/who_and_what. Accessed 20 Jan 2024.
Palaniapan S. Anatomy of a mission statement—plus 5 quality examples. Nectar; 2025. https://nectarhr.com/blog/mission-statement. Accessed 3 Sept 2025.
Penman P. Benefits and drawbacks of unincorporated associations. East Coast Private Membership Association; 2023. https://eastcoastpma.com/benefits-and-drawbacks-of-unincorporated-associations/. Accessed 1 Oct 2025.
Pulcini J, Hanson C, Johnson J. National Organization of Nurse Practitioner Faculties: a 40-year history of preparing nurse practitioners for practice. J Am Assoc Nurse Pract. 2019;31(11):633–9. https://doi.org/10.1097/JXX.0000000000000330. PMID: 31688504.

Royal College of Nursing (RCN). The voice of nursing: now. 2026. https://www.rcn.org.uk/library/Museum-and-Events/Exhibitions/The-Voice-of-Nursing/Now-Information-Stories. Accessed 4 Mar 2026.

Sigma Theta Tau International Honor Society of Nursing. About Sigma. 2026. https://www.sigmanursing.org/why-sigma/about-sigma. Accessed 10 Mar 2026.

Urlando S. How to write association bylaws: 10 steps (+sample). Personify WildApricot; 2023. https://www.wildapricot.com/blog/association-bylaws. Accessed 4 Sept 2025.

Walsh A, Daddario K. The dynamic nature of professional associations: factors shaping membership decisions. J Appl Bus Econ. 2015;17:115–25.

Wheeler K, Partin B. The history of the Kentucky Coalition of Nurse Practitioners and Nurse Midwives. Kentucky Coalition of Nurse Practitioners and Nurse Midwives; 2023.

Wright T. How to write a vision statement. Cascade; 2024. https://www.cascade.app/blog/write-good-vision-statement. Accessed 20 Aug 2024.

Workforce Data Keeping as a Foundation for Policy Implementation and Improvement

Kathy J. Wheeler

1 Introduction

Nurses are accustomed to collecting data and information as they relate to patient care. And they understand the significance of data as it applies to research and evidence-based practice, and how it has the potential to impact systems of care. Nonetheless, advanced practice nursing (APN) and nursing workforce data around the world are riddled with problems in terms of accuracy and completeness. This chapter is a discussion of why APN workforce data is critical to collect and analyze, why there are so many problems collecting this information, and how healthcare interested parties (stakeholders) can improve this professional data keeping.

2 Importance of APN Workforce Data

Workforce data is critical for any profession. In addressing nursing workforce data, the 2021 World Health Organization (WHO) publication titled Global Strategic Directions for Nursing and Midwifery 2021–2025 stated:

> Data on stock and distribution, as well as on education (applicants, faculty, graduates) and employment (vacancies, turnover, migration), are essential to develop effective health workforce policies and to forecast and plan for future needs (WHO 2021, p 12).

Workforce planning is a critical element to ensuring the healthcare system delivers safe, effective care (Smiley et al. 2025, 2). A lack of workforce data makes it very hard for administrators, healthcare systems, policy makers, and providers to make informed decisions and act (Poghosyan et al. 2023).

K. J. Wheeler (✉)
University of Kentucky College of Nursing, Lexington, KY, USA
e-mail: kjwheeler623@gmail.com

K. J. Wheeler, M. Acorn (eds.), *Health Policy for Advanced Practice Nursing: A Toolkit for Implementation and Improvement*, Advanced Practice in Nursing,
https://doi.org/10.1007/978-3-032-03667-4_9

But workforce data is also directly useful to the APN profession. It can help justify spending requests and investment in education and recruitment (Center for Health Workforce Studies 2025). When there are sufficient providers and they are appropriately educated, functioning well, and practicing where needed, the profession benefits from professional standing, sensible workloads, and improved collaboration.

3 Basis for Limitation of APN Workforce Data

Despite the many reasons cited above, nursing and APN workforce data around the world are fraught with limitations. The issue is so pervasive that nearly all nursing and healthcare organizations involved in policy development describe struggles with nursing workforce data, often calling for better information keeping strategies. A partial list of these organizations includes the following: WHO (2021, 2025), International Council of Nurses (2025), Sigma Theta Tau International (2017), Organization for Economic Cooperation and Development (OECD 2023), International Labour Organization (2023), National Academy of Medicine of the United States (formerly Institute of Medicine) (2020), and the National Council of State Boards of Nursing (NCSBN 2024).

There are many reasons for the information limitations, especially for APNs. The nursing profession is complex and multilayered, with nurses and APNs often earning multiple degrees and credentials. Nurses and APNs may work in multiple jurisdictions or institutions. In one jurisdiction/institution, they may work primarily under one credential, while working primarily under another credential in another jurisdiction/institution. Institutions/jurisdictions may or may not harmonize the data. Work hours may vary significantly, making workload comparisons unreliable. This impacts the data if it is being used to plan workload and staffing situations.

For APNs the problems are particularly acute. Some organizations only gather information on nursing, with some only recognizing two categories of nursing, but not advanced nursing. APNs may report themselves as nurses, but nothing beyond that. APN titling has been a significant barrier. If APNs are not regulated and registered beyond the institution where they work, the data is limited.

Obviously, the critical issue is who is gathering the information and why they are gathering the data. International and national organizations are looking for trends. In these situations, the data is based on sampling data, largely reliant on the quality of sampling and the degree of response. The most reliable workforce data comes from professional registries. But not all countries or jurisdictions require nurses or APNs to be registered.

4 Global Efforts to Improve APN Workforce Data

The importance cannot be overstated regarding the many efforts currently underway to counter these issues. Organizations have been working for decades to provide definitions, create common language, and collect nursing data.

4.1 Finding Common Ground for APN Titling and Work

Multiple organizations have devoted significant time to defining nursing, advanced practice nursing, and midwifery, hoping to provide professional clarity and direction. The following list is only a partial list of documents devoted to this effort:

- *ICN Renewing the Definitions of "Nursing" and "a Nurse,"* available at https://www.icn.ch/sites/default/files/2025-06/ICN_Definition-Nursing_Report_EN_Web_0.pdf
- *ICN Guidelines on Advanced Practice Nursing 2020*, available at www.icn.ch/system/files/documents/2020-04/ICN_APN%20Report_EN_WEB.pdf
- *ICN Guidelines on Advanced Practice Nursing: Nurse Anesthetists 2021*, available at https://www.icn.ch/system/files/documents/2021-05/ICN_Nurse-Anaesthetist-Report_EN_WEB.pdf
- *ICM Definition of Midwifery 2025*, available at https//internationalmidwives.org/resources/definition-of-midwifery/
- *RCN New Definition of Nursing 2023*, available at https://www.rcn.org.uk/Professional-Development/publications/rcn-new-definition-of-nursing-research-and-rationale uk pub 011 253

4.2 ICN Work on a Common Nursing Language

A long-term project initiated by the ICN in collaboration with multiple other agencies has been the International Classification for Nursing Practice (ICNP) project. The goal was to provide a structured, consistent vocabulary foundational to nursing that would allow cross-mapping for the purposes of data collection and comparison. The system was to consist of three categories: nursing phenomena (nursing diagnoses), nursing interventions, and nursing outcomes (Warren and Coenen 1998). According to the ICN (2025, para 2), the project will:

- Increase nursing visibility, ensure safety, and enhance quality
- Ensure that nursing is adequately represented in multidisciplinary health information systems
- Ensure that nurses have the information tools they need to meet the changing health and care needs of citizens
- Enhance practice and support policy-making through national information standards

- Support both general and specialist nursing practice across settings
- Ensure that the contribution of nursing is accurately captured in resource management systems
- Support evidence-based practice
- Bring different nursing terminologies together

The project continues today under the auspices of the ICN, with ICNP® materials and research managed, produced, and distributed through SNOMED International, accessible through https://www.snomed.org. Research centers are located around the globe (ICN 2026). For instance, the research center in the United States is located at the University of Minnesota School of Nursing, where the research is aligned with a minimum data set used in the United States (ICN 2026), detailed below. It remains unclear whether this level of common language is useful to a profession that performs advanced skills.

4.3 Nursing and APN Workforce Data: What Do We Know Now?

The most recent and comprehensive nursing workforce report is *The State of the World's Nursing 2025: Investing in Education, Jobs, Leadership and Service Delivery*, by the WHO and ICN. The report relies on country-level data provided by WHO member states. Information was requested for 47 indicators in four focus areas: jobs/employment, education, service delivery, and leadership. Response rates varied from 8% to 100% on indices. Of the 47 indicators, one pertained to advanced practice nursing—whether or not advanced practice roles existed in the country. The report was extremely supportive of advanced practice roles, even listing the development of advanced practice nursing as an emerging policy priority. Nonetheless, the report was limited in presenting details about APNs in relation to workforce issues. This limitation is consistent with recent studies that have attempted to gather APN statistics and found the process wanting due to data keeping hampered by titling, process, or other factors (Wheeler et al. 2022; Maier and Aiken 2016; Heale and Buckley 2015; Pulcini et al. 2010).

5 An Exemplar: The US APN and Nursing Workforce Data

Despite shortcomings in gathering APN data, the United States provides one of the best examples of APN data gathering at multiple levels. Recognizing the need early on, multiple organizations have devoted significant efforts toward the process: solving the APN titling problem by agreeing on a system of regulated, title-protected titles that is supported throughout the United States; developing and applying a minimum dataset system for standardizing workforce data and asking regulators to use as APNs update licensing/registration; and securing workforce data at organizational levels (surveys, studies).

5.1 The Consensus Model for APRN Regulation, Licensure, Accreditation, Certification, and Education

Recognizing that many aspects of advanced practice in the United States were inconsistently regulated across the states, the APRN Consensus Work Group (Advanced Practice Registered Nurse Consensus Work Group) and the National Council of State Boards of Nursing APRN Advisory Committee worked to create a regulatory framework for the entire country. The Consensus Model for APRN Regulation: Licensure, Accreditation, Certification & Education was published in 2008. Under the model, the four APN roles in the United States (nurse anesthetists, nurse midwives, nurse practitioners, nurse specialists) practice and are regulated under the "APRN" term. By 2010, over 48 nursing organizations in the United States endorsed the Consensus Model and started implementation across the country (APRN Consensus Group, NCSBN APRN Advisory Committee 2008). Up to that time, titles, education, licensing, accreditation, and certification varied from state to state, with some components varying within a state. Aside from reducing public and professional confusion, easing employer credentialing, and improving interprofessional collaboration, the process was a significant professional step for APNs (Wagner 2025). The United States is still implementing the Consensus model, but it has been a noteworthy step toward improving workforce data for APNs in the United States.

5.2 Minimum Datasets

Parallel to the above development, there has been a broader effort to standardize workforce data for nursing in the United States. Many organizations have been involved in workforce data collection in the United States, but one particular effort has been aimed at data that is thorough, detailed, and reliable. In 2009, the National Forum of State Nursing Workforce Centers (NFSNWC 2024a) produced and offered a minimum dataset for the purpose of standardizing nursing workforce data. Since then, there have been two revisions, the last being the 2024 National Nursing Workforce Minimum Dataset: Supply, available at https://nursingworkforcecenters.org/wp-content/uploads/2025/02/2024-Supply-MDS-Proposed.vFinal.pdf (NRSNWC 2024b).

The United States is still working to adopt the National Forum's minimum dataset across nursing systems. The newest dataset includes information on time spent providing direct patient care, telehealth, travel nursing, amount of student loans, and well-being. In gathering the data during license renewal periods, the hope is that workforce data will be collected at the jurisdictional level and standardized, allowing comparability. NFSNWC has also produced two additional datasets, one on nursing demand and one on education, to provide data on program applicants, students, and faculty (Oliveira et al. 2024). These last two align well with the Global Strategic Directions for Nursing and Midwifery 2021–2025 of the WHO, as cited above (NFSNWC 2020a, b), available at https://nursingworkforcecenters.org/

wp-content/uploads/2025/07/Nurse_Demand_MDS_RevisedDecember2020.pdf and https://nursingworkforcecenters.org/wp-content/uploads/2025/07/Nurse_Education_MDS_Revised_December2020.pdf.

A new initiative, undertaken by the National Organization of Nurse Practitioner Faculties (NONPF) in the United States was the development of a Doctor of Nursing Practice Nurse Practitioner Minimum Data Set (DNP NP MDS) to standardize data collection and analysis of this group of APNs. After extensive research and development, a multivariable data instrument was produced to collect data on demographics, education, and DNP-NP practice. It is anticipated that this sort of data gathering can support DNP practice and improve patient outcomes and is an example of how a minimum data set can be used to affect policy (NONPF 2022). Permission to use the instrument must be obtained from NONPF, available at https://www.nonpf.org/general/custom.asp?page=DNP_NP_MDS.

6 Organization Level Workforce Data

Another method to obtain workforce data in the United States has been at the professional organization level. Many such organizations have supported this effort as a routine part of their operation, primarily through surveys or other studies, with participants choosing to participate or not and with data safeguarded for privacy, integrity, and confidentiality. For example, the American Association of Nurse Practitioners (AANP) has performed this work on a regular basis, securing comprehensive data about a variety of workforce issues. Every other year, chosen AANP members and nonmembers obtain a survey with questions about practice or a survey with questions on compensation. The data is tallied and then made available, providing information on nurse practitioner characteristics, practice settings, education, and compensation (AANP 2026).

7 Conclusion: Potential Solutions to Improve APN Workforce Data

Obviously the movement toward gathering workforce data for APNs will be complicated, but it deserves the same attention as information gathering for generalist nurses, physicians, and other healthcare providers. Critical steps include the following:

- Recognize APN workforce data and titling limitations exist.
- Recognize gathering APN workforce data is worth the time, expense, and effort to gather and analyze. This may involve convincing interested parties (stakeholders) that APN data needs to be gathered and analyzed as distinct but as a subset of nursing.
- Plan carefully as to what data needs to be collected, how it will be collected, how it will be used, and how it will be protected.

- Build data gathering processes and infrastructure systems that are sustainable and secure.
- Ensure all methods of data collection and analysis meet data protection measures: utilizes informed consent (option to participate/not participate; how data will be used, potentially shared, and stored; confidential and private), meets ethical standards, is protected, and is deidentifiable.
- Consider data-gathering strategies that support the process, such as nurse registries and licensing systems that gather the data during licensing/registration periods and enlisting professional organizations and agencies to participate in the process.

References

American Association of Nurse Practitioners (AANP). Research reports. 2026. https://www.aanp.org/practice/practice-related-research/research-reports. Assessed 14 Mar 2026.

APRN Consensus Work Group, National Council of State Boards of Nursing APRN Advisory Committee. Consensus model for APRN regulation: licensure, accreditation, certification & education. 2008. https://www.ncsbn.org/public-files/Consensus_Model_for_APRN_Regulation_July_2008.pdf. Accessed 1 July 2025.

Center for Health Workforce Studies. The importance of health workforce data in decision making. 2025. https://www.chwsny.org/the-health-workforce/importance-of-data-in-decision-making/#:~:text=Analysis%20of%20basic%20health%20workforce,have%20on%20the%20health%20workforce. Accessed 1 July 2025.

Heale R, Buckley R. An international perspective of advanced practice nursing regulation. Int Nurs Rev. 2015;62(3):421–9. https://doi.org/10.1111/inr.12193.

International Council of Nurses (ICN). About ICNP. 2025. https://www.icn.ch/how-we-do-it/projects/ehealth-icnptm/about-icnp. Accessed 14 Mar 2025.

International Council of Nurses (ICN). ICN-accredited centres for ICNP™ research & development. 2026. https://www.icn.ch/how-we-do-it/projects/ehealth-icnptm/about-icnp/icn-accredited-centres-icnptm-research-development. Accessed 14 Mar 2026.

International Labour Organization. What labour force survey data can tell us about the workforce in the health and social care sector: a review of data from 56 countries. 2023. https://www.ilo.org/sites/default/files/2024-09/What%20labour%20force%20survey%20data%20can%20tell%20us%20about%20the%20workforce%20in%20the%20health%20and%20social%20care%20sector%20-%20A%20review%20of%20data%20from%2056%20countries.pdf. Accessed 1 July 2025.

Maier C, Aiken L. Task shifting from physicians to nurses in primary care in 39 countries: a cross-country comparative study. Eur J Publ Health. 2016;26(6):927–34. https://doi.org/10.1093/eurpub/ckw098.

National Academy of Medicine of the United States. The future of nursing: leading change, advancing health. 2020. https://nap.nationalacademies.org/resource/12956/Future-of-Nursing-2010-Report-Brief.pdf.

National Council of State Boards of Nursing. Workforce: the 2022 national workforce study video transcript. 2024. NCSBN Scientific Symposium. https://www.ncsbn.org/public-files/presentations/transcript_2024scisymp_rsmiley.pdf. Accessed 1 July 2025.

National Forum of State Nursing Workforce Centers (NFSNWC). National nursing workforce minimum dataset: demand—2020 revision. 2020a. Available at https://nursingworkforcecenters.org/wp-content/uploads/2025/07/Nurse_Demand_MDS_RevisedDecember2020.pdf. Accessed 14 Mar 2026.

families within the United States. The authors were interested in whether NPs contributed to higher healthcare costs. This question is often discussed when reviewing policies that impact access to NP care. Therefore, the authors sought to see if costs were indeed a factor. They studied a 2-year cross-section of 85,830 Medicare beneficiaries cared for by NPs and 382,124 beneficiaries whose care was provided by physicians. The results showed the costs associated with NP care were consistently lower across all risk levels. Policymakers can use these findings to support NP roles in healthcare settings, as the financial savings do not compromise the quality of care. Cost-benefit analyses offer an evidence-based approach to making informed decisions about healthcare investments.

2.6 Program Evaluations

Program evaluations systematically assess the effectiveness of healthcare programs and initiatives, providing updated, practical feedback for improvement. This research method is particularly valuable in refining APN educational programs, ensuring they meet the demands of healthcare systems and prepare competent professionals. The American Association of Colleges of Nursing (AACN 2021) has played a pivotal role in leveraging evaluations to promote the continuous improvement of nursing education. By integrating feedback from program evaluations into the 2021 essentials, they demonstrated the importance that educational programs remain responsive to healthcare demands, ultimately influencing policies that govern the educational preparation of APNs. Such evaluations not only ensure program quality but also have broader implications for healthcare policy, as they guide the accreditation process and standard setting in APN education. Data from these program evaluations have been used to advocate for increased federal funding to support NP education, further shaping policies that support workforce development in primary care and other critical areas of healthcare.

2.7 Case Studies

Case studies provide an in-depth look at specific instances of healthcare interventions, offering rich insights into how policies play out in real-world settings. They allow researchers and policymakers to examine the challenges and successes of particular healthcare models, often revealing valuable lessons for broader application. The development of APN roles in Canada's home health sector serves as a case study in how targeted policy interventions can enhance care for vulnerable populations, such as the elderly (Exemplar 2). Case studies are especially useful for illustrating the practical implications of policies, offering concrete examples of what works—and what does not—in healthcare reform (Heale and Butcher 2010).

2.8 Needs Assessment

Needs assessments identify gaps in healthcare services and determine what resources are required to meet those needs. They are often used to inform the development of new programs or policies by highlighting areas of unmet demand. In the context of the COVID-19 pandemic, needs assessments were instrumental in identifying the gaps in vaccination and treatment access for long-term care (LTC) residents (Exemplar 3). The findings led to federal recommendations for ensuring that antiviral therapies are readily available in long-term care facilities. Needs assessments provide essential data for making informed decisions about resource allocation to address critical healthcare issues.

3 Applying Research to Policy: A Toolkit for APNs

In reviewing all of these examples, key steps were identified and can be used as a roadmap to health policy research implementation (Fig. 2). The figure portrays a road with road signs guiding the way. Like with any journey, there are bumps, pitfalls, and challenges that occur along the way. These events can provide learning opportunities to shape the journey towards policy development further. In this image, there are six key steps, as explained and explored through the examples shared in this chapter.

APNs play a critical role in influencing health policy through research. The following toolkit outlines six key steps for leveraging research to affect policy:

1. Identify the problem:

   Clearly define the question or issue you aim to address through policy change. For example, are APNs a viable solution to the shortage of primary care providers?

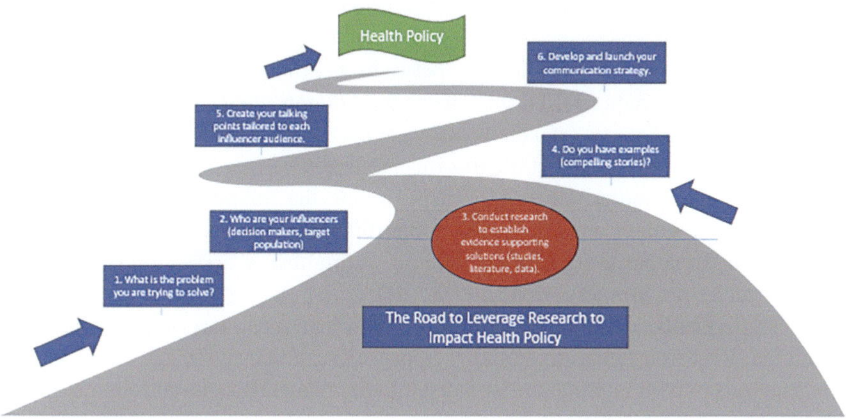

Fig. 2 Roadmap to health policy research implementation

2. Understand your audience:
   Identify the decision-makers who can influence policy. Understanding their values, goals, and priorities is essential to tailoring your research findings effectively.
3. Conduct research:
   Utilize a variety of research methodologies to gather evidence. This can include literature reviews, original studies, or secondary data analysis. Synthesize your findings to present clear evidence that supports policy change.
4. Collect stories and data:
   Combine data with real-life examples to make a compelling case for policy change. Stories can provide context and humanize the issue.
5. Develop key talking points:
   Create concise messages that summarize your research findings and policy recommendations. These "elevator pitches" should be easy to understand and highlight the importance of the proposed changes.
6. Implement a communication strategy:
   Develop a plan to share your findings with decision-makers and interested parties (stakeholders). Whether through personal meetings, letters, or public presentations, choose the communication methods that will have the greatest impact.

4 Exemplar 1—Singapore Implementation Study—Advancing Advanced Practice Nursing: Integrating Research to Shape Policies and Practice in Singapore

Research is crucial to the development of advanced practice nursing (APN) in Singapore. As healthcare evolves, integrating research findings is essential for refining policies and advancing APN practices. APNs, as master's-prepared professionals, undergo rigorous training, including an 18-month program, a 12-month internship, and certification by the Singapore Nursing Board (SNB). However, challenges remain regarding the understanding of APN roles among interested parties (stakeholders), making research vital to bridging these gaps and ensuring evidence-based policymaking.

A key issue in Singapore is the gap between theoretical knowledge and clinical practice for APN graduates. Despite stringent training, there is often a mismatch between interested party (stakeholder) expectations and graduate competencies. Since APN training began in 2003, this misalignment has persisted. In response, an APN development committee was formed to review the competency framework and align education with clinical demands, supporting APN integration into the healthcare system. To achieve the goal to increase the number of APNs to 700 by 2030, which is set by the Ministry of Health (MOH).

APNs frequently collaborate with physicians, which can lead to role misunderstandings. Research helps define APN boundaries and communicate their unique contributions to both nursing and interdisciplinary teams (Brooks and Fulton 2020). Clarifying and prioritizing APN roles is essential to prevent role confusion and overload (Bryant-Lukosius et al. 2004).

Exploratory research on Singapore's APN practice patterns and role expectations (Villeneuve 2017) identified five core domains of APN practice: clinical care, system support, research, education, and leadership. To address gaps between competencies and clinical practice, nine entrustable professional activities (EPAs) were developed, effectively aligning educational and clinical expectations (Woo et al. 2019). These EPAs map the entire APN education process, from the 18-month master's program to the 12-month internship, establishing milestones and levels of entrustment to align interested party (stakeholder) expectations.

While EPAs offer a structured framework for APN development, challenges remain, particularly in standardizing their use across healthcare institutions. Rigorous faculty training is needed to ensure fairness and consistency in evaluations. Ongoing studies are examining the effectiveness of EPAs in preparing APN interns for autonomous practice and certification (Zhou et al. 2022), providing insights into how EPAs support the transition from RN to APN.

Research plays a fundamental role in shaping the future of Advanced Practice Nursing in Singapore. By using evidence-based approaches, policymakers, educators, and healthcare administrators can support APN growth and integration into the healthcare system, ultimately contributing to higher standards of care.

4.1 Exemplar 2—Canada Case Study—Leveraging Data and Outlining Key Steps in Advancing Home Care Services Provided by NPs in Primary Care

Recent overviews of systematic reviews to identify indicators sensitive to the practice of community-based primary care NPs ($n = 44$ reviews) and advanced practice nursing ($n = 117$ reviews) identified important gaps in research examining implementation processes and interprofessional team functioning (Kilpatrick et al. 2024; Kilpatrick et al. 2023). It is essential to identify effective strategies that enhance APN role implementation in teams and care quality.

In Canada, healthcare is under provincial and territorial jurisdiction, and most services are publicly funded (Villeneuve 2017). Healthcare services are determined at the provincial level to meet populational needs. In Québec, Canada, investments have been made in home care services to help older adults remain at home as long as possible (Commissaire à la santé et au bien-être 2024). However, these investments have not kept pace with healthcare costs as they represent only 4.5% of the province's 2022 healthcare budget (Commissaire à la santé et au bien-être 2023a). The need for home care services is increasing because of the growing number of homebound patients who require primary care or complex services (Curioni et al. 2023; Sun et al. 2022). Home care can support homebound patients to remain at home for longer periods, improve quality of life, and reduce hospitalizations, transfers to the emergency department, and healthcare costs (Curioni et al. 2023). Home care services are provided by interprofessional teams that include unlicensed personnel, nurses, social workers, physiotherapists, and physicians. In some jurisdictions, APNs are key providers of home-based primary care (Sun et al. 2022). In facility (Chidambaram 2022). Residents' advanced age, multimorbidity, need for one-on-one care, and shared living spaces contributed to their heightened risk of COVID-19 morbidity and mortality (National Healthcare Quality and Disparities Report 2023). The primary series vaccination was available in the early months of 2021, followed by the availability of the COVID-19 bivalent booster, which targeted the original strain of the virus as well as the Omicron (B.1.1.529) variant. Although the Omicron variant was believed to have lower potential to cause severe illness than earlier variants, the concern to prevent severe infection and unplanned healthcare utilization was still a priority for healthcare providers of older adults. There was a need for strong, consistent public messaging about the importance of the booster vaccination, especially to counter its misconceptions and myths. During this same time, the US Food and Drug Administration (FDA) issued an Emergency Use Authorization (EUA) for Paxlovid (nirmatrelvir/ritonavir) for the treatment of mild-to-moderate COVID-19 in adults (US Food and Drug Administration 2021). Despite the growing concern of COVID-19 infections in LTC facilities, vaccination and treatment practices across the United States were highly variable. There was also a wide knowledge gap among long-term care healthcare providers about the availability and accessibility of COVID-19 vaccination and treatment.

In October 2022, members of the White House COVID-19 Response Team convened a meeting with leaders of healthcare associations nationwide. Association leaders were asked to provide education to their members and other interested parties (stakeholders) about the importance, effectiveness, and accessibility of the bivalent booster vaccination and antiviral therapeutics available to treat COVID-19 infections. During this time, Jennifer Kim, a doctorally prepared gerontological APN, was president of the Gerontological Advanced Practice Nurses Association (GAPNA), the premier professional organization that represents the interests of APNs involved in improving care of older adults.

4.4 The Vax and Pax Toolkit

The Society for Post-acute and Long-Term Care Medicine partnered with GAPNA, the American Association of Nurse Practitioners (AANP), the American Academy of Physician Associates (AAPA), and the American Society of Consultant Pharmacists (ASCP) to develop and disseminate an evidence-based, best practices toolkit for prevention and management of COVID-19 in LTC facilities. Collaboration among these associations was intentional, reinforcing the importance of interprofessional practice in the LTC setting. Collaboration was also important for consistent messaging to patients and healthcare providers. The "COVID-19 Vaccination and Therapeutics in PALTC Toolkit: Resources for Clinicians" ("Vax and Pax" toolkit) was an electronic resource available for free PDF download on all the associations' websites and websites of other interested party (stakeholder) organizations (US Post-acute and Long-Term Care Medicine Society 2023). It included frequently asked questions (FAQs), patient education sheets, standing order templates, flowcharts, and prescribing guides.

4.5 COVID-19 Vaccinations

During the same time the Vax and Pax Toolkit was introduced (fall 2022), the Director of the American Association of Retired Persons (AARP) Policy Center contacted Jennifer Kim to inquire about common vaccination practices in LTC facilities. The Director wanted to learn of APNs' experiences working in LTC facilities with high vaccination rates. A list of LTC facilities in the United States that had 95%+ vaccination rates among residents and staff members was provided for Dr. Kim, who then collaborated with other GAPNA leaders to find organization members who practiced within these facilities. These GAPNA members then participated in focus group sessions led by the Director, which included discussions of clinical practices and variables believed to be associated with facilities with high vaccination rates. A predominant theme in the focus groups was the critical need for APN leadership within the facility. APNs were often the facility champions who promoted vaccination. The Director synthesized important pieces of information from these sessions and shared them with the White House COVID-19 Response Team.

4.6 COVID-19 Therapeutics

During the fall of 2022, a member of the White House COVID-19 Response Team initiated contact with Jennifer Kim, requesting a meeting with GAPNA leaders to gain an understanding of LTC APNs' knowledge and accessibility to Paxlovid (nirmatrelvir/ritonavir) and other antiviral treatments for COVID-19. Dr. Kim formed a team of GAPNA leaders to serve as the organization's spokespersons and also extended an open invitation to all GAPNA members, especially those in the PAC/LTC Specialty Interest Group (SIG), to share their experiences with ordering and administering COVID-19 antivirals. Members consistently shared two significant barriers: (1) misunderstanding of the indication for antiviral therapeutics that it should be reserved for only those with a significant infection; and (2) inability to store emergency doses of antivirals within an LTC facility, leading to long wait times to initiate treatment. Members noted the availability of emergency access to antiviral medications for influenza infections within their respective facilities, raising questions as to why antivirals for COVID-19 infections could not also be available. GAPNA leaders met with members of the White House COVID-19 Response Team to relay these barriers, which they had not been aware. GAPNA leaders also recommended allowance of on-site emergency doses of COVID-19 antivirals, noting the success of this delivery method to expedite initiation of antiviral treatments for influenza infections.

4.7 The Voice of the Gerontological APN

GAPNA's collaboration with the White House COVID-19 Response Team and the AARP Policy Center contributed to the federal government's recommendations to have onsite emergency doses of antiviral therapies for COVID-19 infections available within LTC facilities. Additional APN education about the indication of antiviral therapy for COVID-19 infections was also provided. These recommendations, along with others provided by GAPNA leaders, were included in *The White House Winter Playbook*, published in December 2022 (U.S. Whitehouse 2022).

Antiviral prescriptions in LTC facilities nearly doubled from November 2022 to March 2023, much of which was attributed to the collaboration of GAPNA and other interested party (stakeholder) groups with the White House COVID-19 Response Team. Jennifer Kim and GAPNA leaders continue to collaborate with government interested party (stakeholder) groups and organization leaders via the White House Long-Term Care Leadership Summits to develop strategies for improved respiratory illness vaccinations in long-term care facilities.

5 Conclusion

For APNs to effectively influence health policy, leveraging research is essential. By following the systematic steps outlined in this toolkit—conducting research, engaging with decision-makers, and crafting clear, evidence-based recommendations—APNs can drive meaningful policy changes that improve patient outcomes and healthcare systems. Collaboration with interprofessional teams and policymakers is key to ensuring the successful implementation of research-informed policies.

References

2023 National Healthcare Quality and Disparities Report. Impact of COVID-19 on nursing homes. Rockville: Agency for Healthcare Research and Quality (US); 2023. Available from: https://www.ncbi.nlm.nih.gov/books/NBK600464/. Accessed 10 Oct 2024.

American Association of Colleges of Nursing (AACN). The essentials. 2021. https://www.aacnnursing.org/essentials. Accessed 8 Oct 2024.

Asad Zandi M. Concepts and theories of nursing with a sound heart model. Tehran: Heidari Publication; 2014.

Bradshaw NA. Florence Nightingale (1820–1910): an unexpected master of data. Patterns (N Y). 2020;1(2):100036. https://doi.org/10.1016/j.patter.2020.100036. PMID: 33205102; PMCID: PMC7660360.

Brooks M, Fulton J. Defining the boundaries of advanced nursing practice: a study of role clarity and stakeholder perceptions. Nurs Outlook. 2020;68(1):7–35. https://doi.org/10.1016/j.outlook.2019.07.008.

Bryant-Lukosius D, DiCenso A, Browne G, Pinelli J. Advanced practice nursing roles: development, implementation, and evaluation. J Adv Nurs. 2004;48(5):519–29. https://doi.org/10.1111/j.1365-2648.2004.03234.x.

Candello Solutions by CRICO. A Sea change in U.S. care delivery: an analysis of advanced practice provider and physician malpractice risk. 2023. crico_candello_bmr_apps_seachange_final101223.pdf (hubspotusercontent-na1.net). Accessed 30 Jan 2024.

Chidambaram P. Over 200,000 residents and staff in long-term care facilities have died from COVID-19. KFF Policy Watch. 2022. https://www.kff.org/policy-watch/over-200000-residents-and-staff-in-long-term-care-facilities-have-died-from-covid-19/. Accessed 10 Oct 2024.

Commissaire à la santé et au bien-être. Bien vieillir chez soi-Tome 2: Chiffrer la performance. 2023a. https://www.csbe.gouv.qc.ca/publication/bien-vieillir-chez-soi-tome-1-comprendre-lecosysteme.html. Accessed 10 Oct 2024.

Commissaire à la santé et au bien-être. Horizon 2040: Projection des impacts du soutien à l'autonomie au Québec. 2023b. https://www.csbe.gouv.qc.ca/publication/horizon-2040-projection-soutien-autonomie-quebec.html. Accessed 10 Oct 2024.

Curioni C, Silva AC, Damião J, et al. The cost-effectiveness of homecare services for adults and older adults: a systematic review. Int J Env Res Public Health. 2023;20(4):3373.

Gigli KH, Martsolf GR, Vinci RJ, Buerhaus PI. A cross-sectional examination of the nurse practitioner workforce caring for children in the United States. J Peds. 2023;257:113376. https://doi.org/10.1016/j.jpeds.2023.02.020.

Hassan M. Survey research-types, methods, examples. 2024. https://reesearchmethod.net/survey-research/. Accessed 10 Oct 2024.

Heale R, Butcher M. Canada's first nurse practitioner-led clinic: a case study in healthcare innovation. Nurs Leadersh. 2010;10(3):21–9. https://doi.org/10.12927/cjnl.2010.21939.

Kapu AN, Kleinpell R, Pilon B. Quality and financial impact of adding nurse practitioners to inpatient care teams. J Nurs Adm. 2014;44(2):87–96. https://doi.org/10.1097/NNA.0000000000000031.

Kilpatrick K, Paquette L, Jabbour M, et al. Systematic review of the characteristics of brief team interventions to clarify roles and improve functioning in healthcare teams. PLoS One. 2020;15(6):e0234416.

Kilpatrick K, Tchouaket E, Savard I, et al. Identifying indicators sensitive to primary healthcare nurse practitioner practice: a review of systematic reviews. PLoS One. 2023;18(9):e0290977.

Kilpatrick K, Savard I, Audet L-A, et al. A global perspective of advanced practice nursing research: a review of systematic reviews. PLoS One. 2024;19(7):e0305008.

Nightingale F. Florence Nightingale. Cassandra: an essay. 1979. Am J Public Health. 2010;100(9):1586–7.

Razavi M, O'Reilly-Jacob M, Perloff J, Buerhaus PI. Drivers of cost differences between nurse practitioner and physician attributed Medicare beneficiaries. Med Care. 2021;59(2):177–84. https://doi.org/10.1097/MLR.0000000000001477.

Savard I, Jabbour M, Tchouaket E, Gauthier N, Kilpatrick K. Evaluating the influence of primary healthcare nurse practitioners' interventions in home care on hospitalizations and emergency department transfers. J Eval Clin Pract. 2024;30(3):440–52.

Sun CA, Parslow C, Gray J, Koyfman I, Hladek MD, Han HR. Home-based primary care visits by nurse practitioners. J Am Assoc Nurse Pract. 2022;34(6):802–12.

U.S. Food & Drug Administration. Coronavirus (COVID-19) update: FDA authorizes first oral antiviral for treatment of COVID-19. 2021. https://www.fda.gov/news-events/press-announcements/coronavirus-covid-19-update-fda-authorizes-first-oral-antiviral-treatment-covid-19. Accessed 10 Oct 2024.

U.S. Post-Acute and Long-Term Care Medicine Society. Vax and pax toolkit. 2023. https://paltc.org/sites/default/files/2023-1/Vax%20and%20Pax%20toolkit_11_14_FINAL.pdf. Accessed 10 Oct 2024.

U.S. White House. Winter playbook for nursing homes and other long-term care facilities to manage COVID-19 and protect residents, staff, and visitors. 2022. https://www.whitehouse.gov/wp-content/uploads/2022/12/Winter-Playbook-for-Nursing-Homes-and-Other-Long-term-Care-Facilities-to-Manage-COVID-19-and-Protect-Residents-Staff-and-Visitors.pdf. Accessed 10 Oct 2024.

Villeneuve M. Public policy and Canadian nursing: lessons from the field. Toronto: Canadian Scholars Press; 2017.

Woo BF, Zhou W, Lim TW, Tam SW. Registered nurses' perceptions towards advanced practice nursing: a cross-sectional study. J Nurs Manag. 2019;28(1):82–93. https://doi.org/10.1111/jonm.12893.

Zhou W, Poh CL, Chan HL, Shorey S. Development of entrustable professional activities for advanced practice nurses education. Nurse Educ Today. 2022;116:105462. https://doi.org/10.1016/j.nedt.2022.105462. Epub 2022 Jul 5. PMID: 35839547.

Health Policy for Governance: Regulation, and Professional Credentialing

Advanced Practice Nursing Regulatory Models Around the World

Minna K. Miller

1 Introduction/Background

In an era characterized by an ever-evolving healthcare landscape, the role of advanced practice nurses (APNs) has become increasingly important in meeting the healthcare needs of the population (Miller et al. 2024). The expansion of APN roles into nearly 100 countries worldwide underscores the importance of commensurate development in APN regulation (Almukhaini et al. 2022; De Raeve et al. 2023; Kim et al. 2021; Miller et al. 2024). Both the World Health Organization (WHO) and the International Council of Nurses (ICN) have emphasized the importance of nursing regulation and the need for nurses to be able to work to the full scope of their education and training (ICN 2013, 2020; WHO 2020, 2025). Regulation is broadly defined as "the act of regulating; the state of being regulated" or "a rule or order issued by an executive authority or regulatory agency of a government and having the force of law" (Merriam-Webster n.d.).

The ICN states the purpose of nursing regulation in its position statement:

> laws governing nursing practice are put in place by governments and enforced by regulators to provide mechanisms to ensure as much as possible, that practitioners are safe and competent to practice. The regulatory authority establishes, promotes, and enforces standards for education and practice and by doing so demonstrates to the public, government, employers and other interested parties (stakeholders) that the profession is committed to retaining the public's trust and delivering quality services. Regulation advances public safety and protection through promoting the delivery of safe, ethical and competent care by nurses. The ICN believes that profession-led nursing regulation promotes public protection and quality patient outcomes. Systems of professional regulation are influenced and shaped by the legislative, political, environmental, social, cultural, and professional context in which they are developed. (ICN 2013)

M. K. Miller (✉)
School of Nursing, University of British Columbia, Vancouver, BC, Canada
e-mail: Minnak1@aol.com

K. J. Wheeler, M. Acorn (eds.), *Health Policy for Advanced Practice Nursing: A Toolkit for Implementation and Improvement*, Advanced Practice in Nursing,
https://doi.org/10.1007/978-3-032-03667-4_11

Schober (2016, p. 111) asserts that "regulation is the legitimate and appropriate means whereby order, identity, consistency, and control are brought to a profession." Without regulation, APNs do not have the legal authority to practice in advanced, autonomous roles beyond the scope of practice for a general/registered nurse (Maier et al. 2017). However, there is significant variation in APN role, regulation, education, scope of practice, and licensure by country/region (De Raeve et al. 2023; Elvidge et al. 2024; Ladd et al. 2020; Miller et al. 2024; Scanlon et al. 2019; Wheeler et al. 2022). Largely, this is due to country context-specific APN legislation and professional regulation or authorization that is explicit about APN certification or credentialing (De Raeve et al. 2023; ICN 2020; Miller et al. 2024). ICN has recommended that regulatory mechanisms for APNs include the authority to order diagnostic tests and therapeutic treatment, the authority to diagnose, to prescribe medications, to refer clients to other services and/or professionals, and authority to admit and discharge clients to and from hospital and other services (ICN 2020). Regulatory mechanisms should also include officially recognized title(s) for nurses working as APNs, and legislation to grant and protect the title(s) (e.g., Clinical Nurse Specialist, Nurse Practitioner) (ICN 2020). As stated in the first chapter, it is important to note that in many countries midwifery may be regulated as a distinct profession; this chapter uses "nurse-midwife" only where it is a legally defined nursing-based role. Legislation, regulation, and related regulatory structures that inform APN practice and education are further clarified in Table 1 based on an ICN unpublished credentialing framework described by Schober (2016).

Table 1 Components of regulatory structures

Legislation	Regulation
Definition of APN	Scope of practice definition
Title protection	Standards and guidelines Entry into practice Level of education Practice Assuring competence maintenance Professional conduct
Regulatory body Composition Powers and function Appointment and conditions for office	Processes/procedures for certain regulatory activities Credentialing Providing examinations, reviews, interviews Accreditation of educational programs/ institutions Renewal, suspension, removal, reinstatement of license Hearings, consultations Complaint and disciplinary proceedings
Dealing with other jurisdictions	Communication Reporting
Resources for conducting affairs (power to raise revenue)	Data collection about a credentialee Evaluation of regulatory effectiveness

Reproduced with adaptations from Schober (2016) with permission from Springer Nature

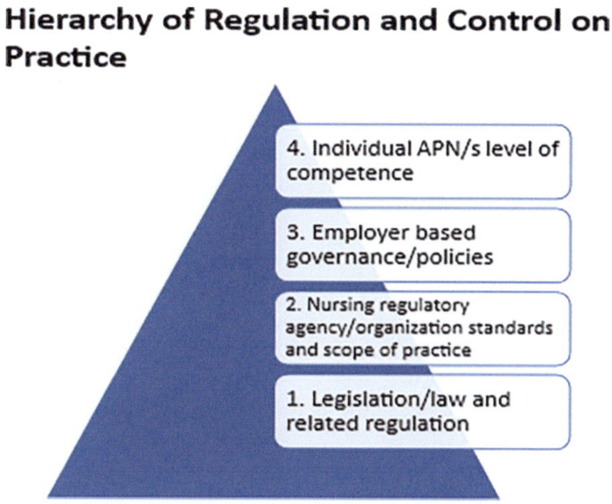

Fig. 1 Hierarchy of APN regulation and control on practice. (Adapted for global context from British Columbia College of Nursing Professionals (2020)

Research has demonstrated that even in the absence of APN-specific legislation/regulation, APNs work to meet individual and population health and healthcare needs and that practice and educational models are outpacing regulatory standards (Ladd et al. 2020). Ultimately, it is the responsibility of each individual APN to practice within her/his own level of competence (Fig. 1).

2 Regulatory Models

Nursing regulatory models exist along a continuum. Some form of nursing regulation is in place in much of the world, although not in all regions or countries, and APN-specific regulation is lagging (ICN 2014; Ladd et al. 2020). Benton et al. (2013) describe five such models with assigned value labels related to professional respect and public safety: (1) no regulation; (2) pure self-regulation; (3) delegated self-regulation; (4) supervised self-regulation; and (5) government-based regulation (Table 2).

Advantages and disadvantages are associated with each model (Benton et al. 2013). Absence of regulation or pure self-regulation have failed to protect the public resulting in professional misconduct, harm and poor patient outcomes (Braithwaite et al. 2007; Motluk 2019). This has led to a shift toward regulatory models with some form of legislative backing or government oversight (Leslie et al. 2023). Not only is there variation in the regulatory models but also in how and by whom the regulations are administered, further impacting APN regulation. Benton et al. (2013) articulate a typology to describe six administrative approaches (Table 3).

Notwithstanding the diversity of nursing regulatory systems, the purpose of these systems has always been to protect and serve the public. The global COVID-19 pandemic necessitated significant regulatory changes, in order to ensure an adequate nursing workforce while also maintaining public safety (Leslie et al. 2023; Ziegler et al. 2024). Post pandemic, health systems everywhere are still struggling

Table 2 Continuum of nursing regulation

Value labels				
1	2	3	4	5
No regulation	Pure self-regulation	Delegated self-regulation	Supervised self-regulation	Government-based regulation
Consumers are empowered to utilize offered services and have the necessary information to make informed decisions and avoid harm	The profession independently establishes and enforces its standards without government involvement	An autonomous board, with legislative backing, develops and administers standards of practice and a code of conduct for the profession, while the government and education body give the board the ability to enforce the code/standards via legislative support	An appointed board develops, administers, and enforces standards of practice and a code of conduct for the profession. Government and education bodies approve these and give the board the authority, through legislative backing, to enforce the code and standards. Enforcement is monitored by a higher power that can intervene if necessary	The government directly controls the development, administration, and enforcement of professional regulation, codes, and standards and may employ professional staff to provide expertise and insight

Adapted from Wheeler et al. (2024) and Benton et al. (2013)

Table 3 Typology describing six administrative approaches

Multi disciplinary single board model	Multi disciplinary model with individual board with shared services	Multi disciplinary model with individual boards	Single board model	Regulatory unit model	Division of powers model
Umbrella legislation covering multiple disciplines with a single governance board	Umbrella legislation covering multiple disciplines with delegated authority to multiple, profession-specific boards that can make policy in a range of areas but share services or accommodation	Umbrella legislation covering multiple disciplines with delegated authority to multiple, independent, profession-specific boards	Profession-specific legislation with delegated power to a single profession-based board	Regulation processes managed by a unit or as part of a government entity, such as the Ministry of Health established through a ministerial or other decree	Division of powers among federal and regional structures or different entities relating to levels of nurses

Adapted from Benton et al. (2013)

to secure a sufficient nursing workforce. The International Council of Nurses has identified the current shortage of nurses as a global health emergency (ICN 2024). In light of nursing and healthcare workforce shortages, the aging population, increasing healthcare needs and costs, noncommunicable diseases, emerging new infectious diseases, and access to care inequalities, the drivers for regulatory reform are changing and the concept of "acting in the public interest" has been redefined (Benton et al. 2019). Acting in the public interest is defined as "A multi-dimensional concept that evolves over time; is context sensitive; and embraces the use of a range of interventions to address the effective, efficient, and safe provision of services to the recipient. In addition, the concept embraces the simultaneous balancing of equity of access to services by the user, while minimizing provider barriers that are proportionate to the level of risk" (Benton et al. 2019, p. 6). Therefore, from a regulatory system redesign perspective, "acting in the public interest" must take into account the costs of regulation, increased efficiency and cost effectiveness, reduction in entry to profession/practice barriers, reduction of barriers to mobility, promoting competition, considering alternatives to the licensure model, be responsive to a highly complex health system, and facilitate regulation proportionate to risk (Benton et al. 2019; Mahat et al. 2023). Within this context, some jurisdictions/countries are embracing Right Touch Regulation (Professional Standards Authority 2015, 2018).

Right Touch Regulation is a model for regulatory decision-making, based on a thorough evaluation of risk, with focus on outcomes and public safety. It assists in determining the minimum regulatory force required to achieve a desired effect. The main strength of risk-based regulation is that when it is used well, it provides a clear, transparent, and rational basis for determining what and how to regulate. When risks are both quantified and qualified, regulation decisions can be described as risk based (College of Registered Nurses of Manitoba [CRNM] 2022, p. 2).

Guiding principles for Right Touch Regulation:

1. Proportionate: Regulators should only intervene when necessary. Response should be appropriate to the risk posed while identifying and minimizing costs.
2. Consistent: Rules and standards must be implemented fairly.
3. Targeted: Regulation should be problem focused and minimize side effects.
4. Transparent: Regulators should be open and keep regulations simple and user-friendly.
5. Accountable: Regulators must be able to justify decisions and be subject to public scrutiny.
6. Agile: Regulators must be visionary, anticipate change rather than looking back to prevent previous crisis from recurring. An agile regulator foresees changes, anticipates the risks as a result of the change, and takes timely action to mitigate the risks (CRNM 2022; Mahat et al. 2023; Professional Standards Authority 2018).

3 Case Exemplars

Case exemplars specific to APN regulatory models in this section provide a snapshot of a variety of APN roles and related regulations in context of five different countries.

3.1 United States of America

The healthcare system in the United States consists of several models, including a not-for-profit, single-payer (Medicare) system for elders who qualify, a not-for-profit joint federal and state program (Medicaid) for low-income individuals who quality, and a mostly for-profit system for others, leaving those who do not qualify for Medicare or Medicaid and cannot afford to pay for services within the for-profit model as potentially uninsured or underinsured. The development and implementation of APN roles in the United States has been driven by need to improve access to healthcare services, with the first records of advanced practice activities by nurses dating back some 100 years (Wheeler et al. 2022).

The United States has the largest regulated APN workforce in the world with 461,000 nurse practitioners (AANP 2025a), 89,000 Clinical Nurse Specialists (NACNS 2021), over 7750 nurse midwives (U.S. Bureau of Statistics 2021) and nearly 50,000 certified registered nurse anesthetists (AANA 2023). Each state regulates its APRNs. The Consensus Model for Advanced Practice Registered Nurse (APRN) Regulation: Licensure, Accreditation, Certification and Education of 2008 (APRN Consensus Work Group and the National Council of State Boards of Nursing APRN Advisory Committee 2008; NCSBN 2025a) was developed to provide guidance for all US states/jurisdictions to adopt uniformity in the regulation of APRN roles. It puts forth the definition of APRN and includes seven main elements:

1. Title: Advanced practice registered nurse.
2. License: APRN license.
3. Identifies four APRN roles: Certified nurse midwife (CNM), certified nurse practitioner (CNP), certified registered nurse anesthetist (CRNA), and clinical nurse specialist (CNS).
4. Education: Graduate degree or postgraduate certificate is required.
5. National certification: APRNs would be expected to pass a nationally accredited certification exam.
6. Autonomous practice: APRNs would be granted authority to practice autonomously without physician supervision/collaborative agreements.
7. Autonomous prescribing: APRNs would be granted authority to prescribe without physician oversight/collaborative agreements.

APRNs are educated and certified in both their role (CNP, CRNA, CNM, CNS) and in one of six population foci (Fig. 2).

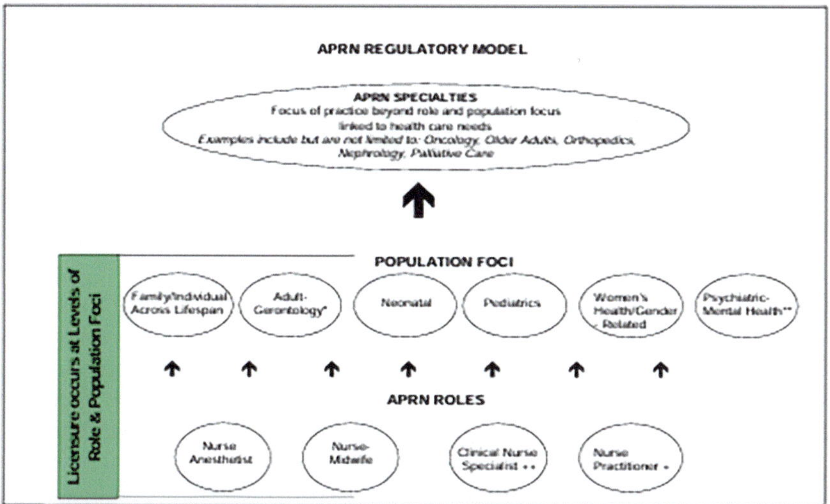

+The certified nurse practitioner (CNP) is prepared with the acute care CNP competencies and/or the primary care CNP competencies. At this point in time the acute care and primary care CNP delineation applies only to the pediatric and adult-gerontology CNP population foci. Scope of practice of the primary care or acute care CNP is **not setting specific** but is based on patient care needs. Programs may prepare individuals across both the primary care and acute care CNP competencies. If programs prepare graduates across both sets of roles, the graduate must be prepared with the consensus-based competencies for both roles and must successfully obtain certification in both the acute and the primary care CNP roles. CNP certification in the acute care or primary care roles must match the educational preparation for CNPs in these roles.

Diagram 1: APRN Regulatory Model

Under this APRN Regulatory Model, there are four roles: certified registered nurse anesthetist (CRNA), certified nurse-midwife (CNM), clinical nurse specialist (CNS), and certified nurse practitioner (CNP). These four roles are given the title of advanced practice registered nurse (APRN). APRNs are educated in one of the four roles and in at least one of six population foci: family/individual across the lifespan, adult-gerontology, neonatal, pediatrics, women's health/gender-related or psych/mental health. Individuals will be licensed as independent practitioners for practice at the level of one of the four APRN roles within at least one of the six identified population foci. Education, certification, and licensure of an individual must be congruent in terms of role and population foci. APRNs may specialize but they can not be licensed solely within a specialty area. Specialties can provide depth in one's practice within the established population foci.

* The population focus, adult-gerontology, encompasses the young adult to the older adult, including the frail elderly. APRNs educated and certified in the adult-gerontology population are educated and certified across both areas of practice and will be titled Adult-Gerontology CNP or CNS. In addition, all APRNs in any of the four roles providing care to the adult population, e.g., family or gender specific, must be prepared to meet the growing needs of the older adult population. Therefore, the education program should include didactic and clinical education experiences necessary to prepare APRNs with these enhanced skills and knowledge.
** The population focus, psychiatric/mental health, encompasses education and practice across the lifespan.
++ The Clinical Nurse Specialist (CNS) is educated and assessed through national certification processes across the continuum from wellness through acute care.

Fig. 2 US consensus model for APRN regulation with roles and population foci. (Figure reproduced from the APRN Consensus Work Group and the National Council of State Boards of Nursing APRN Advisory Committee (2008, p. 10), https://www.ncsbn.org/public-files/Consensus_Model_for_APRN_Regulation_July_2008.pdf). Figure reproduced with permission from the American Association of Colleges of Nursing Board of Directors

Despite the publication of the APRN Consensus Model over 15 years ago, there continues to be variation in APRN regulation and uptake of the APRN model from state to state. For example, nurse practitioners in only 28 (i.e., 27 states and the District of Columbia) of the 50 states have full practice authority (AANP 2025b). Full practice authority means that state-specific practice and licensure laws permit all APRNs to evaluate patients; diagnose, order, and interpret diagnostic tests; and initiate and manage treatments, including prescribing medications and controlled substances, under the exclusive licensure authority of the state board of nursing. This is the model recommended by the National Academy of Medicine and the National Council of State Boards of Nursing. The remaining states have either reduced or restricted practice authority for NPs, as state practice and licensure laws reduce/restrict the ability of NPs to engage in at least one element of NP practice. In these situations, state law requires a regulated collaborative agreement with another health provider in order for the NP to provide patient care, or it limits the setting of one or more elements of NP practice (AANP nd), resulting in a potential barrier to care access and increase in care costs (Xue et al. 2018). National professional organizations and their state-based counterparts play a significant role in advocating for federal and state legislation to align them with the recommendations in the APRN Consensus model. Several states have started to join the APRN COMPACT, which allows APRNs to have one multistate license, in hopes of facilitating professional mobility across state lines once sufficient states join the COMPACT (NCSBN 2025b).

3.2 Canada

Canada has a publicly administered, not-for-profit, universal healthcare system. Provincial and territorial governments, on behalf of the public, have granted the nursing profession the privilege and responsibility to self-regulate through legislation and regulation (CNA 2019). Nursing regulatory bodies have a mandate to regulate nurses to ensure public protection. They achieve this through specific regulatory activities such as establishing requirements for entry into practice, registration, licensure/relicensure, and title protection; articulating, promoting, and enforcing scope and standards of practice; approving APN education programs (master's degree is required); and administering continuing competence and quality assurance programs (CNA 2019).

Canada has two recognized APN roles, the nurse practitioner (NP) and the clinical nurse specialist. CNSs are regulated within the registered nurse's scope of practice, while NPs have title protection and legislation granting authority for independent practice (Miller et al. 2023). NPs are the fastest-growing health profession in Canada and enjoy high public confidence. At present, there are nearly 13,000 licensed NPs in the country working across settings and specialties (Miller et al. 2023; NPAC 2025). Early records for advanced practice nursing date back to the 1890s to outpost nurses who provided primary care services in the isolated areas of the North. In the 1960s, the impetus for incorporating NPs into the national healthcare system was related to the new publicly funded universal healthcare insurance system, an increase in physician specialization away from primary care, and a perceived maldistribution of physicians. Over the past three decades, the driver for increasing NP positions within the healthcare sector has been the primary care crisis and the need to improve access to related services (Miller et al. 2023).

The Canadian Nurses Association played a key role in enhancing the NP role and role integration into the Canadian healthcare system through the Canadian Nurse Practitioner Initiative (CNPI) of 2006 with the publication of related documents, including a toolkit, technical report, and a 10-year retrospective evaluation, recommending a standardized approach to NP education, regulation, and practice across the nation (CNA 2006a, b, p. 42, 43, 44, 2016). Despite these national recommendations, NP scopes of practice vary across provinces and territories (CIHI 2020), while entry to practice requires graduate-level education and passing a written certification examination in each jurisdiction (Miller et al. 2023). More recently, the Nurse Practitioner Association of Canada has emerged as the voice for all NPs in the country, advocating for and reducing barriers to NP practice.

3.3 The Republic of Ireland

Ireland has a publicly funded healthcare system, each resident with a medical card having access to free medical services, public hospital services, prescribed medication, specific dental, optical and aural services, maternity and infant care, and community care and personal social services (Citizens Information 2022). The regulatory authority for nursing and midwifery in Ireland is the Nursing and Midwifery Board of Ireland (NMBI). The board is charged with the protection of the public in its dealings with nurses and midwives and the promotion of high standards of professional education, training, practice, and professional conduct. It is responsible for establishing and maintaining the register of nurses and midwives (NMBI 2017, n.d.-a, n.d.-b, n.d.-c). The Nurses Act 2011 (Government of Ireland 2011) provided for a distinct division of registered advanced nurse practitioners and registered advanced midwife practitioners. In 2018, five nursing and midwifery Rules were enacted (three of them subsequently revised in 2020), creating the legislative framework that allows the NMBI to fulfill its statutory obligations (Government of Ireland 2018; NMBI 2017, 2020).

Advanced practice nursing is defined "as a career pathway for registered nurses, committed to continuing professional development and clinical supervision, to practice at a higher level of capability as independent, autonomous, and expert practitioners" (Irish Association of Advanced Nurse Midwife Practitioners [IAAPNMP] n.d.; NMBI 2017). The first advanced nurse practitioners registered in 2002, and by June 2024, 968 had registered, with a 20% increase from 2023 (IAANMP n.d.; NMBI 2024). The title is protected, and those using the title of registered advanced nurse practitioner have met the nursing and midwifery boards' criteria for registration to enter the advanced practice division of the register (NMBI 2017). Streams of practice include acute, chronic, emergency, midwifery, and primary care settings. The NMBI has established processes and criteria for assessment and approval of programs of education leading to registration (NMBI 2017). A master's degree in nursing or relevant field, related clinical practicum, and registration in the NMBI Prescribers Division are required for registration as an advanced nurse practitioner (NMBI n.d.-a, n.d.-b, n.d.-c). In 2019, the Department of Health published "A Policy on the Development of Graduate to Advanced Nursing and Midwifery Practice," which puts forth a strategic vision for the development of advanced practice services in the country (Department of Health 2019). The aim of the policy is to maximize the nursing and midwifery response to the current and emerging health service challenges and to create a critical mass of advanced practice nurses to address population health needs. A year later, the Office of the Nursing & Midwifery Services Director published the "National Guideline for the Development of Advanced Nursing or Midwifery Practitioner Services" (Office of the Nursing and Midwifery Services Director 2020a, b). It outlines the implementation plan, education plan, and the key people and their roles and responsibilities related to role implementation across health services, from Chief Director of Nursing and Midwifery (hospitals group) to professional and clinical supervisors. In addition, the guideline also explains the plan for monitoring uptake of the guideline and evaluation of its implementation (Office of the Nursing and Midwifery Services Director 2020a, b). The Irish Association of Advanced Nurse/Midwife Practitioners was organized in 2004 to provide support to ANPs and AMPs, promote advanced practice in Ireland, facilitate education and promotion of professional development among advanced practitioners, and network with colleagues beyond Ireland (IAANMP n.d.).

3.4 Australia

Australia has a universal, publicly funded healthcare system, "Medicare," providing free- or low-cost access to medical services, public hospitals, and medicines (Australian Government Department of Health, Disability and Ageing 2025). The shortage of physicians, especially in rural and remote areas, has been the driver for the implementation and development of advanced practice nursing (nurse practitioner role) in the country (Scanlon and Ikobe 2021). After pilot projects with nurse practitioners identified the benefits of NP care, the first NP was accredited to practice in 2000, while it was not until 2005 that the first NP competency standards were endorsed (Scanlon and Ikobe 2021).

The Nursing and Midwifery Board of Australia (NMBA) regulates the practice of nurses and midwives as stipulated by "The Health Practitioner Regulation National Law" (Queensland Government 2009). The NMBA is authorized under this law to endorse the registration of registered nurses as nurse practitioners, recognizing that they have additional qualifications approved by the NMBA, giving the NPs an extended scope of practice (Leslie et al. 2023). To qualify for such endorsement, a registered nurse (RN) must have a current RN license; have at least 3 years or 5000 h of full-time, advanced clinical practice in the past 6 years; complete an NMBA-accredited program or its equivalent, leading to endorsement; and conform to Nurse Practitioner Standards of Practice (NMBA 2025). The Board registers and maintains a registry of nursing and midwifery practitioners; develops standards, codes of conduct, and guidelines for the profession; and publishes statistical reports quarterly of its registrants, with 2900 NPs endorsed/registered in March 2024 (NMBA 2024). NPs are independent practitioners with graduate-level education who enjoy title protection and have the experience, expertise, and authorization to diagnose and manage a variety of acute and chronic conditions across all ages in a variety of settings (Australian College of Nurse Practitioners [ACNP] 2025). They can also prescribe medication, refer clients to hospital or to specialists, and order diagnostic tests (ACNP 2025).

3.5 Singapore

Singapore is a city-state with a publicly funded healthcare system alongside a significant private health sector. The Ministry of Health and its statutory boards are responsible for regulating the healthcare system, with the Singapore Nursing Board (SNB 2025a) in charge of nursing regulation, its scope and functions articulated in the Nurses and Midwives Act 1999. The Board is responsible for the registration and enrolment of nurses, registration of midwives, and certification of advanced practice nurses (SNB 2025b). The current APN workforce consists of 376 certified APNs (Hirshmann 2025).

The APN practice model is a hybrid of 80% nurse practitioner role with direct patient care and care consultation and 20% clinical nurse specialist role focusing on teaching/education, research, and leadership activities (Hirshmann 2025). There are four streams of specialization: acute care (critical care/emergency), medical/surgical (general, adult, pediatrics), community APN (polyclinics, community care), and mental health (inpatient and outpatient psychiatric setting) (Zhou 2024). In order to pursue entry to the APN program, the RN must have an undergraduate nursing degree, 5 years of work experience, and an advanced diploma/specialty training in a certain specialty. SNB has accredited the Master of Nursing program for APN and endorsed the APN education framework. The framework consists of (1) academic study (two semesters), (2) work-based learning (one semester), and (3) integrated APN internship (12 months). Once the nurse has completed the master's degree and internship requirements with related assignments, examinations, and evaluation, she/he qualifies to apply for certification as APN by the SNB (Zhou 2024). Once certified, the nurse is able to use the legally protected title of advanced practice nurse (APN) (Zhou 2024).

4 Tools and Resources

A few tools and resources are available to those interested in or with responsibilities for assessment, design, or redesign of APN regulation. This section introduces four such tools/resources: a leadership framework outlining capabilities necessary for systems transformation and suggested questions for consideration when initiating such change; a template for SWOT (*S*trengths, *W*eaknesses, *O*pportunities, *T*hreats) analysis; assessment of APN regulation questionnaire; and an APN Nursing Self Appraisal Tool.

4.1 The LEADS Leadership Capabilities Framework

Leadership is one of the four domains of APN practice. APNs are leaders within the organization and communities where they work and serve and can lead within their extended spheres of influence. A leadership framework can be a useful tool in leading any initiative or systems transformation toward APN regulation. The LEADS leadership framework represents the collective wisdom of current literature and the capabilities required by leaders dedicated to making meaningful organizational change (Dickson et al. 2007; Vilches et al. 2016). The framework describes the skills, abilities, knowledge, and behaviors required for successful leadership (Dickson et al. 2007; Vilches et al. 2016). The five leadership domains with two related capabilities for each domain are listed in the first two columns of Table 4, while the far-right column highlights key questions to consider prior to embarking on any new project/initiative.

4.2 SWOT Analysis

The SWOT (Strengths, Weaknesses, Opportunities, Threats) analysis provides a structured framework for organizing and analyzing data. In assessing the current state of APN regulation, a SWOT analysis can help identify internal and external factors that may either benefit or hinder a regulatory system design/re-design, allowing the interested parties (stakeholders) and partners to develop strategies that capitalize on the identified strengths and opportunities while addressing the weaknesses and mitigating the threats (Ladd et al. 2020; Teoli et al. 2023). Figure 3 is a template for a SWOT analysis table, highlighting some considerations specific to internal and external factors.

4.3 A Questionnaire to Assess Current State of Advanced Practice Nursing Regulation

Schober (2016) and the International Confederation of Midwives (Pairman and Tumilty 2016, pp. 1–7) have proposed a series of questions to be asked when discussing, assessing, or developing a professional regulatory structure. A selection of these questions has been adapted for APN contexts in Table 5.

Table 4 LEADS in a caring environment leadership capabilities framework

Leadership domain	Leadership capabilities	Questions to ask
Lead self	Is aware of own assumptions, values, principles, strengths, and limitations Takes responsibility for own performance and health Actively seeks opportunities and challenges for personal learning, character building, and growth Models qualities such as honesty, integrity, resilience, and confidence	What is my vision for this project/initiative? What assumptions am I making about what is required? What is my current level of capacity?
Engage others	Supports and challenges others to achieve professional and personal goals Creates engaging environments where others have meaningful opportunities to contribute and ensure that resources are available to fulfil their expected responsibilities Listens well and encourages open exchange of information and ideas using appropriate communication media Facilitates environments of collaboration and cooperation to achieve results	Who does the proposed change impact immediately? What type of team do we need to lead the initiative? How do we support the team to achieve the results we seek?
Achieve results	Inspires vision by identifying, establishing, and communicating clear and meaningful expectations and outcomes Integrates organizational missions and values with reliable, valid evidence to make decisions Acts in a manner consistent with organizational values to yield effective, customer-centric service Measures and evaluates outcomes, compares the results against established benchmarks, and corrects the course as appropriate	Why are we undertaking this initiative? What is currently happening? What evidence do we need? What are the desired results?
Develop coalitions	Creates connections, trust, and shared meaning with individuals and groups Facilitates collaboration, cooperation, and coalitions among diverse groups and perspectives aimed at learning to improve service Employs methods to gather intelligence, encourage open exchange of information, and use quality evidence to influence action across the system Is politically astute and can negotiate through conflict and mobilize support	Who are the key partners who share our goals? Who has a stake in the outcome of this initiative, and how significant? How will we begin to develop the relationships needed to support this initiative?

(continued)

Table 4 (continued)

Leadership domain	Leadership capabilities	Questions to ask
Systems transformation	Thinks analytically and conceptually, questioning and challenging the status quo, to identify issues, solve problems, and design and implement effective processes across systems and interested parties (stakeholders) Creates a climate of continuous improvement and creativity aimed at systemic change Scans the environment for ideas, best practices, and emerging trends that will shape the system Actively contributes to change processes that improve performance and service delivery	What change challenges/ opportunities do we anticipate in undertaking this initiative? What innovative ideas/ practices can we build on? What are the known enablers and barriers?

Adapted with permission from Dickson et al. (2007)
© Copyright 2010 All Rights Reserved-LEADS in a Caring Environment content is subject to intellectual property protection worldwide and is used under license and certification arrangements by the Canadian College of Health Leaders

SWOT- Strengths, Weaknesses, Opportunities, Threats Table

	Advantages	Disadvantages
Internal factors: • Institutional • Organizational • Regulatory	**Strengths:**	**Weaknesses:**
External factors: • Political/policy environment • Sociodemographic context • Health system environment	**Opportunities:**	**Threats:**

Fig. 3 SWOT analysis table

4.4 Advanced Practice Nursing Role Delineation and Self-Appraisal Tool

APN role delineation tools are used to differentiate nursing from advanced practice nursing roles and have been adapted to various country-specific contexts, based on the Strong Model of Advanced Practice (Jokiniemi et al. 2022). A national survey based on the Australian version of the APN role delineation tool was used to develop the Australian Advanced Practice Nursing Self-Appraisal Tool, The ADVANCE Tool (Gardner et al. 2017). This tool includes five domains of advanced nursing practice: clinician care, optimizing health systems, research, leadership, and education. Each domain has a list of APN activities a nurse is to consider and rate the extent of time she/he spends on that activity in the current role, using a Likert Scale

Table 5 Questionnaire for the assessment of APN regulatory system

Questions to explore:
Why is regulation created?
What is regulated (e.g., APNs, educational programs)?
What APN roles exist in your country (e.g., nurse practitioner, clinical nurse specialist, nurse anesthetist)?
What APN roles are regulated in your country?
Who is the regulatory authority that licenses, registers, certifies, approves or accredits APNs, their education programs or related institutions?
Is it a government-approved/sanctioned authority?
Does the same regulatory body regulate other health professions?
What is the composition of the regulatory body (APNs, nurses, physicians, government officials, public representatives, others)?
What is the name of the head of this regulatory body/authority?
What is the education level of the head of the regulatory body/authority?
What is the required APN entry level to practice education/qualification?
Is there a recognized definition of APN in your country?
Does the definition align with the ICN APN definition (7)?
Is there a national health strategy for primary healthcare in the country?
Do nurses in your country hold a protected title (e.g., registered nurse RN)?
Do APNs have protected titles (e.g., NP, CSN, NA)?
Is title protection based on APN-specific legislation/regulation?
Does the nursing/APN regulatory authority/body approve APN education programs?
Does the regulatory authority/body require ongoing professional development activities for APN license renewal?
Is there a mechanism for APN education programs to be accredited?
Do APN regulations include a scope of practice?
Does your country have established entry-level competencies for APN?
Do APNs have autonomous prescriptive authority?
Do regulations include a code of ethics?
Does your country have established standards of practice for APNs?

Adapted from Schober (2016) and Pairman and Tumilty (2016)

(4 very great extent–0 not at all). She/he then calculates the average score for each domain (the higher the score, the more APN activities the nurse is including in current practice role). Research has shown that the minimum mean domain scores to indicate advanced practice is a score of two for clinical practice, optimizing health systems, and education domains, while a score of 1.7 reflects advanced practice for the domains of research and leadership. After this activity, the nurse is to provide rationale and evidence for each domain score by way of description of activities, projects, or portfolios she/he may have been involved with, justifying the average score per domain (Gardner et al. 2017).

5 Summary

This chapter provides an introduction to nursing regulation, common regulatory models, and key components of APN regulatory structures. Case exemplars of APN regulatory models from five countries with established APN roles illuminate the variability that exists in the regulatory frameworks governing APN role regulations across countries/jurisdictions, with the recognition that even greater variability in APN regulations may exist in countries where APN roles are still in development or emerging. This variability can result in lack of standardized education and training, leading to inconsistent qualifications and competencies; variability in scope of practice can further contribute to lack of role clarity and title protection, potentially placing patients at risk of poor outcomes. The tools and resources highlighted in this chapter may prove beneficial for those interested in or tasked with the assessment of existing regulatory models or with the design or redesign of such in their respective jurisdictions.

References

Almukhaini S, Weeks LE, Macdonald M, Martin-Misener R, Ismaili ZA, Macdonald D, Al-Fahdi N, Rasbi SA, Nasaif H, Rothfus MA. Advanced practice nursing roles in Arab countries in the Eastern Mediterranean region: a scoping review. JBI Evid Synth. 2022;20(5):1209–42. https://doi.org/10.11124/JBIES-21-00101.

American Association of Nurse Anesthesiology (AANA). Certified nurse anesthetist fact sheet. 2023. https://www.aana.com/membership/become-a-crna/crna-fact-sheet. Accessed 1 Aug 2025.

American Association of Nurse Practitioners (AANP). A behind-the-scenes look at the 2025 nurse practitioner count. 2025a. https://www.aanp.org/news-feed/a-behind-the-scenes-look-at-the-2025-nurse-practitioner-count. Accessed 6 Jan 2026.

American Association of Nurse Practitioners (AANP). State practice environment. 2025b. https://www.aanp.org/advocacy/state/state-practice-environment. Accessed 1 Aug 2025.

APRN Consensus Work Group & the National Council of State Boards of Nursing APRN Advisory Committee. The Consensus model for APRN Regulation: licensure, accreditation, certification & education. 2008. https://www.aacnnursing.org/Portals/0/PDFs/Teaching-Resources/APRNReport.pdf. Accessed 1 Aug 2025.

Australian College of Nurse Practitioners (ACNP). Learn more about nurse practitioners. Author; 2025. https://www.acnp.org.au/aboutnursepractitioners. Accessed 1 Aug 2025.

Australian Government Department of Health, Disability and Ageing. The Australian health system. 2025. https://www.health.gov.au/about-us/the-australian-health-system. Accessed 1 Aug 2025.

Benton DC, González-Jurado MA, Beneit-Montesinos JV. A typology of professional nurse regulatory models and their administration. J Nurs Regul. 2013;4(2):22–9. https://doi.org/10.1016/S2155-8256(15)30153-8.

Benton DC, Cleghorn J, Coghlan A, Damgaard G, Doumit MAA, George JL, González-Jurado MA, Kwek P-E, Johansen C, Msibi GS, Nyante F, Owyer E, Reed CM, Rodriguez A, Vogt T. Acting in the public interest: learnings and commentary on the occupational licensure. J Nurs Regul. 2019;10(4):S1–S40. https://doi.org/10.1016/S2155-8256(19)30120-6.

Braithwaite J, Healy J, Dwan K. The governance of health safety and quality: a discussion paper. Australian Council for Safety and Quality in Health Care; 2007. https://johnbraithwaite.com/wp-content/uploads/2016/03/Governance_Health_2005.pdf. Accessed 1 Aug 2025.

British Columbia College of Nursing Professionals (BCCNP). Scope of practice for nurse practitioners. 2020. p. 8. https://cnps.ca/wp-content/uploads/2020/03/NP_ScopeofPractice-1.pdf. Accessed 1 August 2025.

Canadian Institute for Health Information (CIHI). Nurse practitioner scopes of practice in Canada, 2020—data table. 2020. https://www.cihi.ca/en/nurse-practitioner-scopes-of-practice-in-canada-2020. Accessed 1 Aug 2025.

Canadian Nurses Association. Canadian Nurse Practitioner Initiative-Implementation and Evaluation toolkit for nurse practitioners in Canada. 2006a. https://albertanps.com/wp-content/uploads/2015/09/toolkit_implementation_evaluation_np_e.pdf. Accessed 1 Aug 2025.

Canadian Nurses Association. Canadian nurse practitioner initiative technical report: legislative and regulatory framework. 2006b. https://1library.net/document/q07rm8xz-practitioner-initiative-technical-legislative-regulatory-framework-technical-practitioners.html#google_vignette. Accessed 1 Aug 2025.

Canadian Nurses Association (CNA). The Canadian nurse practitioner initiative: a 10-year retrospective. 2016. https://ia903103.us.archive.org/30/items/5762376-Canadian-Nurse-Practitioner-Initiative-a-10Year/5762376-Canadian-Nurse-Practitioner-Initiative-a-10-Year.pdf. Accessed 1 Aug 2025.

Canadian Nurses Association (CNA). Advanced practice nursing: a Pan-Canadian framework. 2019. https://hl-prod-ca-oc-download.s3-ca-central-1.amazonaws.com/CNA/2f975e7e-4a40-45ca-863c-5ebf0a138d5e/UploadedImages/documents/nursing/Advanced_Practice_Nursing_framework_e.pdf. Accessed 1 Aug 2025.

Citizens Information (Ireland). Entitlement to health services. 2022. https://www.citizensinformation.ie/en/health/health-system/entitlement-to-public-health-services/. Accessed 1 Aug 2025.

College of Registered Nurses of Manitoba (CRNM). Right touch regulation. 2022. https://www.crnm.mb.ca/wp-content/uploads/2023/09/Right-Touch-Regulation-Guidelines-Nov-2022.pdf. Accessed 1 Aug 2025.

De Raeve P, Davidson PM, Bergs J, Patch M, Jack SM, Castro-Ayala A, Xyrichis A, Preston W. Advanced practice nursing in Europe-results from a pan-European survey of 35 countries. J Adv Nurs. 2023;80(1):377–86. https://doi.org/10.1111/jan.15775.

Department of Health. A policy on the development of graduate to advanced nursing and midwifery practice. 2019. https://www.gov.ie/en/publication/96ce55-a-policy-on-the-development-of-graduate-to-advanced-nursing-and-midw/. Accessed 29 Sept 2025.

Dickson G, Briscoe D, Fenwick S, MacLeod Z, Romilly L. LEADS in a caring environment: health leadership capabilities framework. Canadian College of Health Leaders; 2007. https://pld.cchl-ccls.ca/site/about/about-us/framework?nav=sidebar. Accessed 1 Aug 2025.

Elvidge N, Hobbs M, Fox A, Currie J, Williams S, Theobald K, Rolfe M, Marshall C, Phillips JL. Practice pathways, education, and regulation influencing nurse practitioners' decision to provide primary care: a rapid scoping review. BMC Prim Care. 2024;25(1):182. https://doi.org/10.1186/s12875-024-02350-3.

Gardner G, Duffield C, Gardner A, Batch M. The Australian advanced practice nursing self-appraisal tool. (The ADVANCE tool). Figshare; 2017. Journal contribution. https://doi.org/10.6084/m9.figshare.4669432.v2.

Government of Ireland. Nurses and midwives act 2011. Irish Statute Book. 2011. https://www.irishstatutebook.ie/eli/2011/act/41/enacted/en/html. Accessed 1 Aug 2025.

Government of Ireland. Nurses and midwives (registration) rules. Irish Statute Book; 2018. https://www.irishstatutebook.ie/eli/2018/si/221/made/en/pdf. Accessed 20 Sept 2025.

Hirshmann R. Number of advanced practice nurses in Singapore in 2023- by certification. Statista. 2025. https://www.statista.com/statistics/1082482/singapore-number-of-of-advanced-practice-nurses-by-certification/#:~:text=Number%20of%20advanced%20practice%20nurses%20in%20Singapore%202023%2C%20by%20certification&text=By%20the%20end%20of%202023,holding%20advanced%20practice%20nurse%20certifications. Accessed 1 Aug 2025.

International Council of Nurses (ICN). ICN position: nursing regulation. 2013. https://www.icn.ch/sites/default/files/2023-04/B04_Nsg_Regulation.pdf. Accessed 1 Aug 2025.

International Council of Nurses (ICN). Regulatory board governance toolkit. 2014. https://www.icn.ch/sites/default/files/inline-files/2014_Regulatory_Board_Governance_Toolkit.pdf. Accessed 1 Aug 2025.

International Council of Nurses (ICN). Guidelines on advanced practice nursing. 2020. https://www.icn.ch/system/files/documents/2020-04/ICN_APN%20Report_EN_WEB.pdf. Accessed 1 Aug 2025.

International Council of Nurses (ICN). Recover to rebuild: investing in the nursing workforce for health systems effectiveness. 2024. https://www.icn.ch/sites/default/files/2023-07/ICN_Recover-to-Rebuild_report_EN.pdf. Accessed 1 Aug 2025.

Irish Association of Advanced Nurse/Midwife Practitioners. Position statement: advanced nurse practitioners. n.d. https://www.iaanmp.ie/position-statement. Accessed 1 Aug 2025.

Jokiniemi K, Tervo-Heikkinen T, Peltokoski J, Mikkonen S. Construct validity of advanced practice role delineation tool: a confirmatory factor analysis. Int J Nurs Pract. 2022;28(5):e13064. https://doi.org/10.1111/ijn.13064.

Kim S, Lee TW, Kim GS, Cho E, Jang Y, Choi M, Baek S, Lindsay D, Chan S, Lee RLT, Guo A, Wong FKY, Yu D, Chair SY, Shimpuku Y, Mashino S, Lim G, Bonito S, Rumsey M, Neill A, Hazarika I. Nurses in advanced roles as a strategy for equitable access to healthcare in the WHO Western Pacific region: a mixed methods study. Hum Resour Health. 2021;19(1):19. https://doi.org/10.1186/s12960-021-00555-6.

Ladd E, Miller M, Wheeler K, Wainaina S, Aquirre F, McGrath H, Lee S, Nashwan A, Neary A, Core K. A global SWOT analysis of advanced practice nursing: policy, regulation, and practice. Res Sq. 2020; https://doi.org/10.21203/rs.3.rs-113320/v1.

Leslie K, Myles S, Stahlke S, Schiller CJ, Shelley JJ, Cook K, Stephens J, Nelson S. Regulating during crisis: a qualitative comparative case study of nursing regulatory responses to the COVID-19 pandemic. J Nurs Regul. 2023;14(1):30–41. https://doi.org/10.1016/S2155-8256(23)00066-2.

Mahat A, Dhillon IS, Benton DC, Fletcher M, Wafula F. Health practitioner regulation and national health goals. Bull World Health Organ. 2023;101(9):595–604. https://doi.org/10.2471/BLT.21.287728. Epub 2023 Jun 29. PMID: 37638356; PMCID: PMC10452941.

Maier CB, Aiken L, Busse R. Nurses in advanced roles in primary care: policy levers for implementation. OECD Health Working Papers, No. 98. Paris: OECD Publishing; 2017. https://doi.org/10.1787/a8756593-en. Accessed 1 Aug 2025.

Merriam-Webster. Regulation. Author. n.d. https://www.merriam-webster.com/dictionary/regulation#word-history. Accessed 1 Aug 2025.

Miller M, Prodan-Bhalla N, Marchuk S. The NP role and practice in Canada. In: Thomas SL, Rowles JS, editors. Nurse practitioners and nurse anesthetists: the evolution of the global roles. Switzerland: Springer Nature; 2023. p. 145–55.

Miller M, Roussel J, Rogers M, Lehwaldt D. The global phenomenon of advanced practice nurses. In: Rogers M, Lehwaldt D, Roussel J, Acorn M, editors. Advanced practice nurse networking to enhance global health. Switzerland: Springer Nature; 2024. p. 19–42.

Motluk A. Self-regulation in health care professions comes under scrutiny. CMAJ. 2019;191(33):E926–7. https://doi.org/10.1503/cmaj.109-5790.

National Association of Clinical Nurse Specialists (NACNS). National Association of Clinical Nurse Specialists releases census results (Press release). 2021. https://nacns.org/2021/05/national-association-of-clinical-nurse-specialists-releases-census-results/. Accessed 1 Aug 2025.

National Council of State Boards of Nursing (NCSBN). About the APRN Consensus Model. 2025a. https://www.ncsbn.org/nursing-regulation/practice/aprn.page. Accessed 1 Aug 2025.

National Council of state boards of nursing (NCSBN). APRN compact. 2025b. https://www.aprncompact.com/. Accessed 1 Aug 2025.

Nurse Practitioner Association of Canada. Nurse Practitioners in Canada: making a difference in your health [Infographic]. 2025. https://npac-aiipc.org/nps-in-canada/. Accessed 31 Dec 2025.

Nursing and Midwifery Board of Australia (NMBA). Registrant data: June 2024. 2024. https://www.nursingmidwiferyboard.gov.au/Accreditation/Registrant-Data/Nursing-and-Midwifery-Board%2D%2D-Registrant-Data%2D%2D-June-2024. Accessed 1 Aug 2025.

Nursing and Midwifery Board of Australia (NMBA). Guidelines: for nurses applying for endorsement as a nurse practitioner. 2025. https://www.nursingmidwiferyboard.gov.au/Codes-Guidelines-Statements/Codes-Guidelines/Guidelines-on-endorsement-as-a-nurse-practitioner.aspx. Accessed 1 Aug 2025.

Nursing and Midwifery Board of Ireland (NMBI). Advanced practice (nursing) standards and requirements. Nursing and Midwifery Board of Ireland, Dublin; 2017. https://www.nmbi.

ie/NMBI/media/NMBI/Advanced-Practice-Nursing-Standards-and-Requirements-2017.pdf?ext=.pdf. Accessed 1 Aug 2025.
Nursing and Midwifery Board of Ireland (NMBI). What we do-nurses and midwives act 2011, as amended. Nurses and Midwives Rules; 2020. https://www.nmbi.ie/What-We-Do/Legislation. Accessed 1 Oct 2025.
Nursing and Midwifery Board of Ireland (NMBI). State of the Register, 2024. Dublin: Nursing and Midwifery Board of Ireland; 2024. https://www.nmbi.ie/NMBI/media/NMBI/NMBI-State-of-the-Register-2024.pdf?ext=.pdf
Nursing and Midwifery Board of Ireland (NMBI). What we do: the nurses and midwives act 2011. n.d.-a. https://www.nmbi.ie/What-We-Do/Nurses-and-Midwives-Act-2011. Accessed 1 Aug 2025.
Nursing and Midwifery Board of Ireland (NMBI). Registering as ANP/AMP. n.d.-b. https://www.nmbi.ie/Registration/Add-New-Division/Advanced-Practitioners/Registering-as-ANP-AMP. Accessed 19 Mar 2026.
Nursing and Midwifery Board of Ireland (NMBI). What we do-NMBI's role and key functions. Author; n.d.-c. https://www.nmbi.ie/What-We-Do/Our-Role. Accessed 1 Oct 2025.
Office of the Nursing & Midwifery Services Director. National guidelines for the development of advanced nursing and midwifery practitioner services. 2020a. https://healthservice.hse.ie/filelibrary/onmsd/national-guideline-for-development-of-advanced-nursing-or-midwifery-practitioner-services-2020.pdf. Accessed 1 Oct 2025.
Office of the Nursing & Midwifery Services Director. National guideline for the development of advanced nursing or midwifery practitioner services. 2020b. https://assets.hse.ie/media/documents/ncr/national-guideline-for-development-of-advanced-nursing-or-midwifery-practi_qg4CdWV.pdf. Accessed 1 Aug 2025.
Pairman S, Tumilty E. International Confederation of Midwives regulation toolkit. International Confederation of Midwives; 2016. https://internationalmidwives.org/resources/regulation-toolkit/. Accessed 1 Aug 2025.
Professional Standards Authority. Right touch regulation, revised. 2015. https://www.professionalstandards.org.uk/docs/default-source/publications/right-touch-regulation-2015.pdf. Accessed 1 Aug 2025.
Professional Standards Authority. Right touch regulation in practice: international perspective. 2018. https://www.professionalstandards.org.uk/docs/default-source/publications/thought-paper/right-touch-regulation-in-practice%2D%2D-international-perspectives.pdf?sfvrsn=a5b97520_8. Accessed 1 Aug 2025.
Queensland Government. Health practitioner regulation national law act 2009 (QLD). (2009). https://www.legislation.qld.gov.au/view/html/inforce/current/act-2009-045. Accessed 1 Aug 2025.
Scanlon A, Ikobe R. Global APN case study in spirituality-stories of hope from Australia. In: Rogers M, editor. Spiritual dimensions of advanced practice nursing. Switzerland: Springer Nature; 2021. p. 209–21.
Scanlon A, Bryant-Lukosius D, Lehwaldt D, Wilkinson J, Honig J. International transferability of nurse practitioner credentials in five countries. J Nurse Pract. 2019;15(7):487–93.
Schober M. Professional regulation. In: Schober M, editor. Introduction to advanced nursing practice. Switzerland: Springer Nature; 2016. p. 111–25. https://doi.org/10.1007/978-3-319-32204-9_6.
Singapore Nursing Board (SNB). Who we are. 2025a. https://www.snb.gov.sg/who-we-are. Accessed 1 Aug 2025.
Singapore Nursing Board (SNB). Registers of nurses and midwives/roll of nurses. 2025b. https://www.snb.gov.sg/for-professionals/for-nurses-and-midwives/registers-of-nurses-midwives-roll-of-nurses/. Accessed 1 Aug 2025.
Teoli D, Sanvictores T, An J. SWOT analysis. In: StatPearls. Treasure Island: StatPearls Publishing; 2023. https://www.ncbi.nlm.nih.gov/books/NBK537302/. Accessed 1 Aug 2025.
U.S. Bureau of Labor Statistics. Occupational employment and wage statistics, May 2021-Nurse midwives. 2021. https://www.bls.gov/oes/current/oes291161.htm. Accessed 1 Aug 2025.
Vilches S, Fenwick S, Harris B, Lammi B, Racette R. Changing health organizations with the LEADS leadership framework: report of the 2014-2016 LEADS impact study. Fenwick

Leadership Explorations, the Canadian College of Health Leaders, & the Centre for Health Leadership and Research, Royal Roads University. 2016. https://cchl-ccls.ca/app/uploads/2022/11/LEADS_Impact_Report_2017_FINAL.pdf. Accessed 1 Aug 2025.

Wheeler KJ, Miller M, Pulcini J, Gray D, Ladd E, Rayens MK. Advanced practice nursing roles, regulation, education, and practice: a global study. Ann Glob Health. 2022;88(1):42. https://doi.org/10.5334/aogh.3698.

Wheeler KJ, Miller M, Clark M, Tallum E, Mukuna A, Wainaina S. Health policy and regulation. In: Rogers M, Lehwaldt D, Roussel J, Acorn M, editors. Advanced practice nurse networking to enhance global health, vol. 2024. Switzerland: Springer Nature; 2024. p. 163–88. https://doi.org/10.1007/978-3-031-39740-0_9.

World Health Organization (WHO). State of the world's nursing 2020: investing in education, jobs and leadership. 2020. https://iris.who.int/bitstream/handle/10665/331677/9789240003279-eng.pdf.

World Health Organization (WHO). State of the world's nursing 2025: investing in education, jobs, leadership and service delivery. 2025. https://iris.who.int/server/api/core/bitstreams/a4173924-a18f-49b6-8bd1-9c2a4a098980/content

Xue Y, Kannan V, Greener E, Smith JA, Brasch J, Johnson BA, Spetz J. Full scope-of-practice regulation is associated with higher supply of nurse practitioners in rural and primary care health professional shortage counties. J Nurs Regul. 2018;8(4):5–13. https://doi.org/10.1016/S2155-8256(17)30176-X.

Zhou W. Advancing excellence: the evolution of advanced practice nurse certification in Singapore. Presented at: International Council of Nurses 13th NP/APN network conference, Aberdeen, Scotland; 2024.

Ziegler E, Martin-Misener R, Rietkoetter S, Baumann A, Bougeault IL, Kovacevic N, Miller M, Moseley J, Wong FKY, Bryant-Lukosius D. Response and innovations of advanced practice nurses during the COVID-19 pandemic: a scoping review. Int Nurs Rev. 2024;71(2):250–75. https://doi.org/10.1111/inr.12884.

International Advanced Practice Nursing Roles and Credentialing Methods

Lorna Schumann, Diane Tyler, Jill Wilkinson, Sue Adams, and Nanako Tsukui

1 Introduction and Purpose

It is universally understood that nursing and nurses serve to meet the healthcare needs of the public by improving health conditions of individuals and their communities through greater access to quality care. Accordingly, nursing has evolved and advanced over many decades, resulting in expanded education and practice globally. Credentialing and regulatory models have also evolved conforming to national, regional, and/or institutional healthcare system norms. This chapter expands previous comparisons (ICN 2017) of the four advanced practice nursing roles of nurse anesthetist, nurse midwife, clinical nurse specialist, and nurse practitioner. A table format is used to view condensed information in keeping with the toolkit purpose (Table 1). Countries selected for comparison

L. Schumann (✉)
Washington State University College of Nursing, Spokane, WA, United States

Women and Children's Shelter, Union Gospel Mission, Spokane, United States
e-mail: schumannlorna@gmail.com

D. Tyler
American Academy of Nurse Practitioners Certification Board, The University of Texas at Austin, Austin, TX, United States
e-mail: dtyler@utexas.edu

J. Wilkinson
School of Health, Victoria University of Wellington, Wellington, New Zealand
e-mail: Jill.Wilkinson@vuw.ac.nz

S. Adams
School of Nursing, University of Auckland, Auckland, New Zealand
e-mail: S.Adams@auckland.ac.nz

N. Tsukui
Japan Association for Development of Community Medicine (JADECOM), Chiyoda, Tokyo, Japan
e-mail: Taganana77@gmail.com

K. J. Wheeler, M. Acorn (eds.), *Health Policy for Advanced Practice Nursing: A Toolkit for Implementation and Improvement*, Advanced Practice in Nursing,
https://doi.org/10.1007/978-3-032-03667-4_12

Table 1 Representative sample of advanced practice nursing (APN) roles, titles, and credentialing method (CM) by country

Australia			
Nurse midwife	*Nurse specialist*	*Nurse anesthetist*	*Nurse practitioner*
APN role not present	APN role not present	APN role not present	APN role present
Credentialing method Endorsement by Nursing and Midwifery Board of Australia (NMBA) *Education* Midwife: 3-year Bachelor of Midwifery degree Midwife Practitioner: Alternate pathway for nurses is post-graduate midwifery courses *Titles* (protected) Midwife Midwife practitioner *Role* Midwifery and Nursing are separate professions	*Credentialing method* Endorsement by NMBA *Education* Bachelor of Nursing (master's degree not required) *Title* (not protected) Special RN *Role* Not equivalent to clinical Nurse Specialist	*Credentialing method* Endorsement by NMBA *Education* Varies *Title* (not protected) Specialty Nurse *Role* Assists surgeons, dentists, doctors Not advanced practice level NA role does not exist in Australia	*Credentialing method* Endorsement by NMBA *Education* Master of NP *Title* (protected) Nurse Practitioner *Role* Advanced level, direct clinical practice compliant with NP Standards
References: NMBA (2020, 2025), Open Universities Australia (2026), and Wheeler et al. (2022)			
Canada 2022–2023 Highlights Canadian Council of Registered Nurse Regulators (CCRNR) https://static1.squarespace.com/static/671142bd58709c1e559e8c2a/t/672fd815cef3c73690d5f3ed/1731188760830/ccrnr-highlights-english-2022-2023.pdf			
Nurse midwife	*Nurse specialist*	*Nurse anesthetist*	*Nurse practitioner*
APN role not present	APN role present	APN role not present	APN role present

Credentialing method Midwifery regulated by province/territory Mobility agreement established 2001 *Education* Midwifery bachelor's program *Title* Midwife No nursing title *Role* Midwifery not APN role No national standards	*Credentialing method* Not regulated *Education* Graduate nursing degree *Title* Clinical Nurse Specialist *Role* APN with specialty expertise No defined national competencies, entry-level certification or license for practice	*Credentialing method* Not available *Education* Master's degree NP program for nurse anesthetists *Title* Practitioner-Anesthesia *Role* Exploratory role without certification or licensure	*Credentialing method* Provincial regulation and licensure Certification by exam *Education* Master's degree, graduate-level NP program *Title* Nurse Practitioner *Role* Autonomously diagnose, manage care across lifespan, settings National NP entry-level competencies New NP regulatory model approved that aligns graduate education, NP competencies, with a single national entry-level exam for NPs across Canada
References: CMRC (n.d.), CNA (2026), CAS (2022), CCRNR (2023a, b), and BCCN&M (2026)			
Finland			
Nurse midwife	*Nurse specialist*	*Nurse anesthetist*	*Nurse practitioner*
APN role not present	APN role present	APN role not present	APN role present
Credentialing method Nationally licensed and registered as a nurse and midwife *Education* Midwifery bachelor's degree provides both nurse and midwife preparation *Title* Midwife *Role* Not advanced level	*Credentialing method* Not regulated *Education* Master's or doctoral degree *Title* (not protected) Clinical nurse specialist *Role* Healthcare organizations control job titles and descriptions	*Credentialing method* Not available *Education* Special education in anesthesia or perioperative nursing Graduate education is not required *Title* (unofficial) Nurse anesthetist *Role* Not at advanced nursing level	*Credentialing method* Not regulated *Education* Master's or doctoral degree *Title* (not protected) Nurse practitioner *Role* May have limited right to prescribe medication which is regulated. Limited prescription rights require separate 45 hours of additional education
References Jokiniemi et al. (2021) and FNA (2020)			
Hong Kong			
Nurse midwife	*Nurse specialist*	*Nurse anesthetist*	*Nurse practitioner*
		APN role not present	

(continued)

Table 1 (continued)

Credentialing method Endorsement by Nursing Council of Hong Kong (NCHK). Midwives Council of Hong Kong recognizes advanced nursing practice in Midwifery *Education* Experience Employed as RN in Hong Kong. The role is one of a nurse consultant if it meets specific criteria. Refer to the website for details. www.nchk.org.hk/filemanager/en/pdf/Perioperative_and_Anaesthesia_Nursing_eng.pdf *Title* Advanced Practice Nurse (APN) *Role*	*Credentialing method* 16 specialties endorsed by NCHK: Cardiac, Gerontology, Medical, Medical and Medical Surgical Orthopedics, Management, Community, Primary and Public Health, Mental Health, Emergency Care—two levels, Peri-operative and Anesthesia, Surgical, Gynecology *Education* Experience (Same for any APN) Not all specialties at master's level *Title* APN CNS (former title) *Role* Similar to the role of the Clinical Nurse Specialist in the United States	*Credentialing method* Not available *Title* *Role* NA not available APN Nurse Consultant manages preoperative and perioperative care but does not administer anesthesia	*Credentialing method* Endorsed by NCHK as a specialty *Education* Experience (Same for any APN) *Title* APN Nurse Consultant *Role* APN and Nurse Consultant are highest level of nursing practice
References: NCHC (2010a, b, 2021, 2024) and Jokiniemi et al. (2022)			
Netherlands Dutch Professional Nurse Practitioner Organization. About the nurse practitioner. https://venvnvs.nl/information-in-english/ Professional Competency Framework. Nurse Practitioner. https://storage.googleapis.com/capstone01/venvnvs/2019/06/2019-06-25-Nurse-Practitioner-Professional-Competency-Framework.pdf			

Nurse midwife	*Nurse specialist*	*Nurse anesthetist*	*Nurse practitioner*
APN role not present	APN role (combined with NP)	APN role not present	APN role present
Credentialing method Registration with Royal Dutch Organization of Midwives *Education* Midwives are not nurses 4-year bachelor's midwifery degree *Title* Midwife *Role* Midwives practice independently	*Credentialing method* (See NP) *Education* (See NP) *Title* (See NP) *Role* APN and CNS competencies combined into NP/Certified Nurse Specialist role There are also specialized RNs that are not APNs	*Credentialing method* College Ziekenhuis Opleidingen must recognize NA educational program *Education* In-service diploma in anesthesia required, a nursing preparatory course or degree is not required Training is provided by the College of Hospital Education (CZO) *Title* (not protected) Nurse Anesthetist (nursing degree is not required, but may be obtained) *Role* Provide general or local anesthesia and patient care before, during, after surgical procedures	*Credentialing method* Registration with Commission for Nurse Specialist (formerly Council for Nurse Practitioners) 2 specialties: general/somatic and mental care NPs must register in a national quality registry and renew every five years. *Education* Accredited master's advanced practice nursing program *Title* (protected) Certified Nurse Specialist Nurse Practitioner (formerly) *Role* Independent practice Perform medical exams, diagnose, initiate treatment, refer Limited prescriptive authority
References: VSR (2017), KNOV (2017), AVAG (2014), Council of the European Union (2017), and IFNA (n.d.)			
New Zealand Ministry of Health. The credentialing framework for New Zealand Health Professionals (2010) https://www.health.govt.nz/publications/credentialling-framework-for-new-zealand-health-professionals			
Nurse midwife	*Nurse specialist*	*Nurse anesthetist*	*Nurse practitioner*
APN role not present	APN role present	APN role not present	APN role present

(continued)

Table 1 (continued)

Credentialing method Registration with Midwifery Council of New Zealand *Education* Bachelors of Midwifery *Title* Midwife *Role* Nurse midwifery is not available	*Credentialing method* Not available *Education* Variable, graduate nursing degree not required *Title* (not protected) Clinical Nurse Specialist *Role* Experienced RN with advanced knowledge and specialized clinical expertise	*Credentialing method* Not available *Education* No role available *Title* No role available *Role* No role available	*Credentialing method* Registration with Nursing Council of New Zealand after 4 years of specialty practice and panel review of meeting NP competencies Competency reviewed every three years Annual practicing certificate renewal *Education* Master's degree (or equivalent) *Title* Nurse Practitioner *Role* Independently and collaboratively manage common and complex conditions Prescriptive authority
References: Nurse Practitioners New Zealand (2025), CNSSNZ (2026), and NZCM (n.d.)			
Republic of Ireland Nursing and Midwifery Board of Ireland. Guide information for nurses/midwives applying for NMBI verification of Category 2 or equivalent post-registration qualifications. https://www.nmbi.ie/Education/Verification-of-Postgraduate-Education			
Nurse midwife	*Nurse specialist*	*Nurse anesthetist*	*Nurse practitioner*
APN role not present	APN role present	APN role not present	APN role present
Credentialing method Registry with Nursing and Midwifery Board of Ireland (NMBI) *Education* Bachelors in midwifery, post-graduate certificate or diploma, higher diploma, and master's degree are recognized *Title* Registered Advanced Midwife Practitioner *Role* Provide care for childbearing women, newborns, infants	*Credentialing method* No registry for CNS *Education* master's degree, prepared beyond generalist and specialist nurse *Title* Advanced Nurse Practitioner *Role* RN with advanced expertise in area of practice, includes prescribing medicines and ionizing radiation	*Credentialing method* No registry for NAs NMBI licenses nurses with specialty experience *Education* Nursing degree Graduate degree not required *Title* Nurse Anesthetist *Role* Practice in Recovery, Surgery	*Credentialing method* Registry with NMBI RN for 7 years with 2 years in specialty *Education* Master's Degree *Title* (protected) Registered Advanced Nurse Practitioner *Role* Functions within a collaborative agreement to be accountable and responsible for advanced decision-making in the management of patient care. Prescribing within the scope of the collaborative practice agreement
References: NMBI (2025, 2026a, b, c)			

Singapore Singapore Nursing Board. Nurses and midwives. https://www.snb.gov.sg/publications-and-newsroom/announcements/code-for-nurses-and-midwives/ Ministry of Health Singapore. Guidelines for all healthcare professionals. https://www.moh.gov.sg/ Ministry of Health Singapore. Licensing and regulation. https://www.moh.gov.sg/ Singapore Nursing Board. Advanced Practice Nurse. https://www.healthprofessionals.gov.sg/			
Nurse midwife	*Nurse specialist*	*Nurse anesthetist*	*Nurse practitioner*
APN role present	APN role not present	APN role not present	APN combined
Credentialing method Registered with Singapore Nursing Board (SNB) Valid practicing certificate *Education* Academic program in nursing/ midwifery (such as advanced/ specialist diploma, post-graduate diploma dvaMOH.gov.sg *Title* Registered Midwife Registered Nurse Midwife *Role* Meet needs of mothers and infants Home births not permitted	*Credentialing method* Nurse specialist not registered with SNB *Education* Experience Clinically focused advanced diploma and graduate certificate as specialty training *Title* Nurse Clinician *Role* Independently run clinics for patients with specialty and chronic conditions; no pharmacotherapeutic management Similar to CNS role in United States 17 RN level specialty certifications available https://www.moh.gov.sg/hpp/nurses/career-practices/CareerNPracticesDetails/nursing-	Role not available	*Credentialing method* Registered with SNB Certification (24 specialties: medical-surgical and community) *Education* Experience Clinically focused master's degree in nursing *Title* (protected) Advanced Practice Nurse NP title is not used *Role* Independently run clinics, manage acute/chronic conditions Hybrid model for CNS and NP
References: SNB (2023a, b, 2025) and Singapore Health Professionals Portal (2026)			
South Africa Department of Health, Republic of South Africa. National strategic direction for nursing and midwifery education and practice (2020/21–2025/26). https://www.health.gov.za/wp-content/uploads/2022/02/Nursing-Midwife-National-Strategic-Direction-2020-2021-to-2025-2026-Com.pdf			

(continued)

Table 1 (continued)

Nurse midwife	*Nurse specialist*	*Nurse anesthetist*	*Nurse practitioner*
APN role not present	APN role present	APN role not present	APN role not present
Credentialing method Registered with the South African Nursing Council (SANC) as nurse or midwife *Education* Bachelor's degree or Comprehensive Diploma in Nursing and Midwifery *Title* Nurse and Midwife *Role* Scope of Practice for nurses and midwives	*Credentialing method* Registered with SANC *Education* Post-graduate diploma in specialty *Title* Nurse Specialist *Role* Independent practice within scope	*Credentialing method* Not available *Education* *Title* *Role* Anesthesia is administered by anesthesiologists	*Credentialing method* Complete the paperwork required by the SANC *Education* *Title* *Role* 'Nurse practitioner' refers to all nurses
References: Department of Health, Republic of South Africa (2020), SANC (2012, 2025), and Spijkerman (2021)			
United Kingdom (England, Wales, Scotland, Northern Ireland)			
Nurse midwife	*Nurse specialist*	*Nurse anesthetist*	*Nurse practitioner*
APN role not present	APN role present in Scotland	APN role not present	APN role present

Credentialing Method No credentialling Registration with Nursing and Midwifery Council (NMC) as a registered midwife, but not as an APM as this does not exist currently in all of the UK England has APMs with MSc level degrees *Education* 3-year undergraduate program Postgraduate MSc level award *Title* (protected) Midwife *Role* The APN role does not exist in the UK, but some RNs are midwives. Midwives support pregnant people and their babies before, during and after, childbirth	*Credentialing Method* No credentialling In the UK, this would be a Clinical Nurse Specialist and in Scotland, an Advanced Clinical Nurse Specialist Registered with NMC as a registered nurse (not as a CNS as this does not exist) *Education* Variable as not regulated, BSc or MSc level mainly, some practitioners have undertaken doctoral education, but this is not a requirement for the role *Title* Clinical Nurse Specialist or Advanced Clinical Nurse Specialist (Scotland) *Role* Registered Nurse with specialty clinical practice *Notes* Nursing Revalidation. How to become a clinical nurse specialist UK. (7 Feb 2022). https://nursingrevalidation.co.uk/clinical-nurse-specialist/ These are the following policies for the other countries, but none are specific for CNS England policy https://www.hee.nhs.uk/sites/default/files/documents/multi-professionalframeworkforadvancedclinicalpracticeinengland.pdf (currently being updated and due for publication soon) Wales: https://heiw.nhs.wales/workforce/workforce-development/professional-framework-for-enhanced-advanced-and-consultant-clinical-practice/ Northern Ireland: https://www.health-ni.gov.uk/publications/advanced-nursing-practice-framework	*Credentialing Method* No credentialling If a nurse is in this role they may currently be registered with NMC as a nurse but not NA as we do not have NA in the UK. The General Medical Council (GMC) will be regulating NA/PA roles in future after regulatory reform process is completed and the role is not limited to nursing *Education* Variable National Perioperative Training Programme: Accelerated Anaesthetic Practitioner Programme (NHS Scotland Academy n.d.; RCA n.d.) *Title* Scotland Anesthetic Practitioner might be known elsewhere as PA *Role* Collaborate with anesthetist or act under the direction of the anesthetist, they do not have freedom to act autonomously NA role is not recognized in UK Anesthetic Associate (Physician Associate) only non-physician role allowed to administer anesthesia	*Credentialing Method* No credentialling Registered with NMC as a nurse, NPs are not registered *Education* Masters in advanced practice recommended but varies across countries (not required) *Title* Advanced Nurse Practitioners or Advanced Clinical Practitioners or Advanced Critical Care Practitioner or Advanced Emergency Care Practitioner or Advanced Neonatal Practitioner or Advanced Pediatric Practitioner, and specialties and mental health but there is a move away from the ACP title. The title may also vary slightly between employers, areas and countries as it is not a protected title *Role* RNs working in advanced roles May also be a non-RN such as allied health profession or pharmacist Royal College of Nursing endorses advanced level nursing practice via portfolio mapped to clinical practice, leadership, education, research, and job plan, but this is not mandatory. In England the Centre for Advancing Practice accredits universities and offers credentialing for practitioners Employer governance ensures appropriate job description, role detail *Notes* Credentialing is not mandatory. It is available in England via the Centre for Advancing Practice

References: Scottish Government (2021), NHS England (2022), BARNA (2025), RCN (2024), and Sellers et al. (2022)

(continued)

Table 1 (continued)

United States National Council State Boards of Nursing. APRN Consensus Model (2008). https://www.ncsbn.org/nursing-regulation/practice/aprn/aprn-consensus.page			
Nurse midwife	*Nurse specialist*	*Nurse anesthetist*	*Nurse practitioner*
APN role present	APN role present	APN role present	APN role present
Credentialing method Regulation and licensure by state National certification by examination *Education* Graduate or postgraduate nurse midwifery accredited program *Title* Certified Nurse-Midwife (CNM) *Role* Peri-natal care of women and newborns, limited care of male partners	*Credentialing method* Regulation, licensure vary by state National certification exams not available for all populations *Education* Graduate or postgraduate CNS accredited program in 1 of 6 populations *Title* Clinical Nurse Specialist (CNS) Varies by state *Role* Varies by state and facility Symptom/disease management	*Credentialing method* Regulation and licensure by state National certification by examination *Education* Doctoral nurse anesthetist accredited program *Title* Certified Registered Nurse Anesthetist (CRNA) *Role* Full spectrum of anesthesia-related care for individuals across the lifespan	*Credentialing method* Regulation and licensure by state National certification by examination *Education* Graduate or post-graduate NP accredited program in 1 of 6 populations *Title* Certified Nurse Practitioner (CNP) Varies by state *Role* Clinical care includes health promotion, preventive care, diagnosis and management acute and chronic conditions
References: Tracy and Sandelbach (2023, p. 406)			

have English as the primary language and either plan to or have recently hosted ICN/APN meetings. This work aligns with the 2030 Sustainable Development Goals (SDGs) as expanded roles of nurses and advanced practice nurses continue to improve determinants of health and well-being (Sensor et al. 2021) and achieve other SDGs (ICN 2020). While this chapter looks at the current state of APN roles, progress continues globally as innovative roles emerge and develop to meet everchanging healthcare conditions. A historical overview of APN credentialing methods and a detailed description of the certification by examination method are provided at the end of the chapter.

2 Definitions

Definitions are provided for terms used in the chapter. Where available, the International Council of Nurses (ICN) definitions are provided. Other definitions are included for comparison purposes.

3 Roles

Multiple titles are used for the various roles of advanced practice roles. For the benefit of this chapter, the following definitions are provided.

3.1 Advanced Practice Nurse (APN)

An Advanced practice nurse (APN) is a generalist or specialized nurse who has acquired, through additional graduate education (minimum of a master's degree), the expert knowledge base, complex decision-making skills, and clinical competencies for advanced nursing practice, the characteristics of which are shaped by the context in which they are credentialed to practice (ICN 2020). The two most identified APN roles are clinical nurse specialist (CNS) and nurse practitioner (NP) (ICN 2020).

3.2 Advanced Practice Registered Nurse (APRN)

APRN, as used in the USA, is the title given to a registered nurse who has met graduate nursing education and certification requirements and obtained a license to practice in one of four APRN roles: *certified registered nurse anesthetist (CRNA)*, *certified nurse-midwife (CNM)*, *clinical nurse specialist (CNS)*, and *certified nurse practitioner (CNP)*. APRNs have responsibility and accountability for health promotion and the assessment, diagnosis, and management of patient problems, which includes the use and prescription of pharmacologic and non-pharmacologic interventions. The expanded definition of an APRN with the seven delineated criteria is found on pages 7–8 (APRN Consensus Work Group & NCSBN APRN Advisory Committee 2008).

3.3 Nurse Anesthetist

The ICN definition for *nurse anesthetist* and the APRN Consensus Model (2008) definition of *certified registered nurse anesthetist* are essentially identical.

3.3.1 Nurse Anesthetist (NA)

Nurse Anesthetist (NA) is an advanced practice nurse who has the knowledge, skills, and competencies to provide individualized care in anesthesia, pain management, and related anesthesia services to patients across the lifespan, whose health status may range from healthy through all levels of acuity, including immediate, severe, or life-threatening illnesses or injury (ICN 2021).

3.3.2 Certified Registered Nurse Anesthetist (CRNA)

Certified Registered Nurse Anesthetist (CRNA) is an APRN prepared to provide the full spectrum of patients' anesthesia care and anesthesia-related care for individuals across the lifespan, whose health status may range from healthy through all levels of acuity, including immediate, severe, or life-threatening illnesses or injury. This care is provided in diverse settings, including in-patient and outpatient facilities (APRN Consensus Work Group & NCSBN APRN Advisory Committee 2008).

3.4 Nurse Midwife (NM)

Certified Nurse Midwife (CNM) is an APRN prepared to provide a full range of primary healthcare services to women throughout the lifespan, including gynecologic care, family planning services, preconception care, prenatal and postpartum care, childbirth, and care of the newborn. Care is provided in diverse settings from home, birthing centers, ambulatory care settings, and hospitals (APRN Consensus Work Group & NCSBN APRN Advisory Committee 2008).

Definitions from the International Confederation of Midwives and WHO were reviewed but are directed more at general midwifery, including non-nurse midwives or generalist nurse midwives. Data from these organizations show CNMs make up about 5% of the midwifery workforce. There is limited data on CNMs in advanced roles where graduate education is required (Bryant-Lukosius and Wong 2023). As stated in the first chapter, in many countries, midwifery may be regulated as a distinct profession; this chapter uses 'nurse-midwife or certified nurse midwife' only where it is a legally defined nursing-based role.

3.5 Clinical Nurse Specialist (CNS)

Clinical Nurse Specialist, as defined by ICN (2020), is an advanced practice nurse who provides expert clinical advice and care based on established diagnoses in specialized clinical fields of practice along with a systems approach in practicing as a member of the healthcare team.

Clinical Nurse Specialist, according to the APRN Consensus Model (2008), is an APRN role that integrates care involving the patient, nurse, and system (APRN Consensus Work Group & NCSBN APRN Advisory Committee 2008). Key elements of CNS practice are to create environments through mentoring and system changes that empower nurses to develop caring, evidence-based practices to alleviate patient distress, facilitate ethical decision-making, and respond to diversity. The CNS is responsible and accountable for diagnosis and treatment of health/illness states, disease management, health promotion, and prevention of illness and risk behaviors among individuals, families, groups, and communities.

3.6 Nurse Practitioner (NP)

Nurse Practitioner (NP), as defined by ICN (2020), is an advanced practice nurse who integrates clinical skills associated with nursing and medicine in order to assess, diagnose and manage patients in primary healthcare settings and acute care populations as well as ongoing care for populations with chronic illness.

Certified Nurse Practitioner (CNP), per the APRN Consensus Model (2008), is prepared to diagnose and treat patients with undifferentiated symptoms as well as those with established diagnoses. Both primary and acute care CNPs provide initial, ongoing, and comprehensive care, including taking comprehensive histories, providing physical examinations and other health assessments and screening activities, and diagnosing, treating, and managing patients with acute and chronic illnesses and diseases. This includes ordering, performing, supervising, and interpreting laboratory and imaging studies; prescribing medication and durable medical equipment; and making appropriate referrals for patients and families. Clinical CNP care includes health promotion, disease prevention, health education, and counselling as well as the diagnosis and management of acute and chronic diseases. CNPs are prepared to practice as primary care CNPs and acute care CNPs, which have separate national consensus-based competencies and separate certification processes.

4 Credentialing Methods

Credentialing refers to processes used to designate that an individual, program, institution, or product has met established standards set by an agent (governmental or non-governmental) recognized as qualified to carry out this task. The standards may be minimal and mandatory or above the minimum and voluntary. Licensure, registration, accreditation, approval, certification, recognition, or endorsement may be used to describe different credentialing processes, but this terminology is not applied consistently across different settings and countries (Styles and Affara 1997).

Accreditation is a process of review and approval by a recognized agency by which an institution or program is granted time-limited recognition of having met established standards (Schober and Affara 2006; Cary and Smolenski 2018).

Certification is the formal recognition of knowledge, skills, and experience demonstrated by the achievement of the professional standard set for the APN. (Schober and Affara 2006; Cary and Smolenski 2018).

Education, the formal preparation of the APN, is at a master's degree or beyond that of a generalist nurse (Schober and Affara 2006; Cary and Smolenski 2018).

Endorsement is the approval or recognition by an entity supporting an individual's qualifications to practice.

Licensure is the granting of the authority to practice. The process, sanctioned by law, of granting exclusive privilege to ANPs meeting established standards, allows the APN to practice and to use the specifically protected title of APN (Schober and Affara 2006; Cary and Smolenski 2018).

Portfolio is a method of assessing one's performance, knowledge, and skills by reviewing samples of their work, such as a range of patients or a variety of case studies (Henderson 2019).

Registration, in a basic sense, means that an individual's name has been entered into an official register for people who possess the specific qualifications for APNs. The register is maintained by a regulatory or another official governmental body and usually provides title protection. The register is not a validation of competence for the APN but simply a listing or registration of the position (Schober and Affara 2006; Cary and Smolenski 2018) (Table 1).

5 Historical Basis of APN Credentialing

Historically, credentialing dates to 1000 BC, when the Persian cult of Zoroaster developed a process for licensure of physicians (Medwave 2025). To earn the right to practice medicine in Persian, a person had to successfully treat at least three heretics. If all three lived, the license was granted, but if all three died, the license was denied. This act of credentialing began the system of setting standards to ensure competency for practice.

By the thirteenth century, the 'barber' surgeons at the College de Saint Come, France required physician students to meet specific requirements such as being male, young, and willing to do a year of apprenticeship and pass an examination to get into a medical program. In the 1500s, licensure was required to practice medicine. The practice varied depending on what country and whether you were in a large city or in a rural area. Medical organizations such as the Royal College of Physicians in London were given the power to license and regulate medical practice. The standards of credentialing continued to evolve to protect the public (Medwave 2025).

The first known documentation of nursing as a profession was recorded in 300 AD during the Roman Empire. Hospitals built in each town were staffed by women who assisted doctors. Nurses were credentialed in the nineteenth century with the United Kingdom passing the Nurse Registry Act in 1919 and 2 years later compulsory registration became law (Smith 2023). To become registered, the nurse had to have worked for 3 years in a practice setting (general, pediatric, or mental health) and have adequate knowledge and experience to nurse the sick. There was a supplemental registry for male nurses. In the United States, New York was the first state to require licensing for nurses by establishing the nation's first Nurse Practice Act in 1903. Requirements for licensure were the following: graduating from a nursing school, passing a comprehensive exam, being of good moral character, having knowledge of anatomy and physiology, being experienced in medical, surgical, obstetrical, and practical nursing. The licensee was also expected to be experienced in invalid cookery and household hygiene.

Although nurses have practiced at advanced levels throughout history, the advanced nurse role was officially recognized in the twentieth century. As the nursing profession struggled to define itself and its boundaries, the wars of the twentieth century and the need for nurses to work at an advanced level in times of crises led to advances in practice.

In the United States (United States), registering for lay midwives became a federal law in 1921. Certification for Certified Nurse Midwife began in the 1970s (Stephen 2020). States were encouraged to develop their own legislation for licensure (OHSU CWH 2025).

Dr. Loretta Ford, a nurse, and Dr. Henry Silver, a pediatrician, envisioned a nursing position that would bridge the gap between the physician and the nurse in 1965. Dr. Ford served in the Air Force in World War II and earned a nursing diploma. After the war she served on staff at the Public Health Nursing Service in Boulder, Colorado. She earned a bachelor's in nursing in 1949, followed by a master's in nursing in 1951. In 1955, she was appointed assistant professor of nursing at the University of Colorado and went on to receive her PhD. Dr. Ford and Dr. Silver desired better patient access to quality healthcare, especially for children. This led to the development of the first NP program (AANP 2025). The first master's level program for NPs was established in 1967 at Boston College (Brennan 2020). The first NP certification exam was established in 1974 (OAAPN 2021).

Surgical anesthesia was first used in 1846 at Massachusetts General Hospital in Boston by dentist William Norton and surgeon Jon Warren. Historically, nurse anesthesia began during the American Civil War. The 1880's saw the anesthesia advanced practice specialty blossom. The Certified Registered Nurse Anesthetist (CRNA) credential was established in 1956 in the United States (Franke 2018).

In France, World War II was fought with a lack of anesthesiologists in the battlefield. This issue led to the need to train paramedics and nurses to deliver anesthesia. In 1960, an artifact of competence (sense of self-competence and skill) was developed for nurse anesthetists. In the 1980s, the profession was legally recognized (Franke 2018).

The UK began the movement to the nurse anesthesia role during WW I after seeing the USA NA's deliver anesthesia in France. At the end of the war (1918), classes were formed for nursing sisters who began performing hospital duties. The role was expanded to assist the anesthesiologist in the delivery of anesthesia. An anesthetic nursing service was established in 1981 in France (Franke 2018).

German anesthesiologist supervised nurses in the operating room in delivery of anesthesia. In the 1960s, Germany experienced a severe shortage of anesthesiologists, and nurse anesthetists were used to fill the gap. This led to the development of a 2-year anesthesiology program that included intensive care, post and nursing program (Franke 2018).

With other countries moving forward with the NA role, Sweden followed in 1962, Finland in 1963, and Norway in 1965. The Netherlands followed in 1966 with NAs receiving formal education to deliver anesthesia. The NAs worked primarily under surgeons in the 1960's and then under anesthesiologists. In 1984, the Netherlands Ministry of Health approved the formal training of nurse anesthetists (Franke 2018).

The role of the Clinical Nurse Specialist (CNS) has evolved over time. Florence Nightingale, in her leadership role during the Crimean War, is often credited as the initial CNS. War is often the time when nurses rise to the forefront of care and advance the role of the nurse.

Nightingale's vision of healthcare reform and wound care improved the outcomes for many soldiers. The CNS role as it stands today and in Nightingale's time is based on being an expert clinician, nurse educator, researcher, consultant, and leader in healthcare. At the time of the Crimean War, the terminology of credentialing was not required (Matthews et al. 2020).

Hildegard Peplau has long been credited with the development of the CNS role in the United States She established the first CNS program at Rutgers University School of Nursing in 1956. The focus of the role was psychiatric nursing. Peplau was instrumental in expanding the role to Europe. The role of the Clinical Nurse Specialist has grown significantly since World War II. The United States role began in the 1950s followed by New Zealand and the UK in the 1970s, then Australia and Canada in the 1980s. The role became popular in Finland and Ireland in 2001, followed by Singapore in 2006, the Netherlands in 2008, and Hong Kong in 2009 (Matthews et al. 2020). The title varies within each country, and some countries have the blended role of the CNS and NP.

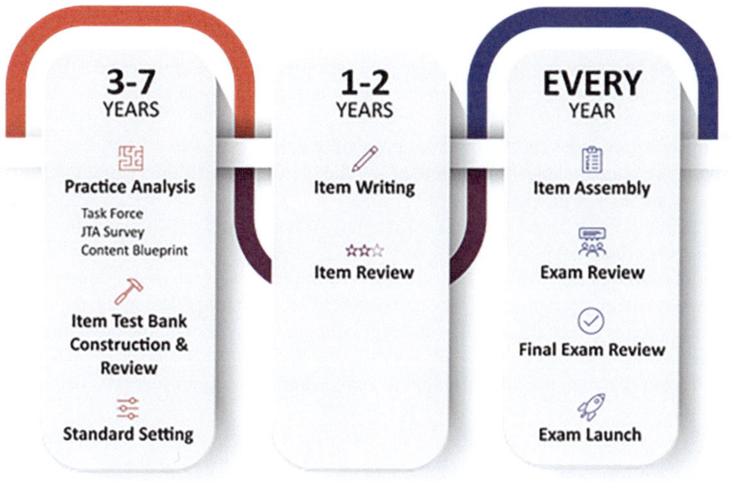

Fig. 1 AANPCB certification examination development process

6 Certification by Examination Exemplar: The United States

Certification by examination from an accredited national nursing certifying body is a component of the credentialing method for APRNs to be licensed to practice in the United States. There are five accredited organizations that offer certification examinations for nurse practitioners at the population level, two organizations certify clinical nurse specialists, one certifies nurse anesthetists, and another one for nurse midwives. Each of these exams is developed and accredited in a similar way. Described here is the methodology used by the American Academy of Nurse Practitioners Certification Board[1] (AANPCB) which offers certification examinations for three of the six NP populations—adult-gerontology, family, and psychiatric mental health.

Like many certifying organizations, AANPCB contracts exam development and exam delivery services with established industry companies. The exam development process is overseen by expert psychometricians and a staff of test developers (see Fig. 1). Computer-based exams are delivered at proctored test-taking centers. The core of a certification program's examination is the role delineation study, also known as a job task analysis (JTA). Several foundational elements must be in place before undertaking a job task analysis (JTA) which are listed in Table 2.

[1] *AANPCB* was founded by the American Association of Nurse Practitioners, formerly the American Academy of Nurse Practitioners, in response to an overwhelming call from the membership to develop a clinical competency-based certification by examination for nurse practitioners. The first examinations for Adult NPs and Family NPs were launched in 1993. As of 17 April 2025, there are over 225,675 AANPCB certifications held by NPs in the United States and Canada.

Table 2 Foundational Elements for Conducting a Job Task Analysis

A clear purpose and need for creating a certification program, such as to create safeguards for protecting the public and to recognize an NP's knowledge, skills, and abilities for competent entry into practice
A defined population to be certified with a scope of practice
Established core competencies for the role or job the certified practitioners are to perform
Established standards of practice
Sufficient demand for certified NPs and sufficient qualified candidates to maintain viability of the certification program
Sufficient interested parties (stakeholders) with a vested interest, such as employers of certified practitioners, academic programs to produce certification exam eligible candidates, consumers who seek the services from certificants, and regulators that may rely on the credential for public protection
The certification organization has sufficient resources and capacity to support a certification program

6.1 Practice Analysis and Test Specifications

For clinical-based roles, the job task analysis (JTA) is commonly known as a practice analysis. It involves a systematic and empirical review of the tasks performed in a job and the knowledge, skills, and abilities needed to successfully perform those tasks. AANPCB selects panels of practicing NPs, referred to as a task force, who are knowledgeable of the role, scope, and standards, clinical competencies, and who represent diverse geographical regions, practice settings, and patients for the certification population focus. Guided by expert psychometricians, the panels identify and define lists of job duties and tasks, and knowledge, skills, and abilities needed to perform the job. Consensus is obtained, then the list is sent to a separate panel to review for accuracy and completeness, which is returned to the task force panel for consideration. The final list is drafted into a survey that asks participants to rate the frequency of task performance, importance to the job, and criticality to safe practice for each of the tasks. The survey is then sent to a large sample of NPs that represent the characteristics of the exam's target population, such as entry into practice NPs. The survey results provide validation of the qualitative data gathered in the previous phases. The data are analyzed, and job tasks are weighted based on frequency, importance, and criticality. The job tasks are also grouped into similar categories, such as those tasks that relate to assessment, or making a diagnosis, creating a plan of care, or evaluating the effectiveness of the plan. The mathematical weighting of the tasks within each category provides the basis for the percentage or number of exam items per category. The categories and the tasks become the exam content outline or test specifications, which is the blueprint for developing the exam forms. Current exam blueprints are available on the AANPCB website (www.aanpcert.org) in the Candidate Handbook.

6.2 Exam Form Development and Administration

Development of an examination form involves five phases: item writing, item review, exam assembly, exam review, and exam publication. There are many types of items that could be used to assess knowledge, skills, and abilities. Currently, AANPCB uses the traditional multiple-choice question with a single correct answer among four response options. It is critical to have sufficient quality items in a test bank. Each item must relate to a specific task on the content outline and meet the qualifications of being a (1) meaningful assessment of a task competency, (2) factually accurate, (3) current, and (4) free from bias. All items must be validated with at least one current reference (within the last 5 years) from an approved list of resources. Certified NPs are invited to participate in item writing training sessions and to submit clinically based questions with the correct answer and three plausible distractors into a remote accessed database. Panels of certified clinical experts are convened periodically to review, revise, and validate items. New exam forms are assembled annually whereby the test developers pull items from the test bank that (1) represent the percentage of items from each content outline category and (2) meet acceptable psychometric parameters. Panels of clinical experts once again convene to review the exam forms to ensure all items are meaningful, accurate, fair, and current. The exams are formatted for 'publication' and delivered electronically via computers at proctored test-taking centers.

6.3 Standard Setting (Passing Point)

The process of setting the passing point or cut score for an examination is called standard setting. This is typically performed only once after a new content outline is developed from the practice analysis. A panel of diverse representative certified, clinical expert NPs and a psychometrician convene to (1) define and achieve consensus on the concept of the minimum acceptable competence of a qualified examination candidate and (2) review each item (or question) on the exam form and estimate the percentage of minimally competent examinees who would answer the question correctly. The percent rating by the panel on each item is tabulated to determine the recommended cut score to be applied for the examination. The concept of minimally competent practitioners is defined as individuals who have capabilities to perform job tasks and responsibilities in a way that meets the minimum requirements of effectiveness, safety, and ethical practice.

6.4 Psychometric Analysis

Each exam item must meet approved statistical parameters to be considered for inclusion on an examination. This step in the exam development process involves psychometric analyses to evaluate each item's difficulty and its ability to discriminate. Difficulty is determined by the percentage of examinees who answered the item correctly; discrimination describes how well an item differentiates high- and low-scoring examinees, which is assessed by the relationship between whether the examinee answered the item correctly and their total exam score. Parameters are set around acceptable ranges of difficulty and desirable discrimination values.

6.5 Accreditation

In the United States to be recognized by the state boards of nursing for licensure, the APRN certification examination must be accredited by either the Accreditation Board for Specialty Nursing Certifications (ABSNC) or the National Commission for Certifying Agencies (NCCA). Both accrediting bodies have similar standards that require certification programs to follow rigorous processes and have policies and procedures addressing governance structure, finance and human resources, psychometrics, error prevention and handling, and maintenance of certification. Achieving accreditation demonstrates that the certification by examination-based program was developed according to accepted credentialing standards.

7 Certification by Portfolio Exemplar: New Zealand

In the 1970s, international advances in nursing practice sparked interest among nurses in Aotearoa New Zealand. Since career advancement was limited to management or education, advanced clinical roles emerged to retain clinical expertise in the workforce.

By 1976, the New Zealand Nurses Association proposed credentialing for senior clinical roles. Two credential levels for specialist and advanced nurses were created over the next decade, requiring peer-assessed portfolios. The Nursing Council of New Zealand later regulated advanced nursing credentialing based on a 1998 Ministerial Taskforce recommendation.

In the 1990s, new clinical career pathways for registered nurses were built on earlier credentialing methods, influenced by Patricia Benner's novice to expert model (Benner 1984). Benner's narrative approach became widely accepted as evidence of clinical competence for advancement.

By 2004, the Professional Development Recognition Programme (PDRP) had been widely adopted in publicly funded health services, linking nurse career levels and pay through a collective agreement. The portfolio is now a standard tool for nurses to demonstrate clinical competence and advance their careers. Completing a PDRP portfolio also fulfills Nursing Council requirements for annual practising certificates, exempting nurses from Council audits.

Under the Health Practitioner Competence Assurance Act (HPCA) 2003, the Nursing Council established the nurse practitioner (NP) scope in addition to enrolled and registered nurse scopes. The Council's duties include setting qualifications, competency standards, and registration processes for each scope, as well as overseeing continuing competence.

Aligned with international standards, nurse practitioners are required to have a clinically focused master's degree and advanced practice competencies. NPs received full prescribing authority in 2014.

7.1 Educational Preparation for Nurse Practitioner Registration in New Zealand

To register as a Nurse Practitioner in Aotearoa New Zealand, applicants must be registered nurses with at least 4 years of practice, hold an approved clinical masters degree for the NP scope, and pass a competency assessment by a Council-approved panel (NCNZ 2017), as outlined by the Nursing Council in the *New Zealand Gazette*.

Clinical master's programs for NP registration are approved by the Nursing Council. Nurses follow a stepwise educational pathway: postgraduate certificate, diploma, then master's program, with the final year comprising an advanced practice practicum under supervision. Required courses include pathophysiology, advanced assessment, diagnostics, pharmacology, prescribing practice, and research skills.

Initially, slow growth in the nurse practitioner (NP) workforce and low registration rates indicated the need for a more coordinated educational approach (Carryer and Adams 2020). The previous system required lengthy portfolios, significant paperwork, in-person assessments, and offered little guidance. Job security was also uncertain, with new NPs often having to create their own roles due to the lack of established positions. These challenges highlighted the need for a more streamlined and supportive NP education and registration process.

In 2016, two universities collaborated to standardize eligibility, practicum design, and clinical hours to meet a 500-hour international minimum. Led by the Chief Nurses Office in the Ministry of Health, this initiative grew into a national training program run by six universities, prioritizing Māori and Pasifika applicants. Ministry funding supports 100 trainee spots per year (120 in 2024), covering university fees, employer reimbursements for supernumerary practice, supervision allowances, and limited travel. Recipients are expected to employ newly registered nurse practitioners.

In their final practicum, students compile portfolios with Nursing Council application documents, including case studies, competence attestations, evidence of professional and leadership activities, development, teaching, and credentials. Once instructors confirm competency, portfolios are submitted electronically for Council review, with most applicants assessed within 1–2 months of graduation.

Although more than 20 years have passed since the first NP registration, the role is still evolving, with only 703 registrants. Growth is hindered by the continued dominance of the biomedical model, regional disparities, limited workforce planning, and insufficient attention to equity. Political influences within and beyond nursing, along with early leadership tensions, further slowed progress (Wilkinson 2008a, b). Nevertheless, ongoing advocacy by NPs is essential for shaping the profession's future, improving education, updating competencies, and streamlining registration processes.

8 Certification by Examination Exemplar: Japan

In 2008, Japan embarked on a groundbreaking journey in healthcare with the initiation of its first graduate education program modeled after the United States (United States) nurse practitioner (NP) system. This pioneering step was primarily driven by the multifaceted challenges faced by the healthcare sector, notably the anticipated demographic shift. Japan, foreseeing a future where over 35% of its population would be aged 65 and above by 2040, recognized an urgent need to adapt its healthcare framework to this changing landscape. Amidst such societal challenges, it was feared the current legal framework, allowing only physicians to make healthcare decisions and provide instructions, might fall short in addressing the diversifying and demanding healthcare needs of that future time. In 2015, the Japan Nursing Association emphasized the significance of timely medical judgment and implementation in home-based care, stating that it is directly related to people's safety and peace of mind. Advocating for an expansion of healthcare providers and implementation of a system for nurses to actively engage alongside individuals, the idea of introducing a qualification akin to the United States nurse practitioner gained prominence as a way to meet evolving healthcare demands.

Initially, this initiative took shape under the banner of the 'Japan NP Council' in 2008. By 2014, it evolved into the 'Japanese Organization of Nurse Practitioner Faculties (JONPF),' a change that underscored the necessity for conducting education at the graduate level. This transition marked a significant step in formalizing and elevating the training and education of NPs to meet international standards. As of 2026, 21 graduate schools across Japan offer NP education programs. These programs are meticulously designed to equip graduates with the requisite skills and knowledge needed in diverse healthcare settings. After completing a two-year master's program, these graduates are eligible to take the JONPF-administered NP qualification exam. This exam is a critical component of the NP credentialing process, ensuring that only qualified individuals are certified to practice. The impact of this initiative has been significant and far-reaching. As of 2024, 984 individuals have successfully passed the qualification exam, marking a notable increase in the number of qualified NPs in Japan (JONPF 2026). These professionals have been instrumental in various healthcare settings, including acute care in hospitals, home care, and elderly care facilities. Their contributions have led to measurable improvements in patient care. For instance, there has been a notable reduction in emergency room visits and unplanned hospitalizations, particularly in the realm of home patient management. This improvement is a testament to the effectiveness of NPs in providing timely and appropriate care, thereby reducing the strain on hospital resources and improving patient outcomes. To maintain and enhance the quality of NP practice, the JONPF has implemented several measures. These include a rigorous program accreditation process, comprehensive NP qualification exams, mandatory five-year license renewals, and targeted training programs for NPs. Additionally, there is a strong focus on information dissemination and training to advocate for the formal regulatory structure of the NP profession in Japan. This aspect is crucial for the long-term success and integration of NPs into the Japanese healthcare system.

Looking back, it was the 2020 landmark collaboration between the JONPF, the Japanese Nursing Universities Council, and the Japan Nursing Association that brought together educators, regulators, and clinicians to create a cohesive effort toward introducing the role. Initially, these organizations had different visions for the NP system, but they eventually aligned their goals with those of the International Council of Nurses (ICN). This alignment was critical in shaping a unified vision for the role of NPs in Japan. It involved envisioning nurse practitioners who could conduct certain diagnoses and treatments autonomously, without the need for direct physician presence. This vision was not only progressive but also necessary for a country facing a significant shift in its social problems. To ensure the success of this initiative, rigorous education standards were established.

Looking to the future, the legal recognition and empowerment of NPs in Japan remains paramount. The goal is to establish a healthcare system where NPs can autonomously provide high-quality care, aligned with international standards. This objective is not only pivotal for addressing the immediate healthcare needs of those such as the aging population but also for ensuring the sustainability and resilience of the healthcare system in the long run. The journey of establishing and integrating the NP profession in Japan has been one of collaboration, adaptation, and innovation. It reflects a broader global trend of evolving healthcare roles to meet the changing needs of societies. As Japan continues to navigate this path, it serves as a model for other countries facing similar demographic and healthcare challenges. The continued development and empowerment of NPs will play a crucial role in shaping a more robust, efficient, and patient-centered healthcare system in Japan.

9 Discussion

The following questions may be helpful in implementing or improving professional credentialing for APNs:

1. How is the decision made to apply a chosen professional credentialing method?
2. What is involved in setting up each type of professional credentialing method?
3. What credentialing models provide the greatest mobility for APNs to meet global healthcare needs?
4. How can the growth of APN educational programs be promoted to develop a stronger global healthcare workforce?
5. What can be done to develop APN educational standards globally?
6. Is there a need for a global consensus model? Would a global consensus model (GSM) improve educational standards, promote uniformity in APN roles, and make movement from country to country standardized?
7. What are the best methods to develop protected APN Sustainable Development titles?
8. What would be the best method(s) employed by APNs to meet Goals, especially # 3 but others too.

Acknowledgments The authors wish to recognize and thank the following country representatives for their review of the advanced practice nurse role content presented in Table 1. Australia: Dr. Beverley Bird; Finland: Krista Jokiniemi; Hong Kong: Dr. Francis Wong; Netherlands: Dr. Jeroen Peters; New Zealand: Deborah Harris; Republic of Ireland: Dr. Daniela Lehwaldt; Singapore: Wentao Zhou; South Africa: Dr. Nonhlanhla Makhanya, Fhumulani Mavis Mulaudzi, and Professor Ntombifikile Mtshali; United Kingdom (Scotland): Colette Henderson. Special thanks to Dr. Madrean Schober and Dr. Daniela Lehwaldt for assisting with finding key informants in the selected countries.

References

Academie Verloskunde Amsterdam Groningen (AVAG). Master of midwifery. 2014. https://www.verloskunde-academie.nl/master-verloskunde/. Accessed 10 Mar 2026.

American Association of Nurse Practitioners (AANP). AANP News. 2025. https://www.aanp.org/news-feed/remembering-dr-loretta-ford. Accessed 13 Mar 2026.

APRN Consensus Work Group & NCSBN APRN Advisory Committee. Consensus model for APRN regulation: licensure, accreditation, certification, and education. 2008. https://www.ncsbn.org/nursing-regulation/practice/aprn/aprn-consensus.page. Accessed 13 Mar 2026.

Benner PE. From novice to expert: excellence and power in clinical nursing practice. Menlo Park: Addison-Wesley; 1984.

Brennan C. Tracing the history of the nurse practitioner profession in 2020, the year of the nurse. J Pediatr Health Care. 2020;34:83–4. https://www.sciencedirect.com/science/article/abs/pii/S0891524519306546/. Accessed 13 Mar 2026.

British Anaesthetic & Recovery Nurses Association. Training to work in anaesthetics: post anaesthetic care unit. 2025. https://www.barna.co.uk/uk-training-courses.html. Accessed 13 Mar 2026.

British Columbia College of Nurses & Midwives (BCCN&M). New NP exam. 2026. https://www.bccnm.ca/NP/applications_registration/exams/Pages/CNPLE.aspx. Accessed 10 Mar 2026.

Bryant-Lukosius D, Wong FKY. International development of advanced practice nursing. In: Tracy MF, O'Grady ET, Phillips SJ, editors. Advanced practice nursing: an integrative approach. 7th ed. St. Louis: Elsevier; 2023.

Canadian Anesthesiologists' Society (CAS). Position statement: Certified Registered Nurse Anesthetists (CRNAs) in Canada. 2022. https://www.cas.ca/CASAssets/Documents/Practice-Resources/Reports-Position-Papers/CRNA-Position-Statement-FINAL-08-22.pdf. Accessed 10 Mar 2026.

Canadian Council of Registered Nurse Regulators (CCRNR). National entry-level competencies for nurse practitioners. 2023a. https://static1.squarespace.com/static/671142bd58709c1e559e8c2a/t/672fdb07719a981d7c5480b7/1731189512640/english-national-np-elcs-final-bibliography-updated-june-2024.pdf. Accessed 10 Mar 2026.

Canadian Council of Registered Nurse Regulators (CCRNR). Nurse practitioner regulation framework implementation plan project. 2023b. https://cannn.ca/wp-content/uploads/2023/05/english-_npr-fipp-project-update-9-final-may-1.pdf. Accessed 10 Mar 2026.

Canadian Midwifery Regulators Council (CMRC). About CMRC. n.d. https://cmrc-ccosf.ca/about-cmrc. Accessed 10 Mar 2026.

Canadian Nurses Association (CNA). Clinical nurse specialists. 2026. https://www.cna-aiic.ca/en/nursing/advanced-nursing-practice/clinical-nurse-specialists. Accessed 10 Mar 2026.

Carryer J, Adams S. Advanced practice nursing in New Zealand. In: Hassmiller SB, Pulcini J, editors. Advanced practice nursing leadership: a global perspective. Switzerland: Springer; 2020. p. 127–40.

Cary AH, Smolenski MC. Credentialing and clinical privileges for the advanced nurse. In: Joel L, editor. Advanced practice nursing: essentials for role development. 4th ed. Philadelphia:

F.A. Davis; 2018. p. 100–15. Cited in ICN 2020. https://www.icn.ch/system/files/documents/2020-04/ICN_APN%20Report_EN_WEB.pdf. Accessed 13 Mar 2026.

Clinical Nurse Specialist Society of New Zealand (CNSSNZ). Position statement: CNS vs. nurse specialist. 2026. https://www.cnssnz.org. Accessed 13 Mar 2026.

Council of the European Union. Council recommendation on the European Qualifications Framework for lifelong learning. 2017. https://eur-lex.europa.eu/legal-content/EN/TXT/HTML/?uri=CELEX:32017H0615(01)&from=EN. Accessed 10 Mar 2026.

Department Health Republic of South Africa. National strategic direction for nursing and midwifery education and practice. 2020. https://www.health.gov.za/wp-content/uploads/2022/02/Nursing-Midwife-National-Strategic-Direction-2020-2021-to-2025-2026-Com.pdf. Accessed 13 Mar 2026.

Finnish Nurses Association (FNA). New roles for nurses: quality to future social welfare and health care services. 2020. https://sairaanhoitajat.fi/wp-content/uploads/2020/01/new-roles-for-nurses.pdf.

Franke E. California Association of Nurse Anesthesiology. A legacy of care and expertise. 2018. https://canainc.org/a-brief-history-of-nurse-anesthesiologists/. Accessed 13 Mar 2026.

Henderson J, editor. Certification: the I.C.E. Handbook. 3rd ed. Washington, DC: Institute for Credentialing Excellence; 2019.

International Council of Nurses (ICN). Nurses' role in achieving the sustainable development goals: international nurses day resources and evidence. Author; 2017. https://www.yorku.ca/unsdgs/toolkit/wp-content/uploads/sites/617/2022/05/Nurses-A-Voice-to-Lead-Achieving-the-SDGs-Report.pdf. Accessed 13 Mar 2026.

International Council of Nurses (ICN). Guidelines on advanced practice nursing 2020. Author; 2020. https://www.icn.ch/system/files/documents/2020-04/ICN_APN%20Report_EN_WEB.pdf. Accessed 13 Mar 2026.

International Council of Nurses (ICN). Guidelines on advanced practice nursing: nurse anesthetists 2021. Geneva: International Council of Nurses; 2021. https://www.icn.ch/system/files/documents/2021-05/ICN_Nurse-Anesthetist-Report_EN_WEB.pdf. Accessed 13 Mar 2026.

International Federation of Nurse Anesthetists (IFNA). The International Federation of Nurse Anesthetists. n.d. https://ifna.org. Accessed 10 Mar 2026.

Japanese Organization Nurse Practitioner Faculties (JONPF). NP certified person. 2026. https://www.jonpf.jp/about/certified_person. Accessed 15 Mar 2026.

Jokiniemi K, Meretoja R, Kotila J. Clinical nurse specialist role and practice in Finland. In: Fulton JS, Holly VW, editors. Clinical nurse specialist role and practice. Advanced practice in nursing. Cham: Springer; 2021. https://doi.org/10.1007/978-3-319-97103-2_9. Accessed 13 Mar 2026.

Jokiniemi K, Chair SY, Wong FKY, Bryant-Lukosius D. Advanced practice role delineation within Hong Kong: A cross-sectional study. Nurs Health Sci. 2022;24(3):679–89. https://doi.org/10.1111/nhs.12964. Epub 2022 Jul 8. PMID: 35699666; PMCID: PMC9545430. Accessed 13 Mar 2026.

Koninklijke Nederlandse Organisatie van Verloskundigen (KNOV). Midwifery in the Netherlands. 2017. https://assets.knov.nl/p/557056/none/PDF%27s/Over%20KNOV/Samenwerken/Midwifery_in_The_Netherlands_versie_2017.pdf. Accessed 10 Mar 2026.

Matthews JH, Whitehead PB, Ward C, Kyner M, Crowder T. Florence Nightingale: visionary for the role of clinical nurse specialist. OJIN. 2020;25(2):Manuscript 1. https://doi.org/10.3912/OJIN.Vol25No02Man01. Accessed 13 Mar 2026.

Medwave. The history of medical credentialing: From ancient times to modern practice. 2025. https://medwave.io/2025/01/the-history-of-medical-credentialing-from-ancient-times-to-modern-practice/. Accessed 13 Mar 2026.

New Zealand College of Midwives (NZCM). How to become a midwife. n.d. https://www.midwife.org.nz/midwives/midwifery-in-new-zealand/how-to-become-a-midwife/. Accessed 10 Mar 2025.

NHS England. Advanced clinical practice in midwifery: capability framework. 2022. https://advanced-practice.hee.nhs.uk/resources/midwifery-resources/midwifery-capability-framework/. Accessed 10 Mar 2026.

NHS Scotland Academie. National perioperative training programme: accelerated anaesthetic practitioner. n.d. https://www.nhsscotlandacademy.co.uk/programmes/national-perioperative-training-programme-accelerated-anaesthetic-practitioner/#whatistheacceleratedanaestheticpractitionerprogramme1%20Royal%20College%20of%20Anesthetists.%20Training%20and%20Careers. Accessed 10 Mar 2026.

Nurse Practitioners New Zealand. Becoming a nurse practitioner (NP) in New Zealand. 2025. https://www.nurse.org.nz/npnz/do-you-want-to-become-an-np. Accessed 10 Mar 2026.

Nursing and Midwifery Board of Australia (NMBA). Fact sheet: advanced nursing practice and specialty areas within nursing. 2020. https://www.nursingmidwiferyboard.gov.au/Codes-Guidelines-Statements/FAQ/fact-sheet-advanced-nursing-practice-and-specialty-areas.aspx. Accessed 10 Mar 2026.

Nursing and Midwifery Board of Australia (NMBA). Professional standards. 2025. https://www.nursingmidwiferyboard.gov.au/Codes-Guidelines-Statements/Professional-standards.aspx. Accessed 20 Mar 2026.

Nursing and Midwifery Board of Ireland (NMBI). State of the register. 2025. https://www.nmbi.ie/Registration/NMBI-state-of-the-Register. Accessed 13 Mar 2026.

Nursing and Midwifery Board of Ireland (NMBI). Standards and guidance. 2026a. https://www.nmbi.ie/Standards-Guidance Accessed 13 Mar 2026.

Nursing and Midwifery Board of Ireland (NMBI). Careers in nursing and midwifery: how to apply. 2026b. https://www.nmbi.ie/Careers-in-Nursing-Midwifery/How-to-apply. Accessed 13 Mar 2026.

Nursing and Midwifery Board of Ireland (NMBI). Guide information for nurses/midwives for NMBI verification of category 2 or equivalent post-registration qualifications. 2026c. https://www.nmbi.ie/Education/Verification-of-Postgraduate-Education. Accessed 13 Mar 2026.

Nursing Council of Hong Kong (NCHC). Voluntary scheme on advanced and specialised nursing practice. 2010a. https://www.nchk.org.hk/en/advanced_specialised_nursing_practice/index.html. Accessed 10 Mar 2026.

Nursing Council of Hong Kong (NCHC). Code of conduct and practice. 2010b. https://www.nchk.org.hk/en/code_of_conduct_and_practice/index.html. Accessed 10 Mar 2026.

Nursing Council of Hong Kong (NCHC). Core-competencies of an advanced practice nurse for perioperative and anaesthesia nursing developed by The Hong Kong Academy of Nursing under the Voluntary Scheme on Advanced and Specialised Nursing Practice. 2021. https://www.nchk.org.hk/filemanager/en/pdf/Perioperative_and_Anaesthesia_Nursing_eng.pdf. Accessed 13 Mar 2026.

Nursing Council of Hong Kong (NCHC). List of local clinical masters in nursing/health science programmes recognised under the Voluntary Scheme on Advanced and Specialised Nursing Practice. 2024. https://www.nchk.org.hk/filemanager/en/pdf/Lists_of_master_programmes.pdf. Accessed 10 Mar 2026.

Nursing Council of New Zealand (NCNZ). Notice of replacement and revocation of notice for nurse practitioners. 2017. https://gazette.govt.nz/notice/id/2017-gs952. Accessed 13 Mar 2026.

Ohio Association of Advanced Practice Nurses (OAAPN). History of NPs in the United States. 2021. https://oaapn.org/2021/06/history-of-nps-in-the-united-states/.

Open Universities Australia. Course results for degrees. 2026. https://www.open.edu.au/courses/degrees?keyword=nursing***. Accessed 13 Mar 2026.

Oregon Health Science University, Center for Women's Health (OHSU CWH). A brief history of midwifery in America. 2025. https://www.ohsu.edu/womens-health/brief-history-midwifery-america. Accessed 13 Mar 2026.

Royal College of Anaesthetists (RCA). Welcome to the Royal College of Anaesthetists. n.d. https://www.rcoa.ac.uk. Accessed 10 Mar 2026.

Royal College of Nursing (RCN). RCN professional development framework: advanced level nursing. 2024. https://www.rcn.org.uk/Professional-Development/publications/rcn-professional-development-framework-advanced-level-nursing-uk-pub-011-127. Accessed 10 Mar 2026.

Schober M, Affara FA. Advanced nursing practice. Oxford: Blackwell Publishing Ltd; 2006. Cited in ICN 2020. https://www.icn.ch/system/files/documents/2020-04/ICN_APN%20Report_EN_WEB.pdf. Accessed 13 Mar 2026.

Scottish Government. Transforming nursing, midwifery and health professions (NMaHP) roles: review of Clinical Nurse Specialist and Nurse Practitioner roles within Scotland. 2021. https://www.gov.scot/publications/transforming-nursing-midwifery-health-profession-nmahp-roles-review-clinical-nurse-specialist-nurse-practitioner-roles-within-scotland/. Accessed 10 Mar 2026.

Sellers C, Penfold N, Gass C, Drennan VM. The experience of working with anaesthesia associates in the United Kingdom and the impact on medical anaesthetic training. Int J Health Plann Manag. 2022;37(5):2767–78. https://doi.org/10.1002/hpm.3502. Epub 2022 Jun 12. PMID: 35690995.

Sensor CS, Branden PS, Clary-Muronda V, Hawkins JE, Fitzgerald D, Shimek AM, et al. Nurses achieving the sustainable development goals: the United Nations and Sigma Theta Tau International Honor Society of Nursing. Am J Nurs. 2021;121(4):65–8.

Singapore Health Professionals Portal. Careers and practices. 2026. https://hpp.moh.gov.sg/career-practice/. Accessed 10 Mar 2026.

Singapore Nursing Board (SNB). Scope of professional nursing and midwifery practice. 2023a. https://isomer-user-content.by.gov.sg/78/9e777f3e-...fessional-nursing-midwifery-practice_2023.pdf. Accessed 10 Mar 2026.

Singapore Nursing Board (SNB). Core competencies of advanced practice nurses. 2023b. https://isomer-user-content.by.gov.sg/78/164d803e-ce80-45ef-82d9-f8154ef89759/core-competencies-of-apn_2023.pdf. Accessed 10 Mar 2026.

Singapore Nursing Board (SNB). Certification as APN. 2025. https://www.snb.gov.sg/for-professionals/advanced-practice-nurse/certification-as-apn/. Accessed 13 Mar 2026.

Smith Y. History of nursing. News Medical Life Sciences; 2023. https://www.news-medical.net/health/History-of-Nursing.aspx. Accessed 13 Mar 2026.

South African Nursing Council (SANC). Advanced practice nursing: SANC's position paper/statement. 2012. https://www.sanc.co.za/advanced-practice-nursing/. Accessed 10 Mar 2026.

South African Nursing Council (SANC). Welcome to the South African Nursing Council. 2025. https://www.sanc.co.za. Accessed 10 Mar 2026.

Spijkerman S. Anaesthetic nurse training in South African and the role of the anaesthetists. S Afr J Anaesth Analg. 2021;27(21):12–4. https://doi.org/10.36303/SAJAA.2021.27.1.2592. Accessed 13 Mar 2026.

Stephen T. The history of midwifery in the United States. Beautiful births. 2020. https://beautifulbirthsmidwifery.com/2020/01/16/the-history-of-midwifery-in-the-united-states/. Accessed 13 Mar 2026.

Styles M, Affara F. ICN on regulation: towards 21st century models. Geneva: ICN; 1997. p. 44.

Tracy MF, Sendelbach S. The clinical nurse specialist. In: Tracy MF, O'Grady ET, Phillips SJ, editors. Hamric & Hanson's advanced practice nursing: an integrative approach. St Louis: Elsevier; 2023. p. 406.

Verpleekundig Specialisten Register (VSR). The profession of the Certified Nurse Specialist: the Nurse Practitioner in the Netherlands. 2017. https://www.venvn.nl/media/zvofiilk/english-additional-information-about-the-certified-nurse-specialist.pdf. Accessed 10 Mar 2026.

Wheeler KJ, Miller M, Pulcini J, Gray D, Ladd E, Rayens MK. Advanced practice nursing roles, regulation, education, and practice: a global study. Ann Glob Health. 2022;88(1):42. https://doi.org/10.5334/aogh.3698. PMID: 35755314; PMCID: PMC9205376.

Wilkinson JA. The ministerial taskforce on nursing: a struggle for control. Nurs Prax N Z. 2008a;24(3):5–16. https://doi.org/10.36951/NgPxNZ.2008.008. Accessed 13 Mar 2026.

Wilkinson JA. Constructing consensus: developing an advanced nursing practice role. Nurs Prax N Z. 2008b;24(3):17–26. https://doi.org/10.36951/NgPxNZ.2008.009. Accessed 13 Mar 2026.

Health Policy for Practice

Advanced Practice Nursing Around the World: Diverse Roles, Shared Challenges, and Pathways Forward

Abigail Kra-Friedman, Gila Zarbiv, Edwin N. Aroke, Jennifer Manning, and Jane Blood-Siegfried

1 Introduction

Advanced practice nursing (APN) care is pivotal in addressing the Sustainable Development Goals (SDGs), specifically, universal access to healthcare and evolving healthcare needs worldwide. As the *State of the World's Nursing 2025* report by the World Health Organization (WHO) and International Council of Nurses (ICN) stated, over 120 countries have established APN roles (WHO and ICN 2025). The *WHO's Global Strategic Directions for Nursing and Midwifery 2021–2025* report emphasizes the need to design and develop nursing policies, particularly to increase advanced education and training for nurses so that more nurses can assume a broader

A. Kra-Friedman (✉)
Selma Jelinek Department of Nursing, Faculty of Life Sciences,
Jerusalem College of Technology, Jerusalem, Israel

Department of Nursing, School of Health Sciences, Ashkelon Academic College, Ashkelon, Israel
e-mail: abbykrafriedman@gmail.com

G. Zarbiv
Department of Health Policy and Management, Ben-Gurion University of the Negev,
Beer-Sheva, Israel

Israel Implementation Science and Policy Engagement Centre (IS-PEC), Ben Gurion University of the Negev, Beer-Seva, Israel
e-mail: gckanal@gmail.com

E. N. Aroke
School of Nursing, University of Alabama at Birmingham, Birmingham, AL, USA
e-mail: earoke@uab.edu

J. Manning
Louisiana State University School of Health and Allied Professions, New Orleans, LA, USA
e-mail: jmanni@lsuhsc.edu

J. Blood-Siegfried
Duke University School of Nursing, Durham, NC, USA
e-mail: blood002@duke.edu

K. J. Wheeler, M. Acorn (eds.), *Health Policy for Advanced Practice Nursing: A Toolkit for Implementation and Improvement*, Advanced Practice in Nursing,
https://doi.org/10.1007/978-3-032-03667-4_13

scope of responsibilities within health systems and impact health outcomes at the individual, local, national, and global levels (WHO 2021).

The International Council of Nurses (ICN) defines an advanced practice nurse (APN) as *"a generalist or specialized nurse who has acquired, through additional graduate education (minimum of a master's degree), the expert knowledge base, complex decision-making skills and clinical competencies for Advanced Nursing Practice, the characteristics of which are shaped by the context in whey they are credentialed to practice…."* (ICN 2020, p. 6).

It is worth noting that this definition, where the master's degree has transitioned from a recommendation to a requirement, is relatively new and, therefore, not yet fully implemented. This has resulted in a multi-layered, complex profession that is attempting to evolve while simultaneously confounding educators and regulators who are trying to keep up with countries where the role is well-established.

As such, this chapter will:

- Identify the complex nature of advanced practice nursing and the policy dynamics related to education, clinical practice, governance, leadership, and research.
- Explore the shared challenges of four APN roles (nurse practitioner, clinical nurse specialist, nurse-midwife, nurse anesthetist) across diverse geographic regions, cultures, and contexts.
- Discuss future directions for policy development, implementation, role expansion, and investment for advanced practice nursing.

2 Education

The education of APNs worldwide is complex and varied, reflecting differences in local healthcare needs, regulatory structures, historical contexts, and resource availability. Although international guidelines advocate for APN education at the master's level or higher, countries vary in their ability to implement this standard. Each role requires a structured curriculum that integrates both didactic and clinical components to ensure competency in advanced practice. Still, the specific pathways, clinical training requirements, and educational structures differ significantly among roles and regions (Wheeler et al. 2022).

There are many advantages to having APNs with advanced degrees and broad educational backgrounds. Graduate-level education enables nurses to acquire higher-level functional skills necessary for practicing as competent clinicians, while also developing expertise in scholarship, research utilization, research generation, health system management, leadership, and mentorship of fellow nurses and new clinicians. Master's level education offers stability within roles and is more consistent than with varied educational entry points. Ultimately, graduate education provides greater professional credibility and autonomy; however, it should also offer an expanded scope of practice, which may be particularly beneficial to rural and underserved communities (Wheeler et al. 2022).

Despite the general push toward master's-level entry for APNs, many practicing APNs globally do not hold graduate degrees. The desire and ability for nurses and countries to move to the master's degree as entry-to-practice is highly complex. The feasibility of implementing a universal master's-level requirement depends on national healthcare priorities, funding, the size of the existing nursing workforce, and the nurturing of nursing leaders. The WHO and ICN *State of the World's Nursing 2025* report emphasizes the need for substantial investments in nursing education to meet this standard, particularly in low- and middle-income countries (WHO and ICN 2025). Investment in multiple educational pathways will be further discussed at the end of this chapter.

NP education focuses on preparing nurses for clinical practice. The credibility and autonomy of the NP role are closely tied to rigorous educational preparation, which includes coursework covering advanced health assessment, pharmacology, clinical reasoning, and leadership (ICN 2020). Countries like the U.S. and Canada require NP-specific master's or doctoral degrees (Wheeler et al. 2022; Bryant-Lukosius et al. 2017), while Israel has developed post-master's courses to qualify NPs (Haron et al. 2019). The competencies required for NP practice vary internationally, with frameworks such as the U.S. National Organization of Nurse Practitioner Faculties (NONPF) model influencing competencies set for other countries developing NP educational pathways (NONPF 2022). In the U.K., APN education has been adapted into broader Advanced Clinical Practice (ACP) roles, with an updated multidisciplinary framework that expands eligibility to non-nursing healthcare professionals (NHS England 2025).

Like NP education, CNS education is grounded in graduate-level training that enhances clinical expertise, leadership, and research application (ICN 2020). Studies consistently demonstrate that CNSs with master's degrees are more effective in implementing advanced practice competencies than those with a bachelor's degree (Fulton 2020). Unlike NPs, whose focus is primarily on direct clinical care, CNSs are often positioned within healthcare organizations as change agents who drive evidence-based practice improvements. These high-level functional skills are central to master's-level CNS education.

Nurse-Midwife education is one of the most variable APN pathways globally. Some countries require dual certification in nursing and midwifery, while others require a master's degree, and still others regulate midwifery independently of nursing (WHO 2024). The International Confederation of Midwives (ICM) advocates for using the *Essential Competencies for Midwifery Practice* (ICM 2019) to set benchmarks for programs that prepare students for entry to practice as midwives and promote high-quality teaching and learning processes. Still, national regulations dictate the level of education required for national certification (Nove et al. 2021). In high-income countries, nurse-midwives often complete graduate education based on the ICM competencies, whereas in other countries, midwifery education may be incorporated into undergraduate nursing education or limited to post-baccalaureate certification programs based on the exact same competencies. The global variation in nurse-midwife education reflects broader differences in maternal healthcare models, available national resources, and regulatory constraints affecting professional autonomy (WHO 2024).

NA education is similarly diverse, with significant differences in entry-level qualifications. In the United States (U.S.), Certified Registered Nurse Anesthetists

(CRNAs) must hold a Doctor of Nursing Practice (DNP) degree, while in Kenya and Ghana, NAs are trained at the diploma or bachelor's level. The International Federation of Nurse Anesthetists (IFNA) has addressed the various pathways by establishing model curricula at certificate, bachelor's, and master's levels, aiming to standardize training across countries (IFNA 2025a, b). IFNA program approval enhances global recognition of NA education and ensures that graduates meet competency standards. The variability in NA education reflects national healthcare needs and the availability of anesthesia providers in different settings (Reisen et al. 2023).

A core component of all APN education is integrating clinical, simulation, and didactic training, building upon foundational nursing knowledge and experience (ICN 2020). Clinical hours vary widely by country and role, ranging from 300 to 1500 hours (Wheeler et al. 2022). For instance, NP education in the U.S. and Italy requires at least 500 supervised clinical hours, while Hungary requires about 1500, and New Zealand mandates at least 300. CNS education similarly varies in clinical practice hours, with the U.S. requiring at least 500 hours (Wheeler et al. 2022) and Canada not having a clearly stated requirement (CNSAO 2025). CNS education specifically emphasizes clinical mentorship and applied research, with graduate-level training ensuring that CNSs can implement evidence-based practice and influence healthcare outcomes at the population level (Fulton 2020).

The integration of clinical simulation in APN education is widely debated, particularly regarding its equivalency to in-person clinical hours (Nye et al. 2018). Simulation provides a controlled environment for students to develop clinical reasoning, technical skills, and decision-making without patient risk. High-fidelity simulations are particularly beneficial for rare or high-risk scenarios that APN students may not frequently encounter in live clinical settings. For example, Nurse-Midwifery students can practice in simulated obstetric emergencies, NA students can simulate complex airway management, and NPs and CNSs can refine diagnostic reasoning in acute care cases. However, critics argue that while simulation enhances competency, it cannot fully replicate the complexities of real-world patient interactions in areas such as communication, adaptability, and bedside manners (Chevalier et al. 2025). The balance between simulation and live clinical exposure varies globally.

In contrast, countries such as the United Kingdom (U.K.) use simulation as a supplement rather than a replacement in urban settings where clinical placements are readily available, emphasizing traditional apprenticeship-based clinical education. Other areas with limited clinical placement opportunities, such as rural Canada, Australia, and parts of Africa, have expanded the use of simulation to address training gaps and a shortage of preceptors. Despite variations in regulation, a hybrid approach—leveraging simulation to strengthen clinical competency while ensuring sufficient real-world practice—is emerging as best practice in APN education worldwide (Diaz-Navarro et al. 2024). The lack of research and quality evidence on simulation education in low- and middle-income countries (LMIC) hinders the development of clear policies and recommendations for regulation.

Preceptorship is another essential element of APN education, requiring a close working relationship between educational institutions and clinical mentors (McInnis et al. 2021). APN students typically apprentice with multiple preceptors to gain diverse clinical experiences. Some preceptors volunteer, while others receive compensation through adjunct faculty appointments, financial incentives, or professional development credits. The availability of qualified preceptors is often a limiting factor in APN education, particularly in regions where APN roles are still developing.

Educational delivery is evolving globally, with a significant shift toward hybrid and online learning models (Ainslie et al. 2021). While traditional in-person education remains dominant, blended programs enable students to maintain employment while pursuing advanced education. These flexible models facilitate local clinical training, increasing the likelihood that graduates will remain in their communities to practice. This approach is particularly beneficial in rural and underserved areas, where APNs are crucial in expanding healthcare access.

While all APN roles share core elements of advanced clinical training, leadership, and evidence-based practice, the educational pathways remain highly dependent on national policies, healthcare structures, and contexts (ICN 2020). The drive toward standardization continues, but complete alignment remains challenging due to differences in healthcare infrastructures, workforce needs, and professional role definitions. Investing in faculty development, clinical preceptorship models, and regulatory frameworks is crucial to supporting the global growth of advanced nursing practice.

3 Clinical Practice

By understanding the similarities and differences in clinical practice among the different APN roles, policymakers and educators can tailor training programs and regulatory frameworks to ensure that APNs are effectively utilized to meet healthcare needs. The continued expansion of APN roles worldwide represents a shift toward more sustainable, accessible, and high-quality healthcare delivery. Table 1 shows a comparison of the various APN roles discussed in this chapter.

While each APN role has distinct responsibilities and scopes of practice, they share common elements of advanced clinical expertise, evidence-based decision-making, and patient-centered care (ICN 2020). The clinical practice of these roles varies significantly across countries and is influenced by regulatory frameworks, healthcare needs, and workforce structures. The following section examines the clinical practice of APNs, comparing and contrasting their roles in various national contexts and highlighting both their shared competencies and distinct contributions.

Table 1 Comparison of aspects of clinical practice advanced practice nursing roles in clinical practice

Aspect	Nurse practitioners (NPs)	Clinical nurse specialists (CNSs)	Nurse-midwives	Nurse anesthetists (NAs)
Focus	Primary, acute, and specialty care	Specialized care, system-level Improvements, role is implemented in three spheres: system, patient, and nurse	Reproductive, maternal, and newborn healthcare	Anesthesia and pain management before, during and after surgical and other medical procedures
Scope	Assess, diagnose, treat, and manage conditions	Direct care, staff education, research, policy, and system	Preconception to postpartum care	Anesthesia administration, pain management, and perioperative care
Autonomy	Varies by country, state, jurisdiction, and facility from full autonomy (New Zealand) to collaboration (Canada, U.K.) to supervision. Some have prescribing authority	Varies by country, state, jurisdiction, and facility. Often hospital-based, leadership-focused, can practice in community and outpatient settings	Varies by country, state, jurisdiction, and facility, from full autonomy (New Zealand, Netherlands, Sweden) to supervision or RN level role (parts of sub-Saharan Africa)	Varies by country. state, jurisdiction, and facility, from full autonomy to supervision
Key contributions	Expand access to care, manage chronic diseases	Improve quality of care and patient outcomes, mentor staff, and lead initiatives	Reduce interventions, improve maternal and neonatal outcomes	Ensure safe anesthesia, expand access to anesthesia, and pain management
Settings	Clinics, hospitals, specialty practices	Hospitals, specialized units	Birth centers, hospitals, and community settings	Hospitals, surgical, obstetric, and emergency units
Global presence	Key roles in the U.S., Canada, parts of Europe, Australia, New Zealand, and select countries of Africa	Key roles in Canada, Australia, Saudi Arabia, Sub-Saharan Africa, Europe, and Asia (Belgium, Germany, Japan, and the U.K.)	Key roles in New Zealand, the Netherlands, Sweden, Scotland, Canada, the U.K., and Australia. Critical in LMICs	Key roles in the U.S., Canada, parts of Europe, Asia, South America, Australia, and Africa
Emphasis	Holistic, patient-centered, preventive care	Patient outcomes, research, implementing evidence-based practice, system enhancement	Midwifery model: childbirth as a physiologic process, holistic well-woman care (U.S.)	Advanced clinical skills, precision, patient safety

Adapted from WHO and ICN (2025), Wheeler et al. (2022), Fulton et al. (2020), WHO (2024), Reisen et al. (2023)

3.1 Nurse Practitioners (NPs)

Nurse practitioners provide comprehensive care across primary, acute, and specialty settings (ICN 2020). Their role integrates elements of nursing and medicine, allowing them to assess, diagnose, treat, and manage acute and chronic conditions. A distinguishing feature of NP practice is its focus on holistic, patient-centered care, emphasizing health promotion, disease prevention, and medical management.

In the U.S., NPs operate under varying degrees of autonomy depending on state regulations (Porat-Dahlerbruch et al. 2024). Some states grant full practice authority, allowing NPs to diagnose and prescribe medications autonomously, while others require physician oversight. In contrast, countries such as the U.K. and Canada mandate a collaborative model, where NPs work alongside physicians in interdisciplinary teams (Bryant-Lukosius and Dicenso 2004). In New Zealand, NPs have full prescriptive authority and function with high levels of autonomy (Htay and Whitehead 2021). These regulatory differences impact the degree to which NPs can serve as primary care providers, particularly in rural and underserved regions where their role is critical for expanding healthcare access.

NPs' ability to manage chronic diseases effectively has been well-documented in research, demonstrating outcomes comparable to, or even exceeding, those of physicians in terms of patient satisfaction, adherence to clinical guidelines, and health outcomes (Kilpatrick et al. 2024). This has led to growing international recognition of the NP role as an essential component of healthcare reform to improve access and quality while reducing costs.

3.2 Clinical Nurse Specialists (CNSs)

Unlike NPs, who provide direct patient care across the lifespan, CNSs specialize in complex clinical areas and focus on system-level improvements (Fulton 2020). Their role encompasses direct patient care, staff education, research application, and policy advocacy. CNSs are particularly valuable in improving healthcare quality, fostering innovation, and mentoring nursing staff to enhance care delivery.

CNS practice varies across healthcare systems. In Canada and Australia, CNSs play a vital role in hospital-based care, particularly in areas such as oncology, critical care, and wound management (CNSAO 2025). Their expertise in evidence-based practice enables them to lead quality improvement initiatives and implement best practices at both the patient and organizational levels. In Sub-Saharan Africa, CNSs have played a crucial role in HIV management (Jones and Cameron 2017). They provide direct patient care while also training nurses and community health workers to enhance healthcare delivery in resource-limited settings.

One key distinction between CNSs and NPs is their primary focus. While NPs often function as primary or specialized care providers, CNSs focus on enhancing patient outcomes through education, research, and system-wide practice improvements. This dual focus on direct and indirect care allows CNSs to bridge gaps in healthcare quality, making them essential in settings where specialized nursing knowledge is needed to drive change.

3.3 Nurse-midwives

Nurse-midwife is the title given to a nurse who has met context-specific education and certification requirements and obtained a license to practice midwifery in a specific jurisdiction. The role is integrated within the APN framework through the regulated nurse-midwife role (ICN 2020).

According to the WHO (2024), midwives and nurse-midwives specialize in sexual, reproductive, maternal, newborn, and adolescent health (SRMNAH) and may provide up to 90% of essential care across this continuum, including preconception, antenatal, intrapartum, and postpartum care. Midwifery models of care are provided by educated, licensed, and regulated midwives who provide primary care for women and newborns and practice autonomously and independently within collaborative interdisciplinary teams (WHO 2024). These models are grounded in a midwifery philosophy that views pregnancy and childbirth primarily as normal physiological processes. Implementing universal access to midwifery models of care has been identified as a strategy to save 4.3 million lives annually by 2035 (Nove et al. 2021).

Globally, the role and autonomy of nurse-midwives vary widely (Small et al. 2025). In some U.S. states, nurse-midwives may have full prescriptive authority and function autonomously or in interdisciplinary care teams, depending on state regulatory models. In contrast, midwifery models of care with clinical autonomy and independence in European countries such as the Netherlands and Sweden are considered the standard, with midwives acting as the primary care providers for women. In all contexts, especially in low- and middle-income countries, midwifery plays a critical role in reducing maternal and neonatal mortality, often functioning within community-based healthcare models to increase access to skilled birth attendance (WHO 2024; ICN 2025).

A substantial body of evidence, alongside global recommendations from the World Health Organization supports the implementation of midwifery models of care as a strategy to reduce unnecessary medical interventions, improve maternal and newborn outcomes, and enhance women's experiences of care (WHO 2024). Yet despite this evidence and growing international momentum, the full implementation of midwifery models of care remains uneven across many contexts and settings, limiting access to high quality, respectful care for women and newborns worldwide (ICM 2025).

3.4 Nurse Anesthetists (NAs)

Nurse anesthetists provide anesthesia and pain management services in a wide range of healthcare settings, including hospitals, ambulatory surgical centers, pain management clinics, radiology clinics, endoscopy centers, obstetric suites, and even dentists' offices (Reisen et al. 2023). They are involved in pre-anesthesia preparation, administering anesthesia, and post-anesthesia care. Their role is critical in ensuring access to surgery with safe anesthesia, particularly in regions where physician anesthetists are scarce.

The level of autonomy and practice authority for NAs also varies significantly across countries (AANA 2025a, b). In the U.S., certified registered nurse anesthetists (CRNAs) can practice autonomously in many states, while others require some level of physician supervision. The trend toward full practice authority has been accelerated by workforce shortages and increased recognition of CRNAs' competencies (Vetter et al. 2025). In Iceland, NAs are indirectly supervised by physician anesthesiologists, with evolving policies allowing them to perform specific anesthesia procedures autonomously. Kenya offers another example where nurse anesthetists are primary providers of anesthesia services in rural hospitals, often working without direct physician oversight due to workforce constraints (AANA 2025a, b).

A unique aspect of NA practice is the strong emphasis on patient safety and technical precision. NAs prioritize patient safety by meticulously monitoring vital signs, advocating for patient-centered care, and collaborating effectively within healthcare teams. Their advanced clinical skills encompass a wide range of responsibilities, including thorough patient assessments, administering diverse anesthesia techniques, mastering advanced airway management, and providing comprehensive pain relief. NAs integrate evidence-based practices, engage in continuous education, and contribute to research to ensure optimal patient outcomes and drive advancements in the field of anesthesia (AANA 2025a, b). Unlike NPs and nurse-midwives, who focus on holistic and long-term patient care, NAs operate in highly specialized, procedure-driven environments where split-second decisions are crucial. The Canadian Medical Education Directives for Specialists (CanMEDS) framework, adopted by the IFNA, outlines NAs' roles as communicators, collaborators, and clinical experts, underscoring the complexity of their practice (IFNA 2025a, b).

4 Comparing and Contrasting APN Clinical Practice

While all APN roles share a foundation in advanced clinical training, evidence-based practice, and patient-centered care, key differences define their scope and impact (ICN 2020). NPs and nurse-midwives provide direct, long-term patient care, with NPs focusing on primary and specialty care across populations and nurse-midwives specializing in reproductive and maternal health. CNSs, in contrast, blend direct patient care with system-level leadership, enhancing healthcare quality through staff development and policy implementation (Fulton 2020). NAs are highly skilled in the technical and procedural aspects of anesthesia administration, focusing on pain management and perioperative care (Reisen et al. 2023).

These distinctions also manifest in regulatory and practice variations worldwide. While NPs, CNSs, and nurse-midwives often function autonomously or in collaborative models, NAs frequently encounter stricter supervision requirements, reflecting the procedural intensity of their work (Wheeler et al. 2022; WHO 2024; Porat-Dahlerbruch et al. 2024). Additionally, midwifery in many countries does not require a nursing degree, and regulatory models exist for both pathways, further conflating the confusion and integrity of the profession.

Despite these differences, the global trend is toward expanding the roles and autonomy of APNs to address healthcare shortages and improve patient outcomes (WHO 2021). Countries with well-integrated APN models demonstrate improved access to care, reduced healthcare costs, and enhanced patient satisfaction (WHO and ICN 2025; Kilpatrick et al. 2024). As healthcare systems continue to evolve, optimizing APN clinical practice through professional development, interprofessional collaboration, and precise regulation is key to maximizing their impact on global health.

5 Governance

As with practice and education, the governance of APNs is layered and complex (ICN 2020). In this toolkit, governance refers to *the framework of authority and accountability that controls APN practice and education.* While APNs share the goal of improving patient care through advanced clinical expertise, the regulatory frameworks, credentialing processes, and scope of practice vary significantly across countries (Wheeler et al. 2022). This diversity reflects differing healthcare needs, resource availability, cultural factors, and the historical development of the nursing profession.

Globally, the regulation of APN roles is influenced by national and regional legislative structures, professional organizations, and accreditation bodies. In countries like Australia and Canada, national or provincial boards such as the Nursing and Midwifery Board of Australia and various provincial nursing bodies in Canada oversee the regulation of APNs, setting standards for education, practice, and continuing professional development. However, even within these countries, significant contextual, provincial, or territorial variations exist, leading to discrepancies in practice autonomy and role clarity (Contandriopoulos and Bertoni 2025).

For example, in Canada, NPs and nurse-midwives may have full practice authority in some provinces, while others impose collaborative agreements or physician oversight. Similarly, in the U.S., the Consensus Model for APRN Regulation standardizes licensure, accreditation, certification, and education, yet state-specific laws still dictate the extent of practice autonomy, particularly affecting CRNAs and nurse-midwives (Wheeler et al. 2022). In contrast, countries like South Africa and Singapore have established dedicated governance bodies for advanced practice roles, such as the Advanced Practice Nurse Accreditation Board in Singapore, ensuring standardized competencies across APN roles.

One significant governance challenge is the variability of educational requirements for APN roles (Wheeler et al. 2022; Small et al. 2025). In high-resource countries like the U.S. and Australia, a master's degree is typically the minimum requirement for advanced practice, with many roles requiring doctoral-level education (ICN 2020). Accredited graduate programs ensure APNs receive advanced clinical training and are prepared for national certification exams. Conversely, in low-and middle-income countries, the path to advanced practice may not always require a master's degree due to limited educational resources. In countries like Botswana and Ghana, APN roles have evolved organically (Seitio and Newland 2008). Initial training is provided at the diploma or certificate level before transitioning to graduate education as capacity builds. This gradual development highlights the need for flexible governance structures that can adapt to resource availability while ensuring quality care.

Title protection and transparent credentialing processes are critical for role recognition and clarity (ICN 2020; Wheeler et al. 2022). Inconsistent use of titles and qualifications can lead to confusion among healthcare providers and patients, thereby undermining the credibility of APN roles. Countries with well-defined credentialing processes, such as the Netherlands and Israel, may experience greater professional recognition and acceptance of APNs within healthcare systems.

The scope of practice for APNs varies widely, influenced by local governance, institutional policies, and national regulations (ICN 2020; Wheeler et al. 2022). While federal laws may establish baseline qualifications and practice standards, local jurisdictions and healthcare institutions often impose additional restrictions. For instance, nurse-midwives in the U.S. may have the legal authority to practice autonomously at the state level; however, institutional policies may require physician oversight, thus limiting their autonomy (Jefferson et al. 2021).

Similarly, CRNAs in the U.S. have full practice authority in many states, allowing them to provide anesthesia care autonomously (Vetter et al. 2025). However, in the U.K., nurse anesthetists fall under the broader category of Advanced Clinical Practitioners (ACPs), with practice authority varying by employer and region. This inconsistency in practice authority can create barriers to professional mobility and affect the integration of APNs into healthcare teams Peacock and Hernandez 2020; Poghosyan and Maier 2022).

Despite organized efforts, significant challenges are likely to remain, particularly in countries with decentralized healthcare systems or underdeveloped governance structures. Inconsistent national policies can hinder the standardization of APN roles, negatively impacting patient care and professional recognition. To be effective, efforts to strengthen regulatory frameworks must consider each country's unique cultural, social, and political context.

In low- and middle-income countries, governance challenges are often compounded by limited educational resources and underdeveloped regulatory structures. APNs in these settings may practice without formal recognition or standardized credentials, leading to variability in the quality of care. For example, in some regions, NPs and CNSs may be trained through residency programs or certificate courses rather than formal graduate education.

Federal governance structures in these countries may be less developed, resulting in gaps in regulation and oversight. This lack of standardized governance can create challenges in ensuring consistent quality of care and professional recognition. However, the gradual development of APN roles, as seen in countries like Botswana and Ghana, demonstrates the potential for successful integration of advanced practice roles even in resource-limited settings (Seitio and Newland 2008).

Integrating governance frameworks across APN roles and countries requires a comprehensive approach that considers each healthcare system's unique challenges and opportunities. Collaborative efforts between national regulatory bodies, professional organizations, and educational institutions are essential for developing standardized frameworks that support the professionalization of APN roles.

Countries with established APN roles can serve as models for developing governance structures in other regions. For example, the regulatory frameworks in Australia and the U.S. provide valuable insights into best practices for credentialing, education, and scope of practice. However, it is essential to adapt these models to local contexts to ensure they meet each country's specific needs (ICN 2020).

Governance of APN roles is a multifaceted challenge that requires navigating diverse regulatory frameworks, educational standards, and professional recognition processes. By integrating best practices and promoting international collaboration, governance structures can be developed that support the growth and professionalization of APN roles worldwide, ultimately improving patient care and healthcare outcomes globally.

6 Research

Research is a pillar of advanced practice nursing (ICN 2020). APNs conduct research to advance clinical practice and improve patient outcomes. Their unique expertise and direct patient care experience position APNs well to investigate critical clinical questions and contribute to the evidence base. APN research may focus on various topics, including patient safety, quality of care, patient satisfaction, cost-effectiveness, knowledge translation, and innovative care delivery models. While there is a large amount of literature on APN practice globally, there is a serious underrepresentation in most WHO world regions outside of North America, the U.K., Australia, and Sweden (Kilpatrick et al. 2024).

Much of the literature that supports APN practice is based on patient satisfaction. While patient satisfaction is important, it does not indicate key system outcomes like decreased hospitalizations, decreased length of hospital stay, or decreased readmissions (Kilpatrick et al. 2024). Thus, further research on patient satisfaction may no longer be necessary; instead, APN research examining systems-wide outcomes might have a greater impact on APN integration (Porat-Dahlerbruch et al. 2024). Multi-disciplinary APN research may also be valuable in demonstrating the systems-level benefits of APN care. This type of evidence can be used to advocate for policy changes, secure funding, and improve patient access to high-quality care. Additionally, APN research can contribute to developing best practices and clinical guidelines, which may help standardize care delivery and improve patient outcomes.

7 Leadership

Effective APN leadership can create a supportive environment where APNs can thrive, advocate for their roles, and deliver high-quality care (ICN 2020). International professional organizations play a vital role in advocating for standardized governance frameworks and promoting best practices. As previously mentioned in this chapter, the International Council of Nurses (ICN), the International Federation of Nurse Anesthetists (IFNA), and the International Confederation of Midwives (ICM) work to harmonize educational and practice standards globally, supporting the professionalization of APN roles. These organizations provide guidelines and resources to help countries develop regulatory frameworks, ensuring safe, high-quality care. Likewise, local professional organizations can provide support for APNs at the national level, advocating for initiatives such as expanding the scope of practice, establishing policies for professional insurance coverage, and creating platforms for continuing education. Strong local leaders promote the value of APNs within healthcare systems and advocate for policies that support their roles (ICN 2020; Wheeler et al. 2022; Porat-Dahlerbruch et al. 2024; Bryant-Lukosius et al. 2017). APN leaders ensure culturally appropriate training and education to meet the needs of their patients and communities.

Developing local leaders sustainably contributes to advocacy that aligns with country resources and current policy. National APN leaders may seek guidance from other professional organizations in other countries. They also may seek advice, guidance, and advocacy from international professional organizations with frameworks for professional development. For example, the ICN's Global Nursing Leadership Institute and the Global Network of WHO Collaborating Centers both support the development of nursing, APN, and midwifery leadership globally (WHO and ICN 2025; ICN 2025).

National workforce leaders provide guidance, support, and mentorship for new APNs, helping them develop their skills and confidence to become future APN leaders themselves (WHO 2025). Additionally, leaders encourage collaborative partnerships between APNs and other healthcare providers to ensure seamless care delivery. APN mentors can motivate APNs to explore innovation and new ways of providing care and embrace technological advancements. By investing in leadership development and creating a supportive environment for APNs, healthcare systems can harness the full potential of these advanced practitioners to improve patient outcomes and enhance the quality of care worldwide (ICN 2024).

8 Policy Implications

8.1 Investment in APNs

It is crucial for stakeholders advocating for advanced practice nursing roles to know key statistics about their significance. The ICN 2024 report, *Our Nurses, Our Future: The Economic Power of Care*, emphasizes the need to invest in APNs for both healthcare improvement and economic growth (ICN 2024). Investing in APNs results in better health outcomes, lower healthcare costs, and a stronger economy. Healthy individuals are better equipped to contribute to their communities and society as a whole. The ICN report reveals that poor health decreases the global economy by approximately 15% of GDP, meaning that enhancing healthcare through investment in advanced practice nursing could help mitigate these losses. APNs are vital in preventing diseases, managing chronic conditions, and reducing unnecessary hospital visits, thus making healthcare systems more efficient and cost-effective (WHO and ICN 2025; ICN 2024).

In addition to improving healthcare, APNs play a significant role in achieving the United Nations SDGs (WHO and ICN 2025). Their efforts directly support SDG 3 (Good Health & Well-being) by making healthcare more accessible and affordable. Given that a large number of nurses are women, investing in APNs also promotes SDG 5 (Gender Equality) by creating more professional opportunities for women. Strengthened healthcare systems contribute to economic growth, aligning with SDG 8 (Decent Work & Economic Growth), while APNs help reduce health disparities, supporting SDG 10 (Reduced Inequalities). By providing care in underserved areas, APNs help make healthcare more equitable and effective.

Both the *State of the World's Nursing 2025* report (WHO and ICN 2025) and the 2024 *Economic Power of Care* report (ICN 2024) underscore the necessity for governments to invest in nursing education, improve salaries, and create supportive work environments. As noted in the beginning of this chapter, as of 2024, over 120 countries have established APN roles, but further investment is essential to enhance APN integration into global healthcare systems (Porat-Dahlerbruch et al. 2025). The demand for APNs varies by country based on their respective healthcare systems, but increasing their availability through training and hiring is critical for achieving the SDGs worldwide.

Investing in APNs is not only a healthcare imperative but also a wise economic strategy (ICN 2024). A well-supported APN workforce leads to improved healthcare, a stronger economy, and a healthier world. Governments need to take action by funding nursing education and expanding APN roles to achieve the global goal of better healthcare for all (Kra-Friedman, et al. 2025).

8.2 Competency-Based Education

The *Global Strategic Directions for Nursing and Midwifery 2021–2025* Report (2021, p. 6) suggests that nurse and midwife graduates should "match or surpass health system demand and have the requisite knowledge, competencies, and attitudes to meet national health priorities." Furthermore, policy priorities must also align with the country's demands and resources. Competencies should be consistent at all levels of education to ensure the best possible health outcomes and system benefits for all. For example, the International Confederation of Midwives recognizes that globally, midwives are regulated to varying degrees of academic education and has thus created a set of core competencies for clinical practice to standardize midwifery curricula (ICM 2019). Similarly, the International Federation of Nurse Anesthetists (IFNA) has developed three curricula for anesthesia programs (IFNA 2025a, b). They differ in program duration and ancillary skills education (level of research, level of clinical leadership, presence/absence of thesis requirement), but the core anesthesia skills are the same, taking into consideration the specifics of the country where they are employed. Both the IFNA curricula and the ICM's competencies are designed to educate students not only at the master's level but also to provide entry points for bachelor's or certificate-trained nurses and midwives.

8.3 Multiple Educational Pathways

Most countries have defined the level of education required based on the unique resources available and cultural expectations (Ng'ang'a and Byrne 2015). For example, the U.S. and Canada require the minimum of a master's degrees to sit for certification exams, and faculty are required to have DNP or PhD level training (Wheeler et al. 2022). Still, in some cases, we must ask ourselves: Can the rest of the world manage that? While standardization is important, the goal is to increase access to healthcare at the level the country can afford. Internationally standardized guidelines may be the final goal, but countries must be allowed to design local educational pathways according to the level of sustainability of the solutions, the resources available, and the nature of local practice.

Some countries' educational structures may neither require nor be able to provide a master's degree for APN roles, let alone doctoral-level education for faculty. Educational structures may be developed to include appropriate requirements for acceptance into schools of nursing, local or international faculty training, curriculum development, or the creation of educational pathways acceptable for certification without a master's degree.

As noted above, investment in resources and support is necessary at every level to develop these structures and build APN capacity (ICN 2024). National and international bridge or sandwich programs that incorporate distance/hybrid/blended education, international partnerships to create certification pathways, and residencies for hands-on learning may enable local practitioners to continue delivering care in their communities while developing the competencies necessary for advanced practice. As regulated educational programs are developed, countries may develop and establish pathways to certify APNs who are already practicing at this level. Aside from increasing the number of APNs, these pathways also ensure that APN faculty and preceptors are available for new programs, allowing students to learn from other APNs as well as physician specialists. Programs like this may also help nurses stay local and avoid relocating internationally after completing their training. This may prevent the "brain drain" and rural disparities in access to healthcare services and thus, health and well-being.

8.4 Low Resource Settings

Rural areas in many countries, including those in Africa, South America, and Asia, may aim to improve healthcare provision by increasing the number of healthcare providers (WHO and ICN 2025; WHO 2021). Since physicians are more likely to practice in urban settings, nurses have become the default healthcare workers, despite a need for more access to advanced training necessary for this critical role (Seitio and Newland 2008).

What does this mean for low- and middle-income countries that struggle with limited numbers of healthcare providers and restricted access to APN education, yet have a strong desire to increase access to advanced practice education for nurses and improve healthcare for underserved populations? Ensuring that nurses have access to the education they need to provide safe and comprehensive care is the best path. The most successful programs have been those that grow over time to sustainably meet the needs of the culture in which they exist.

As capacity grows, APN educational requirements can gradually elevate to the master's level. The ICN *Guidelines for Advanced Practice Nursing* acknowledge and accept that many countries cannot meet master's-level APN practice requirements initially (ICN 2020). Countries should be allowed to follow this continuum and develop the role at their own pace in relation to the available resources. In the meantime, certificate, residency, and diploma programs can support them in ensuring quality, comprehensive healthcare.

Finally, it is important to recognize that, despite a significant need for experienced APNs in various low-resource settings and rural areas to practice and to teach, disparities in educational pathways, regulations, scopes of practice, and credential recognition can hinder their ability to cross state, provincial, or international borders. Although the *Global Strategic Directions for Nursing and Midwifery 2021–2025* Report calls for ethical management of international mobility and migration (WHO and ICN 2025), APNs encounter considerable barriers, including education and credentialing gaps, licensing and certification challenges, and visa and work permit restrictions. However, efforts are being made to improve APN mobility (Peacock and Hernandez 2020; Poghosyan and Maier 2022). Some key initiatives include APRN compact licenses in the US and Mutual Recognition Agreements (MRA) in the European Union, which are working toward establishing common regional standards for APNs. Additionally, global nursing organizations, such as the ICN's Nurse Practitioner/Advanced Practice Nursing Network, advocate for the harmonization of international APN credentials to enhance APM mobility. Furthermore, some countries offer bridging programs, which are short-term courses designed to help foreign APNs meet local requirements.

9 Future Directions

The global landscape of advanced practice nursing presents unique and complex challenges and opportunities, underscoring the need for flexible, culturally relevant strategies that recognize the diverse educational infrastructures, scopes of practice, and regulatory frameworks. Implementation requires critical thinking, flexibility, creativity, and partnership on multiple levels to address conflation and increase resource allocation (Wheeler et al. 2022; Porat-Dahlerbruch et al. 2024). Maintaining APN competencies consistently across all levels of education ensures the best possible health outcomes and system benefits. While some nations, particularly those in high-income countries, have developed robust models of advanced practice that include master's-level preparation, the reality for many low- and middle-income countries is starkly different. In these settings, nurses may be educated at the certificate or diploma level, yet they may perform advanced skills, such as diagnosing and treating patients, due to healthcare shortages. APN advocates should avoid criticizing or imposing unrealistic standards on countries developing this role. Instead, they should provide evidence, offer supplementary education programs, and promote partnerships with countries successful in fostering a culture of hope, inspiration, and practical guidance for advancing advanced practice nursing globally.

One of the central conundrums facing APN development worldwide is the gap between aspirational goals set by organizations and the practical realities on the ground. For example, while many envision graduate-level education as a standard for APN roles, many countries need more foundational steps, or *baby steps*, to support nurses' growth within the systems they work in. Imposing rigid educational requirements where the infrastructure and support systems are not yet in place can hinder progress rather than promote it.

Governance and regulatory structures also play a crucial role in APN development, but the approach must be broad and adaptable. While *regulation* can sometimes feel restrictive, *governance* may provide a more expansive lens, considering institutional, governmental, and educational governance as part of a triangle necessary to support practice. Advancing APN roles is not just about imposing regulation or shifting tasks, but about building capacity—enriching nurses and their education to improve care and outcomes. This perspective is echoed in the 2025 WHO State of the World's Nursing Report, which notes that despite growing evidence on the benefits of APN care, restrictions on nurses' scope of practice represent a missed opportunity to improve health service access, quality, and effectiveness (WHO 2025). Countries that have successfully grown APN roles, such as Kenya and Botswana, have evolved gradually and organically, recognizing their own needs and capacities, and investing in education and health system infrastructure to support APN integration (Seitio and Newland 2008).

At the practice level, APN development cannot be achieved in isolation. Collaborations and partnerships between governments, nursing boards, educational institutions, and healthcare systems are essential. There have been cautionary tales of countries attempting to advance APN without securing support from one or more of these pillars, ultimately delaying progress. The takeaway from these stories is not to discourage, but to provide wisdom on the critical factors that must be in place for sustainable APN growth.

10 In Summary

We conclude with a vision of optimism: regardless of a country's current standing in nursing education and practice, there is a path forward for implementing and improving APN practice. Whether through certificate-level programs or graduate degrees, each step toward expanding APN roles will improve health outcomes, strengthen leadership, and contribute to the global health goals set by the Sustainable Development Goals (SDGs) and Global Strategic Directions for Nursing and Midwifery 2021–2025 (WHO 2021). The key message is that a rising tide lifts all boats—by investing in nursing, particularly APN, countries can meet their health goals, improve access to safe and effective care, and reduce morbidity and mortality worldwide.

References

Ainslie M, Capozzoli M, Bragdon C. Efficacy of distant curricular models: comparing hybrid versus online with residency outcomes in nurse practitioner education. Nurse Educ Today. 2021;107:105146. https://doi.org/10.1016/j.nedt.2021.105146.

American Association of Nurse Anesthesiology (AANA). Professional practice manual. 2025a. https://www.aana.com/practice/professional-practice-manual/. Accessed 20 July 2025

American Association of Nurse Anesthesiology (AANA). Scope of nurse anesthesia practice. 2025b. https://www.aana.com/wp-content/uploads/2023/01/scope-of-nurse-anesthesia-practice.pdf. Accessed 20 July 2025

Bryant-Lukosius D, Dicenso A. A framework for the introduction and evaluation of advanced practice nursing roles. 2004;48(5):530–40. https://doi.org/10.1111/j.1365-2648.2004.03235.x.

Bryant-Lukosius D, Valaitis R, Martin-Misener R, Donald F, Peña LM, Brousseau L. Advanced practice nursing: a strategy for achieving universal health coverage and universal access to health. Rev Lat Am Enfermagem. 2017;25:e2826. https://doi.org/10.1590/1518-8345.1677.2826. PMID: 28146177; PMCID: PMC5288863

Chevalier S, Paquay M, Ghuysen A, Stipulante S. Current state of simulation in advanced practice nursing programs: a survey in French-speaking countries. CSN. 2025;102:101723. https://doi.org/10.1016/j.ecns.2025.101723.

Clinical Nurse Specialist Association of Ontario (CNSAO). Standards of practice for CNS. 2025. https://chapters-igs.rnao.ca/node/2461. Accessed 20 July 2025.

Contandriopoulos D, Bertoni K. What explains interprovincial differences in the uptake of autonomous NP primary care practice? Healthc Policy. 2025;20(3):40–5. https://doi.org/10.12927/hcpol.2025.27601. PMID: 40624864

Diaz-Navarro C, Armstrong R, Charnetski M, Freeman KJ, Koh S, Reedy G, Smitten J, Ingrassia PL, Matos FM, Issenberg B. Global consensus statement on simulation-based practice in healthcare. Adv Simul. 2024;9(1):19. https://doi.org/10.1186/s41077-024-00288-1.

Fulton S. Evolution of the clinical nurse specialist role and practice in the United States. In: Fulton S, Goudreau KA, Swartzell KL, editors. Foundations of clinical nurse specialist practice. 3rd ed. New York: Springer; 2020. p. 1–19.

Fulton S, Goudreau KA, Swartzell KL. Foundations of clinical nurse specialist practice. 3rd ed. New York: Springer; 2020.

Haron Y, Romem A, Greenberger C. The role and function of the palliative care nurse practitioner in Israel. Int J Palliat Nurs. 2019;25(4):186–92. https://doi.org/10.12968/ijpn.2019.25.4.186. PMID: 31013196

Htay M, Whitehead D. The effectiveness of the role of advanced nurse practitioners compared to physician-led or usual care: a systematic review. Int J Nurs Stud Adv. 2021;3:100034. https://doi.org/10.1016/j.ijnsa.2021.100034. PMID: 38746729; PMCID: PMC11080477

International Confederation of Midwives (ICM). Essential competencies for midwifery practice, 2019 update. 2019. https://www.internationalmidwives.org/our-work/policy-and-practice/essential-competencies-for-midwifery-practice.html. Accessed 20 July 2025.

International Council of Nurses (ICN). Guidelines on advanced practice nursing. 2020. https://www.icn.ch/system/files/documents/2020-04/ICN_APN%20Report_EN_WEB.pdf. Accessed 20 July 2025.

International Council of Nurses (ICN). International Nurses Day 2024: the economic power of care. 2024. https://www.icn.ch/sites/default/files/2024-05/ICN_IND2024_report_EN_A4_6.1_0.pdf. Accessed 20 July 2025.

International Council of Nurses (ICN). Global Nursing Leadership Institute. 2025. https://www.icn.ch/how-we-do-it/nna-development-leadership-programmes/global-nursing-leadership-institutetm-gnli. Accessed 20 July 2025.

International Federation of Nurse Anesthetists (IFNA). 2025a. https://ifna.site/about-ifna/. Accessed 20 July 2025.

International Federation of Nurse Anesthetists (IFNA). Standards of education, practice, monitoring and code of ethics. 2025b. https://IFNA.site/app/uploads/2015/08/2012-IFNA-Standards-Codes-2012.pdf. Accessed 20 July 2025.

Jefferson K, Bouchard ME, Summers L. The regulation of professional midwifery in the United States. JNR. 2021;11(4):26–38.

Jones M, Cameron D. Evaluating 5 years' NIMART mentoring in South Africa's HIV treatment programme: successes, challenges and future needs. SAMJ. 2017;107(10):839–42. https://doi.org/10.7196/samj.2017.v107i10.12392.

Kra-Friedman, A., Clark, R., Dutchess, B. et al. Establishing the relationship between nurse practitioner integration and reductions in health disparities; 2025. BMC Nursing. (25,12). https://doi.org/10.1186/s12912-025-04190-7.

Kilpatrick K, Savard I, Audet LA, Costanzo G, Khan M, Atallah R, Jabbour M, Zhou W, Wheeler K, Ladd E, Gray DC, Henderson C, Spies LA, McGrath H, Rogers M. A global perspective of advanced practice nursing research: a review of systematic reviews. PLoS One. 2024;19(7):e0305008. https://doi.org/10.1371/journal.pone.0305008. PMID: 38954675; PMCID: PMC11218965

McInnis A, Schlemmer T, Chapman B. The significance of the NP preceptorship shortage. OJIN. 2021;26(1):Manuscript 5.

National Organization for Nurse Practitioner Faculties (NONPF). Standards for quality nurse practitioner education. 6th ed. 2022. https://cdn.ymaws.com/www.nonpf.org/resource/resmgr/ntfstandards/ntfs_final.pdf. Accessed 20 July 2025.

Ng'ang'a N, Byrne MW. Professional practice models for nurses in low-income countries: an integrative review. BMC Nurs. 2015;14:44.

NHS England. Workforce, training and education: advanced practice. 2025. https://advanced-practice.hee.nhs.uk/mpf2025/capabilities/. Accessed 20 July 2025.

Nove A, Ten Hoope-Bender P, Boyce M, Bar-Zeev S, de Bernis L, Lal G, Matthews Z, Mekuria M, Homer CSE. The State of the World's Midwifery 2021 report: findings to drive global policy and practice. Hum Resour Health. 2021;19(1):146. https://doi.org/10.1186/s12960-021-00694-w. PMID: 34838039; PMCID: PMC8627087

Nye C, Campbell SH, Hebert SH, Short C, Thomas M. Simulation in advanced practice nursing programs: a North American study. CSN. 2018;26:3–10. https://doi.org/10.1016/j.ecns.2018.09.005. ISSN: 1876-1402

Peacock M, Hernandez S. A concept analysis of nurse practitioner autonomy. J Am Assoc Nurse Pract. 2020;32(2):113–9. https://doi.org/10.1097/JXX.0000000000000374. PMID: 32015277

Poghosyan L, Maier CB. Advanced practice nurses globally: responding to health challenges, improving outcomes. Int J Nurs Stud. 2022;132:104262. https://doi.org/10.1016/j.ijnurstu.2022.104262. Epub 2022. PMID: 35633596; PMCID: PMC9040455

Porat-Dahlerbruch J, Ratz S, Ellen M. Development of a taxonomy of policy interventions for integrating nurse practitioners into health systems. Int J Health Policy Manag. 2024;13:8194. https://doi.org/10.34172/ijhpm.2023.8194. Epub 2024 Jan 22. PMID: 39620547; PMCID: PMC11607521

Porat-Dahlerbruch J, Ratz S, Aaron E, Ellen M. Understanding factors affecting the integration of geriatric nurse practitioners into health systems. J Am Assoc Nurse Pract. 2025;35(12):813–25. https://doi.org/10.1097/JXX.0000000000000937. PMID: 37610786

Reisen M, Hoekman J, Björkelund K. Global development of nurse anesthesia education from mid-nineteenth century into today's advanced nursing practice. In: Thomas SL, Rowles JS, editors. Nurse practitioners and nurse anesthetists: the evolution of the global roles. Cham: Springer; 2023. p. 343–65.

Seitio OS, Newland JA. Improving the quality of nurse practitioner education: the case of Botswana. Nurse Pract. 2008;33(3):40–5. https://doi.org/10.1097/01.NPR.0000313002.31328.bc. PMID: 18388834

Small K, Warton C, Fenwick J, Baird K, Homer C, Bradfield Z. The regulation and practice of midwifery prescribing around the world: a scoping review of regulations and literature. Sex Reprod Healthc. 2025;44:101109. https://doi.org/10.1016/j.srhc.2025.101109. Epub 2025 May 15. PMID: 40393113

Vetter L, Maurer D, Zumstein-Shaha M, Hug BL. Global scope of practice of an APN anesthesia: a scoping review. J Perianesth Nurs. 2025;40(3):738–744.e3. https://doi.org/10.1016/j.jopan.2024.07.016. Epub 2024 Oct 24. PMID: 39453349

Wheeler KJ, Miller M, Pulcini J, Gray D, Ladd E, Rayens MK. Advanced practice nursing roles, regulation, education, and practice: a global study. Ann Glob Health. 2022;88(1):42. https://doi.org/10.5334/aogh.3698. PMID: 35755314; PMCID: PMC9205376

World Health Organization (WHO). Global strategic directions for nursing and midwifery 2021–2025. 2021. https://iris.who.int/bitstream/handle/10665/344562/9789240033863-eng.pdf?sequence=1. Accessed 20 July 2025.

World Health Organization (WHO). Transitioning to midwifery models of care: global position paper. Geneva: World Health Organization; 2024. Available from https://iris.who.int/server/api/core/bitstreams/c7d90142-382d-417b-8b56-7189bd855d82/content

World Health Organization (WHO). Global network of WHO collaborating centers. 2025a. https://www.globalnetworkwhocc.com/.

World Health Organization (WHO), International Council of Nurses (ICN). State of the world's nursing 2025: investing in education, jobs, leadership and service delivery. 2025b. Licence: CC BY-NC-SA 3.0 IGO. https://iris.who.int/bitstream/handle/10665/381329/9789240110236-eng.pdf?sequence=1. Accessed 20 July 2025.

Policy in Advanced Practice Nursing Settings Around the World

Barbara Sheer and Patrick Browne

1 Introduction

Healthcare costs around the world have a significant impact on the global economy. In the United States (US) alone, over 18% of the nation's Gross Domestic Product (GDP) is spent on healthcare (Peterson-Kff 2026). These expenses are largely driven by chronic disease and comorbidities, which could be prevented or reduced by primary care (Shrank et al. 2019). In addition, the distribution of healthcare resources is inequitable, with access to care limited to those who can afford it but unavailable to large swaths of the population.

In the 1970s, the World Health Organization (WHO) identified this inequitable distribution of healthcare around the globe as a crisis that is politically, socially, and economically unacceptable. In response, they made a global call with the overarching goal of "health for all." Their vision included a re-allocation of world resources toward more equitable healthcare solutions to be achieved by the year 2000 and proffered primary care as the most central part of a country's healthcare system. While the goal of "health for all" by the year 2000 was aspirational, the concepts derived from their work remain at the forefront of healthcare policy (WHO 2018, 2026).

In 2000, the United Nations continued to promote the advancement of world health, including three distinct healthcare goals within the eight measurable targets for global development known as the Millennium Development Goals (MDGs)

B. Sheer (✉)
University of Delaware, Wilmington, DE, USA
e-mail: sheer@udel.edu

P. Browne
University of Galway, ESNO Associate, European Specialist Nurses Organization, Galway, Ireland
e-mail: Patrick.browne@hse.ie

K. J. Wheeler, M. Acorn (eds.), *Health Policy for Advanced Practice Nursing: A Toolkit for Implementation and Improvement*, Advanced Practice in Nursing,
https://doi.org/10.1007/978-3-032-03667-4_14

(WHO 2018). The MDGs were later replaced by the Sustainable Development Goals (SDGs) in 2015, which continued to include specific healthcare goals of ensuring healthy lives and well-being for all at all ages (WHO 2018). Specific targets within this goal included reducing maternal and child morbidity/mortality, fighting disease, and promoting health, including mental health, for all.

As healthcare policy is enacted, and healthcare systems evolve with efforts to promote these goals, nurses are there. They are essential components of the system and intertwined in all aspects of the care necessary to move toward these healthcare ambitions. Despite their vital importance in the healthcare community, they have not always been supported by national policy and regulation, nor invited to the table to make healthcare policy decisions. Fortunately, there have been advances in this area, resulting in the expansion of advanced practice nurses and an evolution of education, policy, and practice to support their work.

This chapter will begin with a historical perspective, introduce the importance of policy in expanding advanced practice nursing (APN) practice, and describe how the issues of scope of practice, title protection, prescribing, reimbursement, and legislation are intricately related to developing a workforce of advanced practice nurses that can assist with global healthcare goals of "health for all." Unique models employed by different nations will be described, and the collective knowledge and skills needed by APNs to achieve optimal effectiveness in delivering health will be highlighted.

2 Historical Perspective

In the early 1960s, many technological advances emerged that changed the healthcare landscape. These advances introduced expenses contributing to escalating healthcare costs and a workforce shortage in primary care as practitioners transitioned to specialty care. The combination of these forces also created a more imbalanced system where those who can afford these costs and access available providers can receive care, while those who cannot are left out. As noted above, the WHO recognized these disparities as unacceptable and defined a goal of "health for all" (WHO 2018, 2026). Their vision increased emphasis on primary care to promote health, human dignity, and enhanced quality of life. With this shift toward primary care, nurses were ideally positioned to make a difference (WHO 2018).

In the United States, Drs. Loretta Ford (a nurse) and Henry Silver (a pediatrician) understood the need for primary care. They believed that, provided with additional education and skills, public health nurses could meet the needs of the underserved pediatric population (Bruner 2012). What began as a demonstration project at the University of Colorado became the beginning of the nurse practitioner movement. As nurse practitioners were educated, they started filling the gaps in the healthcare system by delivering healthcare to disadvantaged and vulnerable populations who fell through the cracks, thereby increasing access in line with the WHO goals.

The demonstration program was not initially endorsed universally, with resistance arising from physicians, who saw a potential threat, and other nurses in more traditional roles who felt taking on additional skills was beyond the nursing role. Despite this resistance, Dr. Ford, armed with persistence, political acumen, and tenacity, was able to argue that the model deserved a chance, and the University of Colorado eventually embraced the program. As a scientist-practitioner, Dr. Ford was the ultimate advocate for nurses making a difference in healthcare delivery. She collected outcome data, published results, and spoke about the programs success. She collaborated tirelessly with educators, the board of nursing, nursing organizations, and other interested parties(stakeholders) to gain support and acceptance. Drs. Ford and Silver invited interested parties to come to the campus, learn about the program, and experience the difference the pilot program made for the rural pediatric population (Brush and Capezuti 1996).

Word of the program quickly spread across the country. The model was soon replicated by other innovative nurses who believed that the field of nursing could make a significant difference in the healthcare landscape with additional education. Interested parties began to develop and expand innovative nurse practitioner programs to encompass additional specialties, including adult, geriatric, women's health, and family. Most of the initial programs emphasized primary care. Still, the movement also began to advance to acute care settings, eventually including high-tech and specialized environments such as the ICU and emergency care. With this evolution, nurses in intensive care settings found themselves in situations that required an even higher level of assessment and diagnostic skills, and the field soon recognized that a master's degree would be necessary to keep pace with the expanding body of knowledge and increasing responsibilities the advanced nurses were undertaking (Pulcini et al. 2019).

While extremely successful, the rapid expansion of the nurse practitioner movement was not without challenges. Nurse practitioners soon confronted complicated regulation issues, scope of practice, titling, reimbursement, and prescribing. For example, the new scope of practice expanded beyond any healthcare regulation; titling became confusing; service codes and direct reimbursements from third-party payers were nonexistent; and prescribing was managed differently across settings. Some of these challenges continue to persist.

While the advanced practice nurse movement began in the US, international expansion soon followed. The role of advanced practice in nursing emerged as a response to the growing complexity of healthcare demands. In Ireland, the development of ANP can be traced back to the early 2000s, while the UK, comprising England, Scotland, Wales, and Northern Ireland, has a longer history dating back to the 1980s. The policies in both regions have evolved to address changing healthcare needs, professional standards, and the drive for improved patient outcomes (NCPDNM 2005).

Responding to healthcare needs in the United Kingdom (UK), Barbara Stillwell, a nurse practitioner, initiated the first nurse practitioner program at the Royal College of Nursing. This program was designed to meet the primary care needs of British communities, where nurse practitioners worked in collaboration with general medical practitioners (Reis 2016).

To continue to share and collaborate with US nurse practitioners, the first cohort of graduates from this British program was supported to attend a national conference sponsored by the University of Colorado. Here, the UK nurses began a new dialogue of sharing experiences and ideas from an international perspective. Beyond the conference itself, the new nurse practitioners could also shadow experienced American NPs to gain insight into how the role was actualized in the US. The exchange of ideas at this meeting was sufficiently impactful that a joint conference was proposed for 1991. The first US/UK international conference was held in London with the goal of supporting the new British nurse practitioners and establishing nurse practitioners/advanced practice nurses as a substantial force to improve healthcare globally. What started as a one-time event transitioned first to an annual meeting. Then, with each passing year, additional nations sent representatives, significantly increasing the international impact. Additional conferences would soon be held in the UK, Ireland, and Australia. In each conference, nurse practitioners could share experiences, challenges, and resources, and learn from each other. Mentorship was provided, and leadership programs were developed. The group began problem-solving on a global scale and strategizing to assist other nations that were developing new programs (Reis 2016).

As a result of the need for ongoing support and communication on a broader international level, the International Council of Nurses (ICN) developed a nurse practitioner/advanced practice nursing network (NPAPNN), which was launched in 2000. The development of the network itself was an exemplar of how nursing leaders working together with interested parties(stakeholders) can achieve a mutual goal. Specifically, the membership of ICN was initially set up through established enrollment in national member organizations with the expectation that nurses would belong to some national organization. As the nurse practitioner role was emerging worldwide, many nations did not have national organizations that could be managed within this system. Nurse practitioners from the UK and the US collaborated for a few years and shared a mutual identity. Still, if a broader network were to be established, it needed to be inclusive rather than exclusive. The goal was to support and mentor other nations in developing this emerging role. With the assistance of the ICN consultant, the NP leadership of the UK, US, and other interested parties (stakeholders), a new structure emerged for the advanced practice network. The resulting network was open to all NP's and interested parties free of charge. The network emerged as unique within the existing ICN structure through collaboration, knowledge, and negotiations. This was an example of nurses utilizing the political process for a positive outcome (NCPDNM 2005).

Under the auspices of the network, it became easier to communicate and network with nurses from a multitude of nations. This was essential as emerging groups around the world were experiencing similar issues during their individual growing trajectories in the role definition, titling, education, scope of practice, regulation, and reimbursement. The Network began by publishing three documents: a definition of advanced nursing practice, a scope of practice, and competencies. While it was recognized that not all nations with their developing roles could comply with the standards presented, the publications and models espoused represented goals to be attained in the future. This further progressed in developing international collaboration and agreement on the nurse practitioner/advanced practice role (Sheer 2000).

3 Overview of Policy in Practice and Roles Around the World

3.1 Defining Advanced Practice

The concept of "advanced practice" was not universal, and it was important to agree upon a definition of advanced practice that could be applied to all nations. How were nurses with advanced education and in advanced roles different from general nurses? How would this fit into the regulation scheme? Defining advanced nursing practice was a monumental task that the ICN (NP/APN) network undertook. The term "nurse practitioner" was widely accepted in the US, but did not translate globally. Some nurses in the UK were specialists and considered themselves advanced practice nurses. They may have had extensive training in a specific skill and were practicing at a level more advanced than the basic nurse. Nurse-midwives, clinical nurse specialists, and nurse anesthetists also practiced in advanced roles, but the roles were unique, with different skills and training. In Ireland, the concept of advanced practice was more defined and attached to a post initially, rather than the person, although this is no longer the case (NCPDNM 2005).

On the other hand, in developing nations, there were dramatic differences in educational backgrounds as nurses and lay community members in villages were providing significant healthcare without any formal education. To incorporate and clarify issues amongst these very different providers, a consensus was reached with the input of interested parties (stakeholders), and interested parties that the advanced practice nurse (APN) is "a registered nurse who has acquired the expert knowledge base, complex decision-making skills and clinical competencies for expanded practice, the characteristic of which are shaped by the context and/or country in which s/he is credentialed to practice. A master's degree is recommended for entry-level" (Sheer 2000). This definition was the first step in providing a standard to achieve and a direction for future educational programs, legislation, and policy development. The definition would be revised and refined over the years, but it was achieved by nurses working together for a common goal. The next step was to develop competencies and standards for further guidance in education. This required coalitions of educators, practicing nurses, and various other interested parties (stakeholders) from various nations to work together to form a consensus.

3.2 Education

Advanced practice nurses (APNs) education has had to evolve to include additional curricular content based on research and best practice models. Many programs began with post-basic education and then moved to degree status with a standardized curriculum. Other programs or short courses were offered by institutions to allow nurses to practice outside the usual scope and perform advanced skills in their institutions. Still, this training was extremely narrow, as these skills were not transferable to other institutions. There was also a general lack of consistency in standards, with each setting developing its own guidelines. To help resolve these issues, most advanced practice education eventually moved to the university setting with agreed-upon core courses including pathology, pharmacology, and physical assessment. The standardized curriculum would then include specialty courses in the areas of concentration based on settings ranging from primary care to acute care, and age ranges from neonatology to geriatrics. While this solved many problems within specific nations, one education model was unsuitable for all nations. Each nation responded to the need for education in diverse ways, based on opportunity or population needs. The important thread was the need for standardization to be recognized. It was important for nurses to collaborate with other interested parties (stakeholders) and be the prime movers in determining the path toward advancing nursing roles within the healthcare system. The following are examples of the educational evolution in Thailand, the US, Ireland, and the UK.

3.2.1 Thailand

In Thailand, the spark that ignited interest in developing advanced practice nursing education arose from a top-down approach, with the impetus arising from governmental healthcare reform. Specifically, national healthcare reform driven toward universal healthcare coverage was initiated through legislative action, which spurred a need for nursing education. In this example, interested parties (stakeholders) interested in primary care initiatives worked with the Institute of Research and Community Health to increase the number of primary care nurses (Sheer 2000). They established a policy of three levels of care. The first primary care level is at the community medical center, covering 10,000–20,000 individuals and is staffed by a physician, dentist, pharmacist, 3 nurses, and 6 other healthcare professionals. The second level is the community health center covering 5000–10,000 individuals. The third level is the health district covering fewer than 5000 individuals. The second and third levels have 1 to 2 nurses without physicians or dentists. With this scheme, it was estimated that 15,000 nurses would be needed to cover all three levels. In response, nursing schools established 4-month programs to prepare general nurse practitioners to work in the community. The National Health Security Office and Thailand Nursing and Midwifery Council (TNMC) agreed to educate 1000 nurse practitioners in post-basic 4-month programs for a brief time to meet the demand in rural areas as a stopgap measure. The nurses practiced in rural areas, and outcome data was collected regarding their effectiveness. The students in the short-term programs had the opportunity to attend additional programs building on complexity. The outcome data suggested that even the short programs had a positive effect on patient outcomes while they were developing the educational infrastructure on a higher level (Hanucharurnkul 2007). The intent was to discontinue the short-term programs as education moved to the master's level. This is an example of healthcare reform providing an impetus for education. Nurses were able to seize the opportunity to fill a need and work with policyholders to provide a much-needed service to the community.

3.2.2 The United States

By contrast, the expansion of advanced practice nursing education did not originate from legislative action or governmental interest, but rather from the ground-up, grassroots efforts of healthcare visionaries identifying a need and developing solutions to fill that need. Specifically, as previously described, US programs began with the demonstration project at the University of Colorado and evolved into post-baccalaureate certificate programs, master's, and finally to doctoral programs. The evolution took decades and was accomplished by nurses in leadership positions advocating for change and responding to population needs. The initial programs were post-basic certificate programs ranging from 6 months to a year. There was no standardized curriculum, and the quality of graduate experience and competencies varied. The programs were housed in hospitals, colleges, and medical schools. Nurse leaders in the National Organization of Nurse Practitioners (NONPF) developed curriculum guidelines, core competencies, and criteria for evaluation of programs. They also developed a directory of programs (Pulcini et al. 2019). The leadership of the individuals and educational interested parties (stakeholders) of the national organization provided the basis for the standardization of curricula.

3.2.3 Ireland and the United Kingdom

The UK had a similar experience with the growth of advanced practice nursing education sprouting from the academic roots of the Royal College programs. The programs offered at the Royal College of Nursing (RCN) in London were at the post-basic level. The content focused on primary care. The RCN program was later franchised, with the first satellite program offered at the University of Wales in Swansea (Reis 2016). Gradually, the education of nurse practitioners moved to the master's level at multiple universities. In Ireland, however, the education to Advanced Nursing Practice level was initiated at master's level (Castledinc 1994).

In both jurisdictions, the trajectory of nurse practitioner education as a process was determined by the healthcare system infrastructure, population needs, and educational infrastructure. These three examples provide different approaches to establishing educational consistency. It required knowledge of the healthcare system and the needs of the population. Nurses collaborated with other interested parties (stakeholders) to understand the population's needs and discover strategies to provide the healthcare needed within the context of the nation.

As standards of education increased worldwide, it was generally agreed that the essentials for advanced practice include courses in physical assessment, pathophysiology, and pharmacology. General and specialty courses in assessment, diagnosis, and management build upon the core to form the basis for nurse practitioner education.

3.3 Scope of Practice

The scope of practice is a complex issue. On a basic level, it encompasses the range of activities and responsibilities of the advanced practice nurse in a setting within the boundaries of regulation or protocol (Sheer 2000). It is determined in each nation within the context of the population's needs, the healthcare system, and regulations. The scope of practice is defined at the national, state, or institutional level. It is recommended that the scope of practice be flexible and broad to allow for growth. It usually encompasses ethical and cultural conduct, education, experience, and regulation. It further defines accountability and responsibility of the professional (Sheer 2000).

On one level, an institution can allow an advanced practice nurse the authority to undertake specific activities or responsibilities outside the ordinary scope of the basic nurse. This is granted with additional education and competency and may or may not require protocols. The expanded scope of practice is given for practice within the institution and is not transferable to other institutions. Other organizations can offer expanded privileges and the ability to provide care under specific protocols for nurses with additional education. The organization authorizes the authority, but it is not transferable.

On another level, the scope of practice for advanced practice nurses can be state, regional, or national. This may involve educational requirements, licensure, and certification. National organizations can determine the scope of practice, but it is then subject to regulations of individual states or regions or limited to the care of specific populations.

An example from the US demonstrates the complexity of scope of practice issues. National nursing organizations defined the scope of practice for nurse practitioners, which is broad and includes educational, ethical, and professional accountability. For example, the American Association of Nurse Practitioners (AANP) (2022), defined the scope of nurse practitioners as "the professional role in any healthcare setting … which includes but is not limited to assessment; ordering, performing, supervising, and interpreting diagnostic and laboratory tests; making diagnosis, initiating and managing treatment, including pharmacologic and nonpharmacologic treatments; coordinating care; counseling; and educating patients, their families and communities." This scope includes education, accountability, and responsibility, but does not guarantee that all nurse practitioners can practice to the full scope of their authority. The actual ability to practice is determined by regulation in each state. Some states allow full practice authority, while others prohibit certain activities and require protocols or collaborative agreements. A nurse practitioner is required to practice under the state practice act. In this model, a nurse moving from state to state needs to be aware of the nurse practice act in that state. For example, a nurse in one state may have full practice authority and practice independently, while in another state, a collaborating agreement may be required. The Institute of Medicine (IOM) recommended full practice authority for all advanced practice nurses (IOM 2011). Still, not all state regulators have accepted this, and the battle continues on a state-by-state basis. Nurses throughout the states have been networking and collaborating with national organizations, legislators, and other interested parties (stakeholders) to remove barriers and restrictions, but this process requires persistence and patience. Nurses are learning to be politically active and utilizing research and outcomes to make their case in pushing the envelope. The process will continue.

3.4 Title Protection

The use of a title should denote a certain status and responsibility. It may indicate education, licensure, and credentialing (Sheer 2000). In the case of the title Advanced Practice Nurse, there are several titles that can be used for the same position, creating ambiguity and confusion. "Advanced Practice Nurse" is usually a broad title that denotes nurse practitioners, clinical nurse specialists, midwives, and nurse anesthetists. Additional titles are more specific and linked to regulation and licensure. The following are three examples of the use of titles in the US, the Netherlands, Ireland, and the UK.

3.4.1 The United States

In the US, the title of advanced practice nurse is limited to nurse practitioners, clinical nurse specialists, nurse midwives, and nurse anesthetists. It requires graduation from an accredited program with a minimum of a master's degree, passing a certification examination by a national certifying board, and a license beyond the basic registered nursing license. The title is protected by law. While this title of "Advanced Practice Nurse" is straightforward and consistently understood under the auspices of nursing organizations, third-party payers, and national law, each state may require additional titles to designate registration in the state. This inconsistency creates confusion among the interested parties (stakeholders), legislators, and the public. As an example, a nurse practitioner in Pennsylvania will use Certified Registered Nurse Practitioner (CRNP) while another nurse practitioner with the same credentials in a neighboring state will be designated as APN.

3.4.2 The Netherlands

By contrast, in the Netherlands, titling evolved from an informal designation to a formalized protected title. In 2000, the founder of the first nurse practitioner program at Groningen, Dr. Petri Roodbol, awarded the new graduates a pin to designate that they were nurse practitioners. Other programs evolved in the Netherlands at the master's level, focusing on providing direct patient care. As the number of nurse practitioners increased, legislative policies were initiated to regulate practice. By 2002, the Dutch Council for Public Health and Health Care first saw the NP as an important partner in healthcare (Kruth 2024). By 2009, nurse practitioner specialties were officially recognized by the government. By 2021, the capacities of Nurse Practitioners were codified by law through the adoption of a government decree allowing NP's to independently perform tasks formerly deemed in the purview of medicine. The title Nurse Practitioner is protected by law. EU nations, including

Switzerland, Iceland, and Norway, can transfer registration to practice in the Netherlands (Kruth 2024).

3.4.3 Ireland

In Ireland, "Nurse" as a professionally regulated title initially gained legislative protection under the Nurses Registration Act of 1919. Similarly, as additional registers emerged, the Nurses and Midwives Act of 2011 protected these additional titles (Government of Ireland 2011). Nurses in Ireland must achieve a prescribed and regulated Registration before they can call themselves a Registered Advanced Nurse/Midwife Practitioner (NCPDNM 2005).

3.4.4 The United Kingdom

Title protection for nurse practitioners has been debated in the UK since the inception of the first NP program in the 90's. Many attempts have been made to afford the nurse practitioners title protection, but with limited success. Currently, nurse practitioners are covered by basic registration. Over the past decades, the Nursing and Midwifery Council has considered regulating nurse practitioners but has relied on professional codes of conduct instead. This has led to confusion in the UK (Rogers and Gloster 2023). Nurses continue to advocate for title protection.

3.5 Reimbursement: Direct and Indirect

Reimbursement presents another challenge for advanced practice nurses. Nurses may be reimbursed for services directly in the case of independent practice or indirectly through a contract with other professionals. Direct reimbursement is less common throughout the world. In the US, nurse practitioners may receive direct service reimbursement, but this process can be complex. Again, it varies state by state and by insurance companies. In nations with national health insurance, practices are under contracts for services provided to a specific population. When nurses are not directly reimbursed, they become invisible providers. This may decrease their bargaining power in the political arena.

3.6 Relationship of Practice, Education, and Regulation

Practice, education, and regulation are interrelated. The relationship is circular. As the advanced practice role has emerged in response to population needs, education, and regulation, changes in practice were required. In some cases, practice was expanded first, in other cases, regulation was followed by education and practice. Nurses have been innovative in developing new models that can be replicated. To accomplish expansion of services, it is necessary to identify population needs, and develop both appropriate educational curriculum and legislative regulation. Practice often precedes education and regulation. As nurses seek to care for a population, they are often called upon to care for complex healthcare needs. They may be the only providers in a vast geographical area. They may seek additional education to attain the skills needed. They then often find themselves practicing beyond the scope of practice of the basic nurse, so additional regulation is needed. The needs for healthcare in various communities and with underserved populations create opportunities for nurse practitioners and other advanced practice nurses to fill the void. Nurses have seized opportunities. Thailand is an example of how innovative nurses could secure available positions through regulation while developing an adequate educational infrastructure. The US responded to population needs by developing educational programs, followed by regulation. Whether the nurse practitioner movement emerges through education, regulation, or population needs, nurse practitioners must be aware of opportunities. They need leadership skills to take part in the decision-making process, and they need to become politically active to fill the gaps in healthcare and move toward the goal of "health for all."

3.7 Strategies for Political Action

Advanced practice nurses are a substantial force in delivering healthcare. As new roles develop and expand, advanced practice nurses must have the knowledge to understand healthcare's economic, political, and policy dimensions (Buresh and Gordon 2013). Educational programs are focused on clinical expertise and often do not include courses in global leadership and policy, which are necessary in today's environment. Nurses need to become politically competent in developing a toolkit for political action (Buresh and Gordon 2013). This calls for knowledge, leadership, networking, and communication skills.

3.7.1 Knowledge

Advanced practice nurses are experts in providing healthcare. They have the education and experience. Numerous studies have attested to their ability to provide accessible, cost-effective quality care. In the Future of Medicine 2020–2030, the Institute of Medicine (IOM) stated, "that until all advanced practice nurses are permitted to practice to the full extent of their education and training, significant and preventable gaps in access to care will exist" (IOM 2011).

Nurses and their work can be invisible and lack power and authority. Often, titling, scope of practice, and reimbursement obscure their visibility. Nurses must capitalize on their knowledge base and advocate for healthcare. They must know what needs to be accomplished to practice at their educational level and full scope of practice. This involves understanding the population's needs, governance, and the appropriate steps to make changes.

3.7.2 Leadership

Advanced practice nurses must assume leadership positions in local, regional, national, and international healthcare. They need to develop the necessary skills to do this. Leadership can begin by volunteering to take charge of small projects. As they gain confidence in their skills, additional opportunities will follow. These may include appointments to boards or committees or other leadership opportunities.

Aspects of acquiring leadership skills also include mentoring and networking. Finding a mentor with similar goals and values will assist in gaining skills and confidence. Networking with others allows forming coalitions. A place to start is with nursing organizations. The organizations can be local, regional, national, or international. They afford many opportunities to develop leadership skills. Beyond nursing organizations, joining and becoming involved with other organizations interested in healthcare is important. Sharing healthcare knowledge and advocating for healthcare make nurses important members of public organizations. Emphasis on healthcare lends credibility to the profession.

3.7.3 Communication

Moving toward political competency requires the ability to communicate the issues clearly and concisely. Interested parties (stakeholders) are those with power and authority either within or outside an institution, state, region, or nation (Kostas-Polston et al. 2015). They will come to the table with their own values and beliefs. It is important to identify interested parties (stakeholders) and understand their positions on the issues. This requires background research.

It is important to focus on a single most important issue at a time. A strategic plan will assist in narrowing down the scope of the issue. Once the issue has been agreed upon by the core group, others need to be educated. It is important to communicate the purpose of a change, the benefit, and the proposed outcome or the reason for a proposed change. It is important to articulate the healthcare benefits and cost-saving aspects. Change having an economic impact will be viewed more favorably.

Political competency requires using abilities, viewpoints, and values necessary for successful political engagement (Kostas-Polston et al. 2015). It is important to demonstrate how the desired outcome will influence health and healthcare. Enacting change requires a thorough understanding of values and misconceptions of others.

4 Exemplar Policy in Action in Ireland and the United Kingdom

Advanced nursing practice (ANP) plays a crucial role in healthcare systems, enhancing patient care, improving outcomes, and addressing the evolving healthcare landscape. In Ireland and the UK, policies governing ANP have undergone significant transformations in recent years.

Ireland's approach to ANP is characterized by a commitment to enhancing patient care through advanced practice while ensuring high professional standards. The Health Service Executive (HSE) and the Nursing and Midwifery Board of Ireland (NMBI) collaborate to define, regulate, and register ANP roles.

One significant policy development in Ireland is the recognition of various advanced practice roles, including Clinical Nurse Specialist (CNS), Nurse Practitioner (NP), and Nurse/Midwife Prescriber. These roles encompass a spectrum of responsibilities, from direct patient care to leadership, education, and research. The Irish policy framework also emphasizes ongoing professional development, ensuring that ANPs remain at the forefront of evidence-based advanced practice and decision-making.

ANP policies vary across the four nations in the UK but share common foundations. The National Health Service (NHS) in England, NHS Scotland, NHS Wales, and the Health and Social Care in Northern Ireland all recognize and regulate ANP roles.

One prominent feature of the UK's ANP policy is the emphasis on advanced practice education and accreditation. The UK has established specific education and training pathways for nurses aspiring to become advanced practitioners, with a focus on academic qualifications and clinical competence. Like Ireland, the role of ANPs in the UK encompasses clinical expertise, leadership, education, and research, aligning with the broader goals of the healthcare system.

While both Ireland and the UK recognize the importance of ANP in healthcare delivery, there are notable differences in their policy approaches. The UK, with its four distinct geographical NHS healthcare systems, exhibits variations in policy implementation and regulation, reflecting the devolved nature of healthcare governance. In contrast, Ireland's unified policy framework offers a more streamlined approach to ANP regulation.

Moreover, Ireland strongly emphasizes academic qualifications for advanced practitioners, requiring a minimum of a master's-level education for entry into ANP roles. The UK, on the other hand, provides flexibility in educational requirements, allowing experienced nurses to progress into advanced practice through a combination of clinical experience and education.

Advanced Nursing Practice policies in Ireland and the UK demonstrate a commitment to enhancing patient care and addressing the challenges of modern healthcare. While there are similarities, such as the recognition of various ANP roles and a focus on ongoing professional development, differences in educational requirements and policy implementation highlight the unique characteristics of each healthcare system.

As Ireland and the UK continue to navigate the complexities of healthcare delivery, their respective ANP policies will play a pivotal role in shaping the future of nursing practice and contributing to the overall well-being of patients and communities.

5 Exemplar of Policy in Action in the United States

In the US, the scope of practice is regulated by each of the 50 states. Expansion of practice is enacted in a piecemeal fashion, state by state. One state was initiating the first nurse practitioner program in the state. The state had a list of 100 nurse practitioners. Many were practicing more traditional roles involving teaching or school health. Those practicing in an expanded nurse practitioner role were employed by a health maintenance organization (HMO). They were part of a group led by a physician delivering primary care and practicing under the Nurse Practice Act for registered nurses.

With the development of an educational program, the nurse practice act needed to be revised to accommodate expanded practice. The Educational Program Director, the Executive Director of the State Nurses Association, the Executive Director of the State Board of Nursing, and other interested nurse practitioners met biweekly to discuss the changes needed. The group utilized documents published by national organizations. These documents included the scope and standards of practice, quality of care, and competencies of nurse practitioners. The group also networked with other states that had successfully passed model practice acts.

Once a draft was completed, an information packet was developed for legislators and other interested parties (stakeholders). It was a simple bifold pamphlet explaining the role of the nurse practitioner, education, practice locations, and a phone number for additional information. It included photos of a few nurse practitioners in action, particularly with vulnerable populations. A meeting was held with a group of supportive physicians to discuss the proposed regulatory changes and gain their support. The brochure was distributed to legislators and primary care offices for public education, in person when possible. Supportive legislators were enlisted to draft legislation, and others were solicited to support the legislation. Students were enlisted to speak at public forums. The bill was proposed and passed with negotiated restrictions. This was considered a partial win. Over the years, legislation was reintroduced to expand the practice act. This took time and commitment on the part of many. Students became graduates and leaders and continued with political activity.

Many of the program's graduates worked in underserved areas, which strengthened the case when the legislation was reintroduced to reduce restrictions, allow independent practice, and expand prescriptive privileges. Policy steps that ensured success included the following:

- Need for change in regulation
- Identification of interested parties (stakeholders)
- Development of concise materials
- Distribution of materials to interested parties (stakeholders) and the public
- Meetings with additional interested parties (stakeholders) and legislators
- Solicitation of support
- Negotiation on the final regulation
- Continued vigilance and reintroduction later

6 Lessons Learned

During this process, the group learned the value of collaboration and speaking with one voice. Talking points were distributed to ensure consistency in the messaging.

Interested parties (stakeholders) were researched to understand their values and possible concerns about the proposed legislation.

Networking was an important tool. Utilizing national research and documents made the information available on a national rather than a state basis.

Communication with other states that had successfully expanded their practice acts offered some strategies for success.

Including students afforded them leadership opportunities and mentoring from state and national leaders. Students were involved in the process as well as the outcome. They had a sense of ownership and accomplishment, and the value of persistence.

7 Conclusions

Advanced practice nurses worldwide provide quality, accessible, cost-effective care to vulnerable populations. As new healthcare models emerge, advanced practice nurses must be politically active and increase their involvement in regulation, education, and practice decisions. They must have a voice in policy decisions. This chapter aims to highlight the need for advanced skills in policy development. Nurses need to be politically astute as they continue to navigate the complexities of healthcare delivery. Their respective ANP policies will play a pivotal role in shaping the future of nursing practice and contribute to the overall well-being of patients and communities.

References

American Association of Nurse Practitioners (AANP). Scope of practice for nurse practitioners. Author; 2022. https://www.aanp.org/advocacy/advocacy-resource/position-statements/scope-of-practice-for-nurse-practitionershttps. Accessed 29 Jan 2026.

Bruner K. Revolutionary nurse. Coloradan Alumni Magazine; 2012. https://www.colorado.edu/coloradan/2012/09/01/revolutionary-nurse. Accessed 29 Jan 2026.

Brush BL, Capezuti EA. Revisiting "a nurse for all settings": the nurse practitioner movement: 1965-1995. J Am Acad Nurse Pract. 1996;8(1):5–11.

Buresh B, Gordon S. From silence to voice: what nurses know and must communicate to the public. 3rd ed. Ithaca: Cornell University Press; 2013.

Castledinc G. UKCC's standards for education and practice. Br J Nurs. 1994;3(5):233–4. https://pubmed.ncbi.nlm.nih.gov/27907394/. Accessed 29 Jan 2026.

Government of Ireland. Nurses and midwives act 2011. Irish Statute Book of the Office of the Attorney General Electronic Irish Statute Book; 2011. https://www.irishstatutebook.ie/eli/2011/act/41. Accessed 29 Jan 2026.

Hanucharurnkul S. Nurses in primary care and the nurse practitioner role in Thailand. Contemp Nurse. 2007;26(1):83–93. https://pubmed.ncbi.nlm.nih.gov/18041988/. Accessed 29 Jan 2026

Institute of Medicine (IOM). The future of nursing: leading change, advancing health. Washington, DC: National Academies Press; 2011. https://www.nap.edu/catalog/12956/the-future-of-nursing-leading-change-advancing-health. Accessed 29 Jan 2026.

Kostas-Polston EA, Thanavaro J, Arvidson C, Taub LFM. Advanced practice nursing: shaping health through policy. J Am Assoc Nurse Pract. 2015;27(1):11–20. https://journals.lww.com/jaanp/Abstract/2015/01000/Advanced_practice_nursing__Shaping_health_through.5.aspx. Accessed 29 Jan 2026.

Kruth T. Advanced practice nursing in the Netherlands. IAPN; 2024. https://internationalapn.org/2024/06/09/netherlands/. Accessed 29 Jan 2024.
National Council for the Professional Development of Nursing and Midwifery (NCPDNM). A preliminary evaluation of the role of the advanced nurse practitioner. Dublin: NCPDNM; 2005. https://search.library.nuigalway.ie/primo-explore/fulldisplay?docid=353GAL_ALMA_DS2144356230003626&context=L&vid=353GAL_VUJ&lang=en_US. Accessed 29 Jan 2024.
Peterson-Kff Health System Tracker. 2026. http://healthsystemtracker.org. Accessed 29 Jan 2026.
Pulcini J, Hanson C, Johnson J. National organization of nurse practitioner faculties: a 40-year history of preparing nurse practitioners for practice. J Am Assoc Nurse Pract. 2019;31(11):633–9.
Reis T. Introduction to advanced nursing practice – an international focus. Cham: Springer; 2016. https://www.academia.edu/86031584/Introduction_to_Advanced_Nursing_Practice_An_International_Focus. Accessed 29 Jan 2026.
Rogers M, Gloster A. The evolution of the nurse practitioner role and practice in the United Kingdom. In: Thomas S, Rowles JS, editors. Nurse practitioners and nurse anesthetists: the evolution of the global roles. Cham: Springer; 2023. p. 67–80.
Sheer B. International collaboration: initial steps and strategies. J Am Acad Nurse Pract. 2000;12(8):303–8. Available from: https://pubmed.ncbi.nlm.nih.gov/11930449/. Accessed 29 Jan 2026.
Shrank WH, Rogstad TL, Parekh N. Waste in the US health care system: estimated costs and potential for savings. JAMA. 2019;322(15):1501–9. https://doi.org/10.1001/jama.2019.13978. PMID: 31589283. https://web.archive.org/web/20240129021614/https://jamanetwork.com/. Accessed 29 Jan 2024.
World Health Organization (WHO). Health and Well-being. Author; 2026. https://www.who.int/data/gho/data/major-themes/health-and-well-being. Accessed 29 Jan 2024.
World Health Organization (WHO). Millennium Development Goals (MDGs). Author; 2018. https://www.who.int/news-room/fact-sheets/detail/millennium-development-goals-(mdgs). Accessed 29 Jan 2026.

Selected Practice Policy Issues for Advanced Practice Nurses: Scope of Practice, Title Protection, and Prescriptive Authority

Michelle Acorn, Melanie Rogers, Bianca Edwards, Samuel Wainaina, Cecilia Ndungu, Rubi Hickson, Kathy J. Wheeler, Heather McGrath, and Joseph Trinitas

1 Introduction

For advanced practice nurses (APNs) to practice there are numerous policies that need to be in place so the APN can practice effectively and efficiently. While there are many policy issues in practice, this chapter is devoted to three critical policy

M. Acorn (✉)
University of Toronto & Queen's University, Toronto & Kingston, ON, Canada
e-mail: michelleacorn@gmail.com

M. Rogers
University of Huddersfield, Liversedge, West Yorkshire, UK

B. Edwards
North Eleuthera District, Ministry of Health & Wellness, Eleuthera, Bahamas

S. Wainaina
Murungaru Health Center, Naivasha, Kenya

C. Ndungu
Nursing and Midwifery Education, World Continuing Education Alliance, Thika, Kenya

R. Hickson
University of California, San Francisco, CA, USA

National Association of Hispanic Nurses, Rohnert Park, CA, USA

K. J. Wheeler
University of Kentucky College of Nursing, Lexington, KY, USA

H. McGrath
St. James Public Health Services, St. James, Jamaica

J. Trinitas
KCMC University, Moshi, Tanzania

K. J. Wheeler, M. Acorn (eds.), *Health Policy for Advanced Practice Nursing: A Toolkit for Implementation and Improvement*, Advanced Practice in Nursing,
https://doi.org/10.1007/978-3-032-03667-4_15

issues—scope of practice, title protection, and prescriptive authority. This chapter does not address level of autonomy or practice authority (i.e., full practice, reduced practice, restricted practice).

Scope of practice (SOP) refers to the range of "knowledge, skills, and experience" a healthcare professional is expected to possess, while also defining the limitations of practice (HCPC 2021, para 1). SOPs vary by profession, by degree of education and credential, and by geography and regulatory bounds. They allow the professional to practice "safely, lawfully and effectively" (HCPC 2021, para 2). Contained within a legislative and regulatory framework, they provide professional accountability and set standards for practice as well as education (ICN 2010). They are dynamic documents intended to change according to healthcare needs, new knowledge, and advancing technology, thereby requiring periodic review and revision (ICN 2009). Because APNs address an expanded level of care, they need a dedicated SOP that reflects the knowledge, skills, and experience they provide.

Very closely related to SOP is the issue of title protection. Title protection is the restriction of certain professional terms only to those professionals who fulfill certain education and credentialing requirements as specified by the respective nursing law and/or regulation (ANA 2021). Legislation and regulations must take the extra step of providing title protection via separate legal provisions in order to secure title protection, thereby protecting both the profession and the public.

According to the ICN (2021c, p 5), prescriptive authority:

> refers to the level or extent to which a healthcare professional may legally prescribe. Depending on the provisions within the legislation under which the professional is practicing, their prescriptive authority may be broad or limited (Nissen et al. 2015).

Multiple agencies have produced some exemplary documents to assist with implementation and improvement of APN practice policy in all three areas:

- ICN Scope of Nursing and Decision-Making Toolkit 2010 (ICN 2010)
- ICN Guidelines on Prescriptive Authority for Nurses 2021 (ICN 2021c)
- ICN Guidelines on Advanced Practice Nursing 2020 (ICN 2020)
- ICN Guidelines on Advanced Practice Nursing-Nurse Anesthetists 2021 (ICN 2021c)
- ICM International Definition and Scope of Practice of the Midwife (ICM 2024a)
- ICN Code of Ethics for Nurses 2021 (ICN 2021c)

Development in the three areas is assisted when policymakers can also access model rules, regulations, and practice acts, easily accessible via Internet searches. One example is the National Council of Boards of Nursing Model Act of 2021 which, among other components, provides definitions and titles for nursing roles; scopes of practice; composition, powers, duties, and financial responsibilities of boards of nursing; and licensure processes. In the U.S., such a model provides guidance as boards of nursing update nursing laws and regulations.

2 Scope of Practice

2.1 Background and Context

The International Council of Nurses (ICN) has published guidelines on Advanced Practice Nursing and Nurse Anesthetists (ICN 2020, 2021a). According to the ICN APN guidelines, the Clinical Nurse Specialist (CNS) scope of practice extends beyond the generalist and specialized nurse in terms of both advanced expertise, role function, mastery of a specific specialty, and accountability due to their sophisticated nursing and health care knowledge. CNSs function as expert clinicians in a specialty and are leaders in advancing evidence-informed nursing practice by teaching, mentoring, and consulting (ICN 2020). Both direct and indirect levels of care core competencies have been determined. Direct CNS care interactions with patients, families, and groups focus interventions on prevention, maintenance, and alleviation in efforts to improve quality of life. They integrate advanced holistic knowledge for nursing diagnosis, wellness, self-care, diseases as well as prescribing (ICN 2021b) and order therapeutics (ICN 2020). CNSs also utilize data and knowledge to design, implement, and evaluate nursing interventions (ICN 2020). Indirect CNS care occurs through activities that influence patient care, including serving as a consultant in managing complex care problems, achieving quality outcomes with the interprofessional team, providing leadership, developing programs, and evaluating outcomes (ICN 2020).

The ICN APN Guidelines acknowledge that the NP scope of practice differs from the generalist nurse in terms of level of accountability and responsibility. The ICN position for Nurse Practitioners (NPs) scope of practice recognizes that NPs possess graduate-level advanced health assessment and critical decision-making, diagnostic and clinical management skills that include health promotion and disease prevention and pharmacology. NPs practice delivering expert direct clinical care and focus on providing a range of health services by managing individual families and population healthcare needs. NPs are licensed credentialed clinicians with broader levels of autonomy and work collaboratively with other professional teams. NP practice may include direct referrals and integrate education, research, and leadership (ICN 2020).

According to the International Confederation of Midwives (ICM), the scope of practice of "the midwife is recognized as a responsible and accountable professional, who works in partnership with women to give the necessary support, care and advice during pregnancy, labor and the postpartum period, to conduct births on the midwife's own responsibility and to provide care for the newborn and the infant. This care includes preventative measures, the promotion of normal birth, the detection of complications in mother and child, the accessing of medical care or other appropriate assistance, and the carrying out of emergency measures" (ICM 2024a, b). Policy and guidelines for advance practice nursing including nurse midwives should be further defined and delineated due to the cross-functional overlap between nursing and midwifery at the advanced practice level.

The World Health (WHO) Global Strategic Directions for Nursing and Midwifery policy priorities can be advanced with the APN scope of practice optimization, education, leadership, and especially through service delivery supporting improved population health outcomes across systems (Acorn 2021). A national and global call to action to leverage APN to enhance universal health coverage (UHC) and primary care and to remove impeding barriers for maximal scope of practice impacts are needed (Acorn 2021, Acorn 2023a, Acorn 2023b).

2.2 Ontario, Canada Scope of Practice Exemplar

The Canadian Health Institute for Health Information acknowledges NPs as the only title protected advanced practice nurses in Canada. Their scope of practice varies across the ten provinces and three territories across Canada. In 2024, 7477 NPs were employed in direct patient care in Canada. NPs are key contributors to the safe delivery of care across health systems. They integrate clinical skills associated with nursing and medicine to assess, diagnose, and manage patients in a variety of health care settings. Notable variations in scopes of practice for NPs across Canada exist in 30 of the 38 identified activities such as independent therapeutic management, pharmacotherapy, treatment and advanced interactions, and other advanced activities. For example, NPs possess full hospital privileges in Ontario, Manitoba, British Columbia, the Northwest Territories, and Nunavut, allowing them to admit, treat, and/or discharge hospital patients; these activities are out of scope in Quebec and restricted in the remaining provinces. The COVID-19 pandemic has highlighted the importance of collecting scope data to better support policy initiatives such as workforce migration to respond to capacity needs (CIHI 2020).

Due to primary health care workforce shortages and uneven access to care especially in rural, northern, and remote communities, the provincial government launched the NP Initiative in 1994 to address both the education and employment needs of NPs. In 1995, the Council of Ontario University Programs in Nursing (COUPN) began offering the Primary Health Care Nurse Practitioner (PHCNP) education program at ten university schools of nursing.

This author was President of the Nurse Practitioners Association of Ontario when Bill 179, also known as the Regulated Health Professions Statute Law Amendment Act, 2009 received Royal Assent December 2009, passing Bill 179. The new Act amended 26 health-related statutes including the Nursing Act, 1991 (RNAO 2011). The scope of practice for NPs endured years of advocacy and robust research to inform a shift away from a list-based scope of practice approach to care from diagnosing, to ordering medications, lab tests, and diagnostic imaging with the expansion of autonomous controlled acts for NP practice. Narrow list-based diagnosis and prescribing has fully evolved to safe and efficient, broad-based, autonomous scope of practice and comprehensive access to care. Stop gap measures were undertaken until enabling and empowering policy barriers were eliminated. The association utilized bridging scope of care mechanisms such as medical directives and delegation of acts authorized by physicians previously.

Significant progress has been made but a few barriers to full integration and practice of NPs remain across the health system. In Ontario, Canada as of February 2024, a major policy scope of practice barrier remaining is amendment of the Mental Health Act enabling NPs to complete mental health forms across health systems. Organizational culture to fully optimize, utilize, and support NPs to function at the top of their scope for their full value add is key. Enablement is crucial for patient outcomes, building staff capacity, retention, and building a critical mass of NPs for clinical leadership and addressing health solutions. Regulation and legislation policy amendments provincially and federally have expanded scope of practice for NPs related to the prescribing of controlled substances such as opioids and the assessment and provision of Medical Assistance in Dying.

Ontario, Canada has established and funded the first Nurse Practitioner Led Clinics (NPLCs) innovating enhancing access to primary care. The 27 NPLCs unique governance model boasts 51% of the board representatives as NPs, to optimize scope of practice beyond clinicians, leveraging them as clinical leaders and decision makers (NPAO 2025).

The role and scope of practice of NPs in Long Term Care (LTC) homes has evolved significantly but varies across countries. During the COVID -19 pandemic, Medical Directors in LTC homes in Ontario, Canada, were advised by their Medical Association to work virtually. In response, an Emergency Management Act issued by the government in 2020 enabled NPs to work as Medical Directors in LTC homes (McGilton et al. 2021; Ontario MOH 2025), until the Long-Term Care Act is amended. The NP scope of practice to act as Attending NPs optimizing the care for residents, families and building team capacity momentum is building and advocacy for further dedicated funding in ongoing.

Ontario, Canada showcased NP hospital admission with NPs functioning as Most Responsible Provider. The NP has primary responsibility and accountability for the care of a patient within the hospital and across the care trajectory including admission, treatment, and discharge (Acorn and Byers 2020). The MRP responsibilities for patient care upon admission include comprehensive history taking, provisions for ordering diagnostic tests, prescribing medications and treatments, rendering provisional diagnosis, regular care monitoring, documentation during hospital care until discharge, ensuring on call coverage, thorough completion of medical record upon discharge, linking to relevant community primary care providers and resource services, or referrals to specialists for transfer of accountability and responsibility. Hospital professional staff by-laws, credentialing, and privileging require amendments to be inclusive of NPs. Accountability and reporting structures for NPs currently align with the medical advisory council of privileged staff. Leveraging the role of the chief nurse executive (CNE) to oversee NP and nursing quality of care in hospitals was paramount. The CNE holds a strategic role to leverage senior executive nursing leadership and support infrastructures for nursing success and sustainability. The CNE role ensures NP appointments and performance reviews are relevant for patient needs and appropriate for the NP role. The Lakeridge Health NP-Led Hospital Model of Care in Whitby, Ontario was the first pioneering hospital to showcase care delivered by NPs as the MRP and granted full admitting rights through organizational support since July 2012. NP competence and population needs should be the driver of meaningful change (Acorn 2015). Five years after the NP as MRP model of care in hospitals in Ontario was implemented, minimal uptake in the adoption or integration of this role had occurred. A framework for the process of adoption of NP as MRP can be described utilizing Rogers Diffusion of Innovation Model. Diffusion is the process where the attributes of the innovation are communicated (knowledge, persuasion, decision, implementation, confirmation), resulting in a timeline related to adoption (innovators, early adopters, early majority, later majority, laggards). Successful innovation diffusion and reduced uncertainty facilitate adoption in four key areas: innovation characteristics, effective communication channels, decision-making steps and the social system characteristics. Evaluation of the outcomes of NP as MRP model is improved if population and institution specific (Hurlock-Chorostecki and Acorn 2017).

2.3 United Kingdom Scope of Practice Exemplar

This exemplar briefly discusses the scope of practice for nurse practitioners in England which is one of four countries in the United Kingdom (U.K.). NP roles began to evolve in the late 1980s initially in primary care before developing in all areas of clinical practice. The Royal College of Nursing (RCN), a union and professional body for nursing, developed the first scope of practice for NPs in 2008, this was updated in 2012 and then in 2018 (RCN 2012, 2018).

In England, the title *Advanced Nurse Practitioner* (ANP) is commonly used by nurses who are educated at master's level in clinical practice and have full autonomy and authority to assess, diagnose, and treat patients in all clinical settings. The only restriction for ANPs' scope of practice is maternity care, which must be provided by a midwife or medical doctor (RCN 2024). The scope of practice whilst generic in nature identifies specific domains within its scope including:

- Providing autonomous decision making
- Ensuring accountability for own practice
- Assessing and managing patients who present with undifferentiated and undiagnosed presentations
- Making diagnoses and managing patients
- Prescribing independently
- Performing public health screening
- Admitting and referral rights
- Working collaboratively with other health care professionals
- Providing leadership
- Engaging in research and education

In 2017, England moved from allowing only nurses to fulfil advanced practice roles to a multi-professional approach for advanced practice, meaning all healthcare professionals are able to train to work at an advanced level, utilizing the four pillars of practice: clinical practice, leadership and management, education, and research (NHS 2017). In England, the commonly used term for all health professionals working at an advanced level is *Advanced Clinical Practitioner* though many nurses still use the ANP title.

In England, NP development started in the 1980s with Barbara Stilwell pioneering the role (Stilwell 1988) followed by the RCN establishing the first NP training in the 1990s, which later became an accredited program (Rogers and Gloster 2023). At this time, there was no scope of practice to follow as an NP. The training comprised 1 day at university with the rest of the training occurring in clinical practice. The fees for training were paid by the government, and trainees received salaries. The NP apprentice was expected to see *all comings* throughout an 18-month diploma. Primary care appointments were every 10 min though this author negotiated that 15 min were needed in order to bring together "the best of nursing with the best of medicine", thereby offering holistic care to patients.

Lack of prescribing, lack of referral rights, and no NP scope of practice started causing problems. In those early days, NPs stood outside the physician's room until they were free to write the prescription or complete the referral. Prescribing rights began to develop in 2001; however, the formulary was limited to few medications, and physician colleagues were still needed to sign prescriptions (DH 2005, 2006, 2010). However, independent prescribing has evolved, and there are now no restrictions on what can be prescribed and no more standing outside a door asking another clinician to sign prescriptions. NPs are now fully accountable for the prescribing decisions made.

This author found a unique way to not only improve the referral situation but also impact NP isolation and networking. National NP forums were developed, resulting in discussions on clinical practice, education, and leadership. After physicians began rejecting referrals from NPs hospital consultants and physician specialists were invited to the forum discussions. The physicians were impressed with the NP knowledge, experience, and expertise. Not only did the physicians start accepting the referrals they started teaching some of the sessions and consulting more with the NPs.

A final key challenge is the lack of regulation of advanced practice roles and title protection. In 2012, the RCN moved from the title of NP to ANP in order to recognize the advanced level of practice. However, until just recently, the nurse regulator, the Nursing Midwifery Council (NMC), had not seen the need to regulate the role; therefore, there is no title protection or regulation in the U.K. Ongoing challenges relate to the lack of regulation and title protection. For that reason, at the time of this writing, the NMC is again looking at regulation of the ANP role. Other challenges include a lack of educational standardization however this will be addressed if regulation occurs.

2.4 Bahamas Midwifery Scope of Practice Exemplar

In the Bahamas, an archipelago of around 700 islands and cays, healthcare delivery faces unique challenges but continues to be strengthened with the collaboration of the Nurses Association of the Commonwealth of the Bahamas (NACB), the Ministry of Health and Wellness (MOHW), and other interested parties (stakeholders) in health. The healthcare infrastructure is managed by the Ministry, which operates under two fundamental entities: the Department of Public Health (DPH) and the Public Hospitals Authority (PHA). The DPH oversees a vast network of healthcare services, including six health centers/polyclinics, 18 main clinics, and eight satellite clinics spread across the inhabited islands. Additionally, both Nassau and Freeport, Grand Bahama, are served by a mix of public and private clinics. The PHA is responsible for public hospitals, including a geriatric and mental health/rehabilitation center. There are private hospitals in both cities in The Bahamas. Additionally, private medical centers are strategically placed on some islands. These facilities form the backbone of healthcare provision in the country.

Approximately 195 nurses and nurse midwives are employed across the public hospitals and clinics within this comprehensive healthcare system, contributing to various essential services. However, a notable challenge in the sector is the lack of complete data on the total number of nurses and midwives, partly due to the non-mandatory nature of annual nursing license renewals. This gap in data presents a hurdle in fully understanding the workforce dynamics and needs within the Bahamian healthcare system. Despite critical services, including antenatal and postnatal care, roles often go unrecognized and under-compensated. The call for standardizing midwifery education and improving workforce retention through better conditions and remuneration resonates with the Bahamian context. The new Nurses and Midwives Act offers a framework for addressing these issues, but its success hinges on effective implementation.

2.4.1 Legislative Evolution and Its Impact

Nurses in The Bahamas previously practiced under the Nurses and Midwives Act of 1971. A newly passed Nurses and Midwives Act was finalized on May 22, 2023, heralding a transformative era for nursing and midwifery in The Bahamas. It introduces the Advanced Practice Nurse (APN) role, encompassing Midwives, Nurse Anesthetists, Clinical Nurse Specialists, and Nurse Practitioners, expanding their scope of practice significantly. This legislation mandates annual licensing by the Bahamas Nursing Council, requiring evidence of continuous professional development for re-licensure. It updates terminology, raises entry-level requirements, establishes a Bachelor of Science in Nursing as the entry-level for registered nurses, and provides for temporary licensing of Nurse Interns. This act is a monumental step toward modernizing and enhancing the nursing and midwifery professions. Its activation will be through the Ministry of Health.

It is anticipated that the new regulation and recognition will lead to enhanced service to patients, improved professional identity, better infrastructure (i.e., better records accessibility and telehealth via more extensive, more reliable Internet service; accessible ultrasound machines), enhanced recruitment and retention of nurses and midwives, leadership development, and better state funding for community health promotion initiatives. Hopefully, ongoing and structured collaboration between the Bahamas Midwives Association, the Director of Nursing, the Ministry of Health and Wellness, and the Bahamas Nurses Association can result in better compensation, career ladders, safer work environments, and more effective training programs for nurses and midwives so they can care for patients in the manner that optimizes healthcare across the Bahamas.

2.5 Kenya, Africa Scope of Practice Exemplar

In Kenya, the APN role has undergone significant evolution over the years, adapting to the changing needs of society and the healthcare system. This evolution has been driven by a variety of factors, including the need to address health challenges, increase healthcare accessibility, and improve the quality and affordability of healthcare services. The contribution has not been solely limited to providing direct healthcare services but also playing crucial roles in shaping health policies, improving healthcare systems, and advocating for patient welfare.

The initial scope of practice for Kenyan midwives and nurses was written in 1997, followed by updates in 2007 and 2021. A scope of practice for advanced nurses and midwives, as defined by the ICN advanced practice definitions (master's level), is in progress (Ministry of Health 2022). Nonetheless, considerable advanced care is provided through certificate, diploma, or bachelor's degree-trained nurses and midwives.

Over the years, several critical meetings were held to discuss strategic approaches to the implementation of APN initiatives in Kenya. In 2018, the Nursing Council of Kenya met with several universities and deans of schools of nursing to discuss APN education, resulting in program development at multiple universities. That same year other meetings were held to authorize the first edition of the Scope of Practice for Nurse Anesthetists (NCK 2018), launched in 2019 (KRNA 2019).

Despite these significant steps, there were concerns about APN development and progress. APN education was not standardized, and those individuals with degrees beyond a bachelor's degree struggled to find well-established clinical positions (Msuya et al. 2017), with many moving into exclusively management or education roles (East et al. 2014). These professional issues and the recognition that one of the best ways to meet the Kenya Health Policy Framework 2014-2030, achieve universal health coverage, and attend to population needs was to undertake a gap analysis. Ndirangu-Mugo and colleagues published *Scopes of Practice for Advanced Practice Nursing and Advanced Practice Midwifery in Kenya: A Gap Analysis* in 2024, specifically to identify opportunities and threats toward smoothly integrating APNs into the Kenya healthcare system. Table 1 presents gap analysis findings and insights into what factors need attention in order to ensure APN role implementation and improvement and may be useful for other countries undertaking similar introduction and development of the role.

Table 1 Facilitators and barriers to APN role implementation in Kenya

Facilitators	Barriers
Kenya health policy framework (p 4) Standard in place to provide equitable and high-standard healthcare to all Kenyans, including those in rural and underserved areas (including reproductive and emergency care)	Financial support in education and training (p 5) Lack of faculty Lack of preceptors Lack of clinical sites (i.e., competing with medical residents in hospitals) Despite educational preparation tendency to assign these workers to work not reflective of the preparation
Strategic partnerships and Alliance (p 4) Ongoing growth in APN programs in Africa History of financial and technical support by Western countries for the role	Lack of regulation for advanced practice (p 5) Lack of regulations through registration, licensure, and scope of practice for any nurses other than certificate-, diploma-, and bachelor's degree-trained nurses and midwives Situation results in graduate-and PhD/DNP-educated nurses and midwives serving in exclusively administrative or education roles
Contribution to sustainable development goals (SDGs) (p 4) APNs have the potential to contribute to multiple SDGs through access to health promotion, preventive services, and curative services APNs have the potential to contribute to other SDGs by ensuring education, gender equality, decent work, economic growth, and reduced inequalities for those educated in nursing and the population served	Opposition from the medical profession (p 5) Opposition by medical associations
Leadership (p 4) Despite educational preparation (i.e., strategic partnerships and alliances, implementation of evidence, mentorship, quality improvement, collaboration, community involvement) the nursing profession rarely serves in positions of leadership	Structural challenges (p 6) Lack of APN programs Lack of locally trained and practicing APNs Limited succession plans to produce local capacity for nurses moving to advanced training
Early steps toward institutionalization (p 5) Progress already made toward role integration (e.g., two universities offering programs of study and clinical hours consistent with global standards)	
Population needs (p 5) Substantial portions of population have limited resources and limited access to providers Population growing in rural and underserved areas Need for capacity building	

Ndirangu-Mugo et al. (2024). Access article to view sources for above conclusions

3 Title Protection

The ICN, representing over 130 national nursing associations and millions of nurses worldwide, has released numerous position statements, updated in 2012, advocating for the legal protection of the title *nurse*. According to the ICN, this title should be used exclusively by authorized individuals practicing nursing to protect the public, employers, and nurses themselves from unqualified individuals assuming the role of a *nurse*. The ICN emphasized that the absence of formal title protection could lead to individuals practicing nursing without the necessary competency. The organization further recommended that anyone unlawfully using the title *nurse* should face criminal, civil, and/or administrative repercussions, along with those who aid them (ICN 2012a).

The same principle applies to advanced practice nursing, with regulatory bodies needing to provide the same protection via jurisdictionally determined terms. Title protection for APNs maintains the integrity of the profession. The APN role is a growing trend worldwide, and its development and adoption vary among countries (Chun et al. 2021; Scanlon et al. 2022; Sheer and Wong 2008; Wheeler et al. 2022). A study authored by Wheeler et al. (2022, p 16), an online survey with 325 respondents representing 26 countries, found that title protection was a critical professional issue, regardless of geographic mobility, with half of the countries reporting no title protection for APNs. The same study concluded that each jurisdiction must narrow the title and codify it along with scope of practice. In the hope of clarifying terms and roles, international organizations have taken the lead, generating the following documents:

- ICN Guidelines on Advanced Practice Nursing 2020 (ICN 2020)
- ICN Guidelines on Advanced Practice Nursing-Nurse Anesthetists 2021 (ICN 2021c)
- ICM International Definition and Scope of Practice of the Midwife (ICM 2024a, b)

The International Council of Nurses Nurse Practitioner/Advanced Practice Nursing Network's research indicates that approximately 70 countries have either implemented or are introducing the APN role. Additionally, it was found that about 70% of hospitals have some form of advanced nursing practice (Parker and Hill 2017).

APNs' role is increasingly diverse, with a highly adaptable and effective approach to addressing emerging health challenges (Poghosyan and Maier 2022). Current issues are driving the incorporation of APNs into new delivery models, given rising healthcare costs, an aging population, improved health promotion, chronic disease prevention and management, and physician shortages (Bryant-Lukosius et al. 2017).

In several countries, like Australia, Canada, France, and the Netherlands, APNs have the authority to provide treatment and prescribe medications (Mackavey et al. 2024; Sheer and Wong 2008). With the expansion of APN scope of practice to full practice authority, APNs in the U.S. are now licensed and authorized to assess patients, diagnose their conditions, order and interpret diagnostic tests, and initiate and manage treatments. This includes prescribing medications and controlled substances under the licensure authority of a state board of nursing (ANA 2025; Boehning and Punsalan 2023; Kleinpell et al. 2022). As the role of APN continues to grow globally to meet healthcare demands, advocates argue that title protection of the APN must be prioritized.

3.1 Ensuring Public Safety, Achieving Public Trust, and Upholding Professional Integrity

Title protection, as defined by the American Nurses Association (ANA), refers to restricting the use of the title to only those individuals who have fulfilled the requirements for licensure. It is a protection for the public against unethical, unscrupulous, and incompetent practitioners (ANA 2021). The ICN position statement on protecting the title *nurse* ensures accountability and responsibility for maintaining competence and practicing within their scope of practice (ICN 2012a, b).

Without title protection, anyone can claim to be an APN, potentially misleading the public about their qualifications to provide care. Not having title protection can lead people to provide misinformation and falsely state that they are APNs. In the absence of legal restrictions, implementing title protection becomes crucial to ensure patient safety, prevent confusion, and uphold the integrity of the nursing profession. Professional representation is essential for identifying duties, responsibilities, and compliance with practice standards.

Licensed/registered/regulated APNs are required to adhere to the standards established by a licensing/registration/regulation body. This body ensures that APNs have attained the necessary level of education, competency, and regulatory compliance for their specific scope of practice to ensure patient safety (Flook 2003). The licensing agency has the authority to take disciplinary actions in case of law and regulation violations. APNs are accountable to their patients, the nursing profession, and the licensing board and must comply with the regulations set by the governing body (Flook 2003; Kugler et al. 2011).

Title protection will ensure that only qualified healthcare professionals meeting the highest legal and professional standards can use designated titles. APNs are entrusted with the care of patients and are expected to adhere to the highest ethical and professional standards. When individuals publicly identify themselves as APNs, patients and families can engage and trust that they will receive competent, safe, and reliable care. The public has the right to know who is providing care and that they are who they state they are. Transparency regarding healthcare providers is crucial for patient safety because patients are vulnerable since they often share intimate information about their illnesses or diseases. Title protection helps safeguard patients' rights and ensures they receive the best and highest level of care and are protected from unethical and incompetent providers.

Protecting the title of APN is paramount to ensure that only APNs can identify as APNs. The underpinnings of the APN profession are the trust in a patient-provider relationship, a high level of education and skill, delivering compassionate care, bridging the gap between patients and the healthcare system, and advocating for patients.

The Gallup Poll's Most Honest and Ethical Professions survey has ranked the nursing profession as the most *trusted* profession in America for 22 consecutive years (Brenan 2023). Nurses and APNs cultivate public trust by conscientiously adhering to their code of ethics. This social obligation solidifies the profession's credibility by underscoring the promise to provide and advocate for patient safety, prioritize respect and compassion, and maintain integrity and professionalism. According to the ICN Code of Ethics for Nurses (2021c), nurses and nursing students are expected to adhere to ethical values, responsibilities, and professional accountabilities that define and guide ethical nursing practice across various roles. Sections 1.1–1.4 (ICN 2021c p 9) are crucial for ensuring the welfare and safety of society in relation to healthcare providers.

Section 1.1:

Nurses' primary professional responsibility is to people requiring nursing care and services now or in the future, whether individuals, families, communities, or populations (hereinafter referred to as either 'patients' or 'people requiring care').

Section 1.2:

Nurses promote an environment in which the human rights, values, customs, and religious and spiritual beliefs of the individual, families, and communities are acknowledged and respected by everyone. Nurses' rights are included under human rights and should be upheld and protected.

Section 1.3:

Nurses ensure that the individual and family receive understandable, accurate, sufficient, and timely information in a manner appropriate to the patient's culture, linguistic, cognitive, and physical needs, and psychological state on which to base consent for care and related treatment.

Section 1.4:

Nurses hold in confidence personal information and respect the privacy, confidentiality, and interest of patients in the lawful collection, use, access, transmission, storage, and disclosure of personal information.

3.2 United States (U.S.) Title Protection Exemplar

In the U.S., the regulating bodies for nursing and advanced practice are at the state and territorial level. This resulted in geographical variations in terms of APN titling, scope of practice, and credentialing. This variation was confusing to patients, policy makers, insurers, data keepers, and researchers. For APNs and organizations that served multiple states and across state borders, the situation was particularly cumbersome, especially during emergency situations. This led to a multi-agency, multi-year effort to produce a list of recommendations related to APN regulation, specifically on licensure, accreditation, certification, and education (LACE), referred to as the Consensus Model for APRN (Advanced Practice Registered

Nurse) Regulation, published in 2008 by the work of the APRN Consensus Work Group and the National Council of State Boards of Nursing APRN Advisory Committee. Endorsed by 48 U.S. associations, a key recommendation centered on titling for APNs, hopefully leading to title congruency throughout the U.S. and simplifying licensure. Key elements of the Consensus Model include:

- Titling: Advanced Practice Registered Nurse (NCSBN 2025, para 1).
- License: Holds an APRN license (NCSBN 2025, para 1).
- Four roles: Certified Nurse Midwife (CNM), Certified Nurse Practitioner (CNP), Certified Registered Nurse Anesthetist (CRNA), Clinical Nurse Specialist (CNS) (NCSBN 2025, para 1).
- Education: completion of postgraduate education is required (NCSBN 2025, para 1).
- National Certification: APRNs must pass a nationally accredited certification exam (NCSBN 2025, para 1).
- Autonomous Practice: APRNs are granted authority to practice autonomously without physician oversight such as collaboration/supervisory agreement (NSCBN nd para 1).
- Autonomous Prescribing: APRNs are granted authority to prescribe without physician oversight such as collaborative/supervisory agreement.
- Population Foci: APRNs are educated and certified in both their role (see above) and one of six population foci: family/individual across the lifespan, adult-gerontology, women's health/gender-related, pediatrics, neonatal, psychiatric/mental health. The adult-gerontology and pediatric population may be further delineated as primary or acute (NCSBN 2025, para 2).
- Specialty Preparation: preparation in a specialty is optional but if an APRN chooses to do so the specialty builds on the APRN role/population-focused (IOM 2011). For instance, a family nurse practitioner could choose to seek an additional certification in diabetes, infection control, palliative care, or dozens of other specialty certifications.

The document went on to specify implementation strategies for the model, including details for boards of nursing, accreditors, certifiers, and educators (IOM 2011). Once fully adopted, it is thought that the Consensus Model will allow multistate licensure via an APRN Compact. The model demonstrates the critical nature of titles and role classifications, and the hard work it took to standardize terms and defining elements.

4 Prescriptive Authority

4.1 Background and Context

The ICN recently published guidelines on advanced practice nursing and prescriptive authority for nurses (ICN 2020, 2021a, b). The ICM updated similar guidelines for midwives in 2024. Nurse prescribing has existed for over 50 years in some regions and jurisdictions of the world. Prescribing is a complex process that requires in-depth understanding of clinical pharmacology and disease, clinical judgement to weigh the risks and benefits of treatment. It is differentiated from supplying or dispensing of medication and its administration to patients (ICN 2021b). Prescriptive authority refers to the level or extent to which a nurse may legally prescribe ranging from broad prescriptive authority to limited prescriptive authority. Health care workforce policies supporting nurses to their level of education and skills improve job satisfaction and may advance nursing recruitment and retention strategies (ICN 2021b).

A review of the literature demonstrates evidence supporting nurse prescribing (ICN 2021b). Nurses practice with varying but high levels of prescribing autonomy safely in a range of settings. Prescriptive authority for nurses can improve effective and efficient service provision, integrate patient care, increase professional satisfaction, and improve the quality of health services. Three categories of nurse prescribing include independent prescribing, dependent supplementary prescribing, and structure prescribing protocols. A strong clinical background and clinical knowledge are foundation to effective prescribing practices, regardless of the level of nurse as a general or advanced practice registration (ICN 2021b).

A global advanced practice nursing review of systematic reviews was conducted in 2024. A total of 24 reviews were identified. Prescribing was captured under provider indicators. APNs, NPs, and CNSs in both primary and acute care were studied. Prescribing activities include medications, systemic anticancer therapy, blood tests, laboratory tests, weight loss pharmaceuticals, rescue medication, and opioids. Equal to statistically significant results favoring prescribing interventions are evident (Kilpatrick et al. 2024).

The World Health (WHO 2021) Global Strategic Directions for Nursing and Midwifery policy priorities can be advanced through nurse prescribing, education, leadership, and service delivery supporting improved population health outcomes across systems (Acorn 2021). ICN prescribes a global call to action to leverage nurse prescribing to enhance universal health coverage (UHC) and primary care and to remove impeding barriers for maximal impact (ICN 2021b; Acorn 2023a, b).

Access to the scope of practice or the controlled act of prescribing is fundamentally a paradigm shift and tipping point for APNs to optimize comprehensive access to care. Once prescriptive authority is granted, access to the rest of the advanced practice scope of practice really opens up including autonomous broad independent prescribing, diagnosing, and ordering diagnostics. Supportive health system policy, enabling practice environments, and ensuring optimizing quality education for public safety and timely access to care are essential for scaling up and scaling out APN prescribing.

4.2 Jurisdictional Prescribing Policy Toolkit Recommendations

1. Conduct a literature review and environmental scan to capture prescribing standards, competencies, and health workforce solutions to meet primary health care. Target evidence-informed population needs-based realities that could leverage

advanced scope of nursing practice prescribing contributions that embed your country data as well as local to global implementation.[MA1]

2. Create a high-level draft document of your proposed prescribing policy solution targeting improved access to care and patient experience.

A *SBAR* format is helpful to succinctly summarize advance practice nurse prescribing (S-situation, B-Background, A-Assessment, R-Recommendation).

3. Align your prescribing policy with organizational and political health priorities. Garner support with both government and bureaucratic staff, including the government chief nursing/midwifery officer and the ministers of health and education.
4. Build allies to bolster buy-in and support with the regulator, educators, unions, employers, and associations. Letters of support are helpful that delineate collaboration.
5. Embed outcome measures such as data on number of APNs who completed prescribing education, number of prescribers, improvements in access to care, saved emergency room visits, broad classes of medications prescribed such as immunizations, reproductive health, antibiotics, antihypertensives, diabetic, and cholesterol-lowering medications.
6. Identify APN prescriber champions to garner and sustain support in both educational institutions for training and preceptor/mentors. Capture prescribing scale and spread across organizations and sectors for implementation and sustainability.
7. Optimize appropriate prescribing best practices, which also includes deprescribing for patient safety and cost savings.

The list of prescribing competencies and resources is extensive, a few are listed below:

- *Standards for Prescribers—The Nursing and Midwifery Council.* https://www.nmc.org.uk/standards/standards-for-post-registration/standards-for-prescribers/
- *Royal Pharmaceutical Society's Competency Framework for All Prescribers—The Nursing and Midwifery Council* (RPS 2025) https://www.nmc.org.uk/standards/standards-for-post-registration/standards-for-prescribers/royal-pharmaceutical-societys-competency-framework-for-all-prescribers/
- *Registered Nurse Prescribing in Primary Health and Specialty Teams* (NCNZ 2022) https://www.nursingcouncil.org.nz/Public/NCNZ/nursing-section/Registered_nurse_prescribing_in_primary_health_and_specialty_teams.aspx
- *Journal of Prescribing Practice—Analysing the Competency Framework for all Prescribers* (Hall and Picton 2020) https://www.prescribingpractice.com/content/better-practice/analysing-the-competency-framework-for-all-prescribers

This last article, Hall and Picton (2020), is especially helpful as it provides multiple education and support frameworks for individuals and systems involved in prescribing to patients, including the framework cited above by the Royal Pharmaceutical Society (Fig. 1).

The Consultation	Patient	Prescribing Governance
1. Assess the patient		7. Prescribe safely
2. Consider the options		8. Prescribe professionally
3. Reach a shared decision		9. Improve prescribing practice
4. Prescribe		10. Prescribe as part of a team
5. Provide information		
6. Monitor and review		

Fig. 1 Competency framework for prescribers. (Adapted from Hall and Picton (2020), RPS (2025))

4.3 National Prescribing Experiences

4.3.1 Canadian NP Prescribing Policy Exemplar

Nurse Practitioners (NP) are the only title-protected advanced practice nurses in Canada. The scope of practice related to prescribing varies across the ten provinces and three territories across Canada. In 2024, 7477 NPs were employed in direct patient care in Canada, the majority in either community health agencies (33%) or in hospitals (34%). The overall supply of NPs licensed to practice in Canada grew at a rate of 10%, representing the largest percentage increase compared with other regulated nursing types. The majority (95%) of NPs were educated in Canada (CIHI 2025). Nearly all were educated in Canada (CIHI 2020).

Prescribing pharmacotherapy is considered full scope of practice and authorized for NPs across Canada except British Columbia (CIHI 2020). Prescribing controlled substances is restricted in New Brunswick, Quebec, and Alberta (CIHI 2020). Prescribing medical supplies has existing restrictions in Ontario and Saskatchewan.

Fong et al. (2015) highlighted NP prescribing from an international perspective. She found that NPs tend to prescribe to provide care in underserved populations and require good systems literacy to practice across complex systems. The key themes identified related to NP prescribing include barriers to prescribing, confidence in prescribing, and the unique role of NPs in prescribing medicines. Across all countries, further research into the organizational and financial conditions and climates in which NPs prescribe are needed to better understand their true prescribing capacity and inform future prescribing policy.

4.3.2 Jamaica APN Prescribing Policy Exemplar

The NP role was developed in Jamaica in the 1970s, with a master's degree required as of 2002.

The nurse anesthetist role developed in the 1980s, with a master's degree required as of 2007 (IAPN 2024). Registered Midwives in primary health care settings were allowed to prescribe contraceptives interdependently according to their scope of practice. But, outside of that, prescribing was limited to medical doctors (Lai 2018). With the emergence of new disease patterns and treatment modalities, discussions commenced regarding prescribing by other health professionals. As a result of an acute shortage of medical doctors especially in the rural areas in the 1970s, there were extensive deliberations between the Ministry of Health, the Nursing Council of Jamaica, the Nurses Association of Jamaica, and the University of the West Indies exploring the expanded role of the nurse.

In 1977, a cohort of 25 students, eighteen family nurse practitioners and seven pediatric nurse practitioners commenced the 1-year certificate program. Upon completion of their training, NPs were allowed to prescribe interdependently. All prescriptions written by NPs required the signature of the medical doctor.

During the early 1980s, the Nurse Practitioners encountered several challenges. Some pharmacists had issues dispensing medications that were prescribed by them. These unfavorable conditions fueled the draft of a protocol which highlighted the drugs that NPs were allowed to prescribe. Although NPs were well prepared as advanced practice nurses, the issue of not being able to prescribe independently proved to be a challenge. On many occasions, in the absence of the medical doctor, the clients had to return the following day or be referred to another site as the NP present, though competent, could not write the prescription.

Clients and members of staff verbalized satisfaction with the care offered by NPs. Nonetheless, ongoing agitation by members of the medical fraternity deepened as they questioned the educational preparation of NPs to take on the role of prescribing (Lai 2018). The challenges faced by the NPs in the execution of their duties led to the migration of some NPs.

As ongoing agitation by NPs regarding their inability to offer comprehensive care ensued, the Nursing Council of Jamaica, the legislative arm of the nursing profession, set up a Working Group in 2014. The members had the responsibility to formulate the competencies, scope of practice, and standards for Advanced Practice Nurses in Jamaica using the ICN framework. Nurse prescribing formed an integral component of this document. Over the years, numerous Ministers of Health sought to engage the relevant interested parties (stakeholders) regarding the issue of nurse prescribing. Some members of the medical fraternity continued their quest in their disapproval regarding nurse prescribing.

Following an analysis of the increased incidence of noncommunicable diseases and increased life expectancy, in December 2021, a committee was set up by the Ministry of Health and Wellness to review the scope of practice and competencies for APNs. Prescriptive rights for NPs and registration details were included in this mandate. The Committee was chaired by a medical doctor, and the other members included the Chief Nursing Officer, President for the Nurses Association of Jamaica, an Advanced Practice Nurse (Heather McGrath), and the Registrars for the Nursing, Pharmacy and Medical Councils (Allen 2022).

The APNs organized two focus group discussions with clients who were served by NPs and medical doctors in the primary health care setting. The aim of these discussions was to garner the clients and medical doctors' perspectives regarding granting of prescriptive rights to NPs. These discussions yielded positive results for the NPs. The clients reported that they were more satisfied with the care delivered by the NPs, and the medical doctors supported the request to grant prescriptive rights to NPs. A resolution was drafted by a Senior Doctor who attended the Focus Group Discussion. This document was used to facilitate the support of over seventy medical doctors working in the primary health care setting across Jamaica.

In November 2023, the Minister of Health and Wellness reported that Government officials had supported the request for NPs to prescribe independently from an approved list of drugs from the Vital, Essential Necessary (VEN) list in the public health system. Included in this mandate was the registration and licensure of family nurse practitioners and mental health psychiatric nurse practitioners as APRNs. Each NP would be given a unique number (Linton 2023). Though the Ministry of Health also approved registration and licensure for nurse anesthetists no additional prescriptive authority was granted (MOHW 2023).

There are currently approximately sixty NPs in Jamaica, which include Family Nurse Practitioners and Mental Health Psychiatric Nurse Practitioners. Of this number, the majority of the NPs are working in the Primary Health Care setting.

Nurse prescribing in Jamaica is carried out mainly by NPs who are prepared at the master's level. The level of autonomy differs across health regions. Plans are at the advanced stages to allow Nurse Practitioners to prescribe independently in the Public Sector.

4.3.3 Tanzania APN Prescribing Policy Exemplar

The Tanzania Nursing and Midwifery Council (TNMC) is a professional body that has the mandate to protect the public's health and safety through regulation of education, licensure, and practice (TNMC n.d). In 2014, the Council revised the scope of practice for nurses and midwives, codifying roles and functions as described in the Nursing and Midwifery Act of 2010. This comprehensive document sets out the full range of functions that nurses and midwives will be trained to undertake (Mtema 2014).

This scope of practice provides guidance and job descriptions for each category of nursing practice. The following categories are authorized to fully function and provide nursing care as stipulated by the Act of 2010; (1) Certificate in Nursing/Midwifery (also referred to as an enrolled nurse/midwife); (2) Diploma in Nursing/Midwifery (also referred to as a registered nurse/midwife); (3) Advanced Diploma in Nursing/Midwifery; (4) Bachelor's degree in nursing Midwifery Sciences; (5) Master's degree in nursing/Midwifery; and (6) Doctorate Degree or PhD in Nursing Midwifery.

The Nursing and Midwifery Scope of Practice also includes public health nurses, pediatric nurses, psychiatric nurses, operating theatre nurses, nurse anesthetists, ophthalmic nurses, and nurse tutors and lecturers. All these forms of nursing professionals practice within their scope and level of education preparations. In the country, general nurses can prescribe when they have undergone training on prescribing. NPs may initiate prescriptions on their own authority based on circumstances. They also have more involvement in disease management as experts in areas such as maternal and child health, where they run programs in the Ministry of Health.

Tanzania Nurses and Midwifery Council granted authority to nurses to prescribe in certain situations, for example, “In the absence or shortage of a medical doctor, the nurse shall prescribe medicines, perform minor surgical procedures, and carry out other complex tasks requiring special knowledge” (TMTZ 2014). Nurses are not licensed to prescribe or dispense medication in terms of their scope of practice, except in circumstances where they have had special training (Msuya et al. 2017). Nurses are allowed to prescribe medicine for some acute, chronic, and emergency conditions.

The African Health Professions Regulatory Collaborative Program (ARC) has played a pivotal role in shaping the regulatory landscape, enabling nurses to advance and broaden their scope of practices. This expansion has empowered nurses to acquire competencies and skills, allowing them to deliver safe and tailored healthcare to diverse populations. Notably, the inclusion of Nurse Initiated and Management for Antiretroviral Therapy (NIMART) for HIV or AIDS, endorsed by the World Health Organization (33), within the regulatory norms established by ARC, has significantly augmented the capacity of the nursing workforce.

The enhanced capacity is essential for improving access to HIV care (Dynes et al. 2016). The introduction of a Task Sharing policy in Tanzania as many African countries have opened up new avenues for nurses to broaden their prescriptive roles (Msuya et al. 2017). Nurses are trained to prescribe specific medications for combating HIV/AIDS, tuberculosis (TB), malaria, mental health conditions, as well as in palliative care (Zuber et al. 2014). This policy expanded roles to nurses who reside in rural areas to have more authority and power to manage and treat health conditions under primary care disease management guidelines (Msuya et al. 2017). This policy was developed to address challenges encountered by nurses working in resource-limited areas, where there is shortage of physician (Crowley and Mayers 2015). The successful implementation of a task shifting policy allowed nurses and other nonphysician professionals to prescribe certain medication under legal authorities. For example, policy gives legal authority for nurses to prescribe medication in response to HIV/AIDS, TB, malaria, mental health, and palliative care treatment. Nurses were trained to initiate antiretroviral therapy (ART) in their respective areas of work. This expanded role has not only motivated more nurses to undergo training but has also facilitated their ability to provide medications to patients, families, and communities at large.

The increasing acceptance of APNs in Tanzania is a game changer for nurses to widen their scope of practice in different areas. APNs acquire extensive knowledge, skills, and competencies in assessment, diagnostic evaluation, and pharmaceutical management. ANP in Tanzania are nurses trained at master’s or doctoral level. ANP may demonstrate their prescriptive competencies in a situation in the absence of medical personnel. In most working environments, ANPs practice their advanced role in specific conditions; this means that their scope is still narrowed and challenged by many factors such as inadequate legal framework support (Msuya et al. 2017). Despite their educational and intensive years of experiences, APN professional experience challenges barriers or difficulties while implementing their roles. It is recommended that the respective authority revises and updates the current scope of practice to reflect current needs and abilities of APN professionals. APNs are underutilized in prescribing because of the limited scope of practice. To maximize the contribution of ANPs, it is imperative to eliminate barriers and broaden their scope of practice in line with their education and professional experience. The recommended enhancement to the ANP curriculum involves incorporating advanced pharmacotherapeutic courses, which will provide additional knowledge on principles of drugs and application of those principles in clinical practice. Furthermore, the course will explain diagnostic and treatment reasoning and rational drug selection, while providing useful clinical pearls from experienced practitioners including monitoring aspects.

A purposeful and conscientious effort is required to review and update the education, prelicensure, and legal standard procedures for Advanced Practice Nurses (APNs). This transformative process is crucial, emphasizing the need for a deliberate decision-making approach. It is important to note that nurses do not seek to establish dominance or superiority in professional roles; rather, their focus should be on fostering collaboration, partnership, and teamwork among nursing practitioners and other professions. The key objective is to create a healthcare environment that values a collective and interdisciplinary approach to patient care. This approach aims to dismantle any existing barriers that impede the seamless provision of holistic healthcare. Through intentional efforts to enhance APN education and align legal standards with contemporary practices, we can cultivate an atmosphere where professionals work collaboratively, ensuring the highest standards of patient care and promoting a unified and cohesive healthcare system.

5 Securing Scope of Practice, Title Protection, Prescriptive Authority, and Authorization for Other APN Services

A lot of groundwork, consensus building, meetings, and decision-making must take place before authorizing bodies take the steps to define advanced practice for a jurisdiction. Authorizing bodies defining and regulating nursing customarily provide a set of rules and regulations that are generally taken together to be thorough, cohesive, and directive. For instance, in the U.S., each state generally has a board of nursing (or some close variation of that) that oversees the creation and adherence to a nurse practice act (NPA) and, though there is some variation, generally that act includes (Russell 2017, p 19):

- definitions
- authority, power, and composition of a board of nursing
- educational program standards
- standards and scope of nursing practice
- types of titles and licenses
- protection of titles
- requirements for licensure
- grounds for disciplinary action, other violations, and possible remedies

The NPA is generally considered the legal authorization (law), periodically updated, and supported by a variety of regulations, which are also periodically updated. This rule-writing process is complex but related professions do have a chance to comment, with legislators providing final authorization. Nursing boards and councils all around the world provide similar direction for the professionals under their purview, hopefully taking up the task for APNs.

References

Acorn M. Nurse practitioners as most responsible provider: impact on care for seniors admitted to an Ontario hospital. Int J Nurs Clin Pract. 2015;2:126. https://doi.org/10.15344/2394-4978/2015/126.

Acorn M. Commentary: the future of advanced practice nursing: what's next for Canada and the world? Nurs Leadersh (Tor Ont). 2021;34(4):79–85. https://doi.org/10.12927/cjnl.2021.26686

Acorn M. Commentary: Investing in advance practice nurses is a global health system solution. Int Nurs Rev. 2023a;70(1):97–9. https://doi.org/10.1111/inr.12804.

Acorn M. What is your global nurse leadership policy literacy? Nurse Leader. 2023b;21(1):56–60. https://doi.org/10.1016/j.mnl.2022.10.

Acorn M, Byers D. Integration of advanced practice nursing roles in Canada. In: Staples E, Pilon R, Ram H, editors. Canadian perspectives on advanced practice nursing. 2nd ed. Toronto: Canadian Scholars' Press; 2020. p. 50–60.

American Nurses Association (ANA). Title "nurse" protection. 2021. https://www.nursingworld.org/practice-policy/advocacy/state/title-nurse-protection/. Accessed 1 Oct 2025.

American Nurses Association (ANA). Advanced practice registered nurse. ANA; 2025. https://www.nursingworld.org/practice-policy/aprn/. Accessed 1 Oct 2025.

Boehning AP, Punsalan LD. Advanced practice registered nurse roles. In: StatPearls. Treasure Island: StatPearls Publishing; 2023. PMID: 36944002. https://www.ncbi.nlm.nih.gov/books/NBK589698/. Accessed 1 Oct 2025.

Brenan M. Nurses retain top ethics rating in the U.S. but below 2020 high. Gallup; 2023. https://news.gallup.com/poll/467804/nurses-retain-top-ethics-rating-below-2020-high.aspx. Accessed 1 Oct 2025.

Bryant-Lukosius D, Valaitis R, Martin-Misener R, Donald F, Pena LM, Brousseau L. Advanced practice nursing: a strategy for achieving universal health coverage and universal access to health. Rev Lat Am Enfermagem. 2017;25:e2826. https://doi.org/10.1590/1518-8345-1677.2826.

Canadian Institution for Health Information (CIHI). Nurse practitioner scopes of practice vary across Canada's provinces and territories. CIHI; 2020. Accessed 1 Oct 2025.

Canadian Institution for Health Information (CIHI). Nurse practitioners. CIHI; 2025. https://www.cihi.ca/en/nurse-practitioners. Accessed 1 Oct 2025.

Chun CK, Wong FKY, Wang SL, Chen W. Examining advanced nursing practice in Hong Kong and Guangzhou. Int J Nurs Sci. 2021;8:190–8. https://doi.org/10.1016/j.ijnss.2021.03.001.

Crowley T, Mayers P. Trends in task shifting in HIV treatment in Africa: effectiveness, challenges and acceptability to the health professions. Afr J Prim Health Care Fam Med. 2015;7(1):1–9. https://doi.org/10.4102/phcfm.v7i1.807.

Department of Health (DH). Improving patients' access to medicines: a guide to implementing nurse and pharmacist independent prescribing within the NHS in England. London: Department of Health; 2005. Accessed 1 Oct 2025.

Department of Health (DH). Scoping study of supplementary prescribing. London: Department of Health; 2006. Accessed 1 Oct 2025

Department of Health (DH). Advanced level nursing: a position statement. London: Department of Health; 2010. Accessed 1 Oct 2025.

Dynes M, Tison L, Johnson C, Verani A, Zuber A, Riley PL. Regulatory advances in 11 sub-Saharan countries in year 3 of the African Health Profession Regulatory Collaborative for Nurses and Midwives (ARC). J Assoc Nurses AIDS Care. 2016;27(3):285–96. https://doi.org/10.1016/j.jana.2015.11.004.

East LA, Arudo J, Loefler M, Evans CM. Exploring the potential for advanced nursing practice role development in Kenya: A qualitative study. BMC Nurs. 2014;13(1):1–11. https://doi.org/10.1186/s12912-014-0033-y.

Flook DM. The professional nurse and regulation. J Perianesth Nurs. 2003;18(3):160–7.

Fong J, Buckley T, Cashin A. Nurse practitioner prescribing: an international perspective. Nurs Res Rev. 2015;5:99–108. https://doi.org/10.2147/NRR.S56188.

Hall K, Picton C. Analysing the competency framework for all prescribers. J Prescr Pract. 2020;2:122–8. https://www.prescribingpractice.com/content/better-practice/analysing-the-competency-framework-for-all-prescribers.

Health & Care Professions Council (HCPC). Scope of practice. HCPC; 2021. https://www.hcpc-uk.org/standards/meeting-our-standards/scope-of-practice/. Accessed 1 Oct 2025.

Hurlock-Chorostecki C, Acorn M. Diffusing innovative roles within Ontario hospitals: implementing the nurse practitioner as the most responsible provider. Nurs Leadersh (Tor Ont). 2017;30(4):60–6. https://doi.org/10.12927/cjnl.2017.25448

Institute of Medicine (US) Committee on the Robert Wood Johnson Foundation Initiative on the Future of Nursing, at the Institute of Medicine. The future of nursing: leading change, advancing health. Washington (DC): National Academies Press (US); 2011. https://www.ncbi.nlm.nih.gov/books/NBK209870/. Accessed 1 Oct 2025.

InternationalAdvancedPracticeNursing(IAPN).AdvancednursingpracticeinJamaica.IAPN;2024.https://internationalapn.org/tag/nurse-anesthetist/. https://internationalapn.org/tag/nurse-anesthetist/.

International Confederation of Midwives (ICM). ICM essential competencies for midwifery practice. ICM; 2024a. https://www.internationalmidwives.org/wp-content/uploads/EN_ICM-Essential-Competencies-for-Midwifery-Practice-1.pdf. Accessed 1 Oct 2025.

International Confederation of Midwives (ICM). International definition and scope of practice of the midwife. ICM; 2024b. https://internationalmidwives.org/resources/international-definition-of-the-midwife/. Accessed 1 Oct 2025.

International Council of Nurses (ICN). Regulation 2020: an exploration of the present: vision for the future. ICN; 2009. Accessed 1 Oct 2025.

International Council of Nurses (ICN). Scope of nursing practice and decision-making framework toolkit. ICN; 2010. Accessed 1 Oct 2025.

International Council of Nurses (ICN). Position statement: Protection of the title "nurse". ICN; 2012a. https://www.icn.ch/sites/default/files/2023-04/B06_Protection_Title_Nurse.pdf. Accessed 1 Oct 2025.

International Council of Nurses (ICN). Position statement: Scope of nursing practice. ICN; 2012b. https://www.icn.ch/sites/default/files/inline-files/B07_Scope_Nsg_Practice.pdf. Accessed 1 Oct 2025.

International Council of Nurses (ICN). Guidelines on advanced practice nursing. ICN; 2020. https://www.icn.ch/system/files/2021-07/ICN_APN%20Report_EN.pdf. Accessed 1 Oct 2025.

International Council of Nurses (ICN). Guidelines on advanced practice nursing: nurse anesthetists. ICN; 2021a. https://www.icn.ch/system/files/documents/2021-05/ICN_Nurse-Anaesthetist-Report_EN_WEB.pdf. Accessed 1 Oct 2025.

International Council of Nurses (ICN). Guidelines on nurse prescribing. ICN; 2021b. https://www.icn.ch/system/files/2021-09/ICN_Nurse_prescribing_guidelines_EN_WEB.pdf. Accessed 1 Oct 2025.

International Council of Nurses (ICN). The ICN code of ethics for nurses. ICN; 2021c. https://www.icn.ch/sites/default/files/inline-files/ICN_Code-of-Ethics_EN_Web.pdf. Accessed 1 Oct 2025.

Kenya Registered Nurse Anesthetists (KRNA). Launch of the official KRNA scope of practice. KRNA; 2019. https://krna.org/launch-of-the-official-krna-scope-of-practice/. Accessed 1 Oct 2025.

Kilpatrick K, Savard I, Audet L, Constanzo G, Khan M, Atallah R, Jabbour M, Zhou W, Wheeler K, Ladd E, Gray D, Henderson C, Spies, McGrath H, Rogers M. A global perspective of advanced practice nursing research: A review of systematic reviews. PLoS One. 2024;19(7):e0305008. PMID: 38954675; PMCID: PMC11218965.

Kleinpell R, Myers C, Likes W, Schorn M. Breaking down institutional barriers to advanced practice registered nurse practice. Nurs Adm Q. 2022;46(2):147–3.

Kugler EC, Burhans LD, George JL. Removal of legal barriers to the practice of advanced practice registered nurses. N C Med J. 2011;72(4):285–8.

Lai C. Prescriptive rights for the family nurse practitioner. Medical Association of Jamaica; 2018. https://www.majdoctors.com.

Linton L. Law to be amended to provide prescriptive rights to APRNs. 2023. https://jis.gov.jm/law-to-be-amended-to-provide-prescriptive-rights-to-aprns/. Accessed 1 Oct 2025.

Mackavey C, Henderson C, de Zwart van Leeuwen W, Maas L, Ladd A. The advanced practice nurse role's development and identity: an international review Int J Adv Pract 2024; 2(1): 1–16. https://doi.org/10.12968/ijap.2024.2.1.36

McGilton KS, Krassikova A, Boscart V, Sidani S, Iaboni A, Vellani S, Escrig-Pinol A. Nurse practitioners rising to the challenge during the coronavirus disease 2019 pandemic in long-term care homes. Gerontologist. 2021;61(4):615–23. https://doi.org/10.1093/geront/gnab030.

Ministry of Health (Kenya). National nursing and midwifery policy: Towards excellence in nursing and midwifery services for all 2022–2032. 2022. https://repository.kippra.or.ke/server/api/core/bitstreams/3b3a6563-a55d-4d14-8a90-f855427aabbf/content. Accessed 1 Oct 2025.

Ministry of Health and Wellness (MOHW). Cabinet give approval for prescriptive rights for advanced practice registered nurses. MOHW; 2023. https://www.moh.gov.jm/cabinet-gives-approval-for-prescriptive-rights-for-advanced-practice-registered-nurses/. Accessed 1 Oct 2025.

Msuya M, Blood-Siegfried J, Chugulu J, Kidayi P, Sumaye J, Machange R, Mtuya CC, Pereira K. Descriptive study of nursing scope of practice in rural medically underserved areas of Africa, South of the Sahara. Int J Afr Nurs Sci. 2017;6:74–82. https://doi.org/10.1016/j.ijans.2017.04.003.

Mtema N. Tanzania: scope of practice for nurses ready. AllAfrica: Tanzania Daily News (Dar es Salaam); 2014. https://allafrica.com/stories/201411130465.html.

National Council of State Boards of Nursing (NCSBN). APRN consensus model. 2025. https://www.ncsbn.org/nursing-regulation/practice/aprn.page. Accessed 1 Oct 2025.

National Health Service (NHS). Multi-professional framework for advanced clinical practice in England. NHS; 2017. https://hee.nhs.uk/sites/default/files/documents/Multi-professional%20framework%20for%20advanced%20clinical%20practice%20in%20England.pdf. Accessed 1 Oct 2025.

Ndirangu-Mugo E, Kimani RW, Onyancha C, Mutwiri BD, May B, Kambo I, Tallam E, Koech N, Mukuna A, Henderson C, Shumba CS. Scopes of practice for advanced practice nursing and advanced practice midwifery in Kenya: a gap analysis. Int Nurs Rev. 2024;71(2):276–84. https://doi.org/10.1111/inr.12947.

Nissen L, Lynne T, Bettenay K. Optimising registered nurse and midwife prescriptive authority in medicines, poisons and therapeutic goods regulatory mechanisms in Queensland. Queensland University of Technology; 2015.

Nurse Practitioners Association of Ontario (NPAO). Nurse practitioner-led clinics. 2025. https://npao.org/nplcs/. Accessed 1 Oct 2025.

Nursing Council of Kenya (NCK). Scope of practice for nurse anaesthetists. Facebook. 2018. https://www.facebook.com/NursingCouncilKenya/posts/the-nursing-council-of-kenya-held-a-stakeholder-engagement-meeting-during-the-va/2051618875128197/. Accessed 1 Oct 2025.

Nursing Council of New Zealand (NCNZ). Registered nurse prescribing in primary and specialty teams. NCNZ; 2022. https://www.nursingcouncil.org.nz/Public/NCNZ/nursing-section/Registered_nurse_prescribing_in_primary_health_and_specialty_teams.aspx. Accessed 1 Oct 2025.

Ontario Ministry of Health. Attending nurse practitioners in long-term care homes initiative funding policy. Ontario Ministry of Health; 2025. https://www.ontario.ca/page/attending-nurse-practitioners-long-term-care-homes-initiative-funding-policy. Accessed 1 Oct 2025.

Parker J, Hill MN. A review of advanced practice nursing in the United States, Canada, Australia, and Hong Kong Special Administrative Region (SAR), China. Int J Nurs Sci. 2017;4(2):196–204. https://doi.org/10.1016/j.inss.2017.01.022.

Poghosyan L, Maier CB. Advanced practice nurse globally: responding to health challenges, improving outcomes. Int J Nurs Stud. 2022;132:104262. https://doi.org/10.1016/j.ijnurstu.2022.104262.

Registered Nurses Association of Ontario (RNAO). Nurse practitioners are ready for bill 179. From Michelle Acorn August 7, 2011. 2011. https://rnao.ca/sites/rnao-ca/files/NPAO_-_Nurse_Practitioners_are_Ready_for_Bill_179.pdf. Accessed 1 Oct 2025.

Rogers M, Gloster A. The evolution of the nurse practitioner role and practice in the United Kingdom. In: Thomas S, Rowles J, editors. Nurse practitioners and nurse anesthetists: the evolution of the global roles. Paris: Springer; 2023. p. 160–81.

Royal College of Nursing (RCN). Advanced nurse practitioner: an RCN guide. London: RCN; 2012.

Royal College of Nursing (RCN). RCN standards for advanced level nursing practice, advanced nurse practitioners, RCN accreditation and RCN credentialing. London: RCN; 2018.

Royal College of Nursing (RCN). Advanced practice standards. London: RCN; 2024.

Royal Pharmaceutical Society (RPS). Royal Pharmaceutical Society's competency framework for all prescribers. RPS; 2025. https://www.nmc.org.uk/standards/standards-for-post-registration/standards-for-prescribers/royal-pharmaceutical-societys-competency-framework-for-all-prescribers/. Accessed 1 Oct 2025.

Russell KA. Nurse practice acts guide and govern: update 2017. J Nurs Regul. 2017;8(3):18–25.

Scanlon A, Murphy M, Smolowitz J, Lewis V. Advanced nursing practice and advanced practice nursing roles within low and lower-middle-income countries. J Nurs Scholarsh. 2022;55:484–93. https://doi.org/10.1111/jnu.12828.

Sheer B, Wong FKY. The development of advanced nursing practice globally. J Nurs Scholarsh. 2008;40(3):204–11.

Stilwell B. Patients attitudes to a highly developed extended role: the nurse practitioner. Recent Adv Nurs. 1988;21:82–100.

Tanzania Nursing and Midwifery Council (TNMC). Scope of practice for nurses and midwives in Tanzania. TNMC; 2014.

Tanzania Nursing and Midwifery Council (TNMC). Who we are? n.d.. https://www.tnmc.go.tz/who-we-are/.

Wheeler KJ, Miller M, Pulcini J, Gray D, Ladd E, Rayens MK. Advanced practice nursing roles, regulation, education, and practice: a global study. Ann Glob Health. 2022;88(1):1–21. https://doi.org/10.5334/aogh.3698.

World Health Organization (WHO). Global strategic directions for nursing and midwifery 2021–2025. WHO; 2021. https://apps.who.int/iris/bitstream/handle/10665/344562/9789240033863-eng.pdf. Accessed 1 Oct 2025.

Zuber A, McCarthy CF, Verani AR, Msidi E, Johnson C. A survey of nurse-initiated and-managed antiretroviral therapy (NIMART) in practice, education, policy, and regulation in east, central, and southern Africa. J Assoc Nurses AIDS Care. 2014;25(6):520–31. https://doi.org/10.1016/j.jana.2014.02.003.

Advanced Practice Nurses and Reimbursement: Direct and Indirect

Sandra Leyan Castillo and Gene E. Harkless

1 Introduction

The World Health Organization (WHO) has predicted future shortages in the healthcare workforce, exacerbating global health inequities and disparities (WHO 2025). The shortage is further exacerbated by the mismatch between education and employment opportunities as health systems are slow to adapt to population needs as evidenced by the less than rapid adoption and utilization of advanced practice nurses (APNs) who have demonstrated their ability to provide high-quality, frontline services. Notably, nursing is the fastest-growing healthcare profession globally (Goodson et al. 2001). APNs are poised to play an important role in addressing these inequities and predicted shortages (Wheeler et al. 2022). They are prepared to provide high-quality primary and specialty care but often run into roadblocks negotiating wages and salaries and/or setting up indirect or direct payment systems for their services. Payment for APN services is essential if APNs are to play an important role in ameliorating the predicted shortage and maldistribution of highly qualified health professionals (Wheeler et al. 2022). Obtaining equitable, dependable reimbursement for professional services is a fundamental matter for advanced practice nurses worldwide. Understanding different reimbursement models for APN services across the globe is essential to ensure APN practice continues to grow economically and in market strength in order to meet critical healthcare needs. This chapter will define direct and indirect reimbursement, describe common types of reimbursement, and discuss considerations on how to negotiate reimbursement.

S. L. Castillo (✉)
NEW Health – Mass General Brigham, Cambridge, MA, USA
e-mail: sleyan@mgb.org

G. E. Harkless
University of New Hampshire, Alton, NH, USA

K. J. Wheeler, M. Acorn (eds.), *Health Policy for Advanced Practice Nursing: A Toolkit for Implementation and Improvement*, Advanced Practice in Nursing,
https://doi.org/10.1007/978-3-032-03667-4_16

2 Types of Reimbursements in Healthcare

The intricacy of reimbursements for healthcare is that there is no universal system that applies to every country. The mechanisms of payment for APN services are varied and depend on the country's healthcare system and that includes the regulatory environment for APNs and the availability of payment through public or private insurance schemes or consumer's self-pay. Most APNs still work as employees under a traditional wage/salary model. How the employer bills or receives payment for the APN work is often based on a fee-for-service model but may include other health system-determined processes such as population-based capitation, outcomes-based pay-for-performance, and other models such as diagnosis-based payment and relative value units. Within each of these systems, an essential issue is whether the APN is identified as the billing provider and the payment is assigned to the APN providing the service, or if the billing or payment system is set up only in the physician or health system's identity. In the first instance, this is a direct reimbursement process as the APN receives payment under the identity of the APN. The funds may go to the employer of the APN if the APN is not self-employed, but the financial accounting ascribes that payment to the work product of the APN. Indirect reimbursement for APN services is when the billing entity does not ascribe the service to the APN but rather to another provider, most likely a physician.

2.1 Fee-for-Service

The primary model for reimbursement for services is fee-for-service through direct or indirect billing. In fee-for-service, the employer or provider bills for the services and is reimbursed after the care is provided. The challenge for APNs in this model is the question of what services an APN can be reimbursed for and what the compensation will be within and across countries. The payment can come from the individual receiving services or through a third-party such as through insurance. The fee-for-service model has the potential to encourage the provision of more and more services in that the business incentive is to maximize profit by generating more revenue. Most often in a fee-for-service model, the APN receives a wage or salary that has been negotiated by the provider.

The fee-for-service reimbursement amounts are often determined by private or government health insurance schemes and often there is no fee-for-service parity among different healthcare providers (Kyeremanteng et al. 2019). As more APNs in the United States (U.S.) and around the globe move toward full practice authority, including full prescriptive authority, reimbursement parity is a key priority. Reimbursement parity occurs when payment is based on the service, not on who is providing the service.

Reimbursement parity continues to be a problem within the U.S. healthcare system, often varying by state, type of insurance, and reimbursement law. For instance, under Medicare (federal insurance for those over 65 years of age and other eligible groups including those with severe disabilities and end-stage renal disease) to receive pay parity with physicians, APNs must provide the service under "incident to" requirements, otherwise referred to as indirect billing. To receive 100% of the physician fee schedule for an APN-provided service, a physician must be physically present in the practice, the patient must have an established relationship with the physician, the service being provided by the APN must not be addressing a new diagnosis, and the bill for the service must be submitted under the physician's billing number. The APN service is then not attributable to the APN, and the APN service remains hidden in the insurance records. In the U.S., APNs can bill Medicare under their own provider number, otherwise known as direct billing, but their practice then receives only 85% of the physician reimbursement fee. Notably, for Medicaid (joint federal and state insurance for those with limited income and resources), payment equity among different states varies, but in the majority of the 50 states, the Medicaid payment is the same across different healthcare professionals providing the same service (KFF 2023). For instance, the New Hampshire Medicaid Program pays the same for physician or APN services, while other states may pay lower rates for APN services.

As most APNs continue to work as employees within a healthcare system, usually the employer bills and collects for the APN services and pays the APN salary. In Australia, this coexistence of both salary and fee-for-service reimbursement for APNs is evident. Most Australian APNs work in the public healthcare sector where they have fixed salaries by the government. In primary care, APN employers can bill through their national Commonwealth Government Medicare Benefits Schedule (MBS). This means that the APN employers can bill under their name, receive 85% of the scheduled fees for a limited range of services and the revenue goes directly to the healthcare institution that provides a fixed salary for the APNs. These constraints pose a barrier to expansion of the NP role (Woods and Murfet 2015).

Where insurance programs are rare, fee-for-service reimbursement may not pass through a third-party insurer. As an example, in Kenya, private practice nurses, regulated by the Kenyan government, are able to provide services as independent, private practice nurses (East et al. 2014). Supporting the movement of nurses and APNs into the healthcare marketplace to address unmet community needs has been the social franchise model (Na). This model brings together private healthcare providers, often nurses, into a network that uses a commercial branding identity to achieve a social cause, rather than a financial goal (Syengo and Suchman 2020). Within the franchise, the providers are expected to provide specific services and are supported with training, branding, and monitoring to do so, with the aim of continuous quality improvement. As a direct payment model, the private practice nurse within a franchise model collects fees directly as the practice delivers important health services.

One notable fee-for-service franchise model is South Africa's Unjani Clinic initiative (Johnson and Johnson 2018). The Unjani Clinics aims to empower Black female professional nurses as entrepreneurial nurses to provide first-level primary care for underserved communities. The Unjani Clinics are nurse-led and nurse-owned facilities. Initial funding for the infrastructure and operating capital is provided to set up the clinic with the fee-for-service model achieving financial sustainability within 1 year. Nurses must apply for participation in the program, and the site selection is based on an assessment of commercial viability along with a community survey of at least 200 respondents to determine the primary healthcare needs for that location. Importantly, Unjani clinics act as an economic driver as the Unjani nurses become employers and create new jobs as the clinic needs grow to include assistants, administrators, and security guards. This nurse-led primary care model has empowered nurses to be successful businesspeople providing financial sustainability for their families and professionally rewarding careers.

2.2 Capitation

Capitation is another reimbursement model that along with all the other reimbursement mechanisms discussed here, can be direct, that is; the payment is done and received under the APN's identity or indirect meaning that the capitation is negotiated and received under another provider, usually a physician. Capitation is a prospective payment system in which the amount paid for every patient enrolled is predetermined. In two-tiered capitation, practice or the individual clinician receives a fixed payment to treat a fixed number of patients. The rate is usually calculated by providing a certain amount of funding on a per patient per year basis. As an example, in the U.S., with a patient group of 2000 and the capitation fee of $400 per year per patient, the practice would receive $800,000 to provide all contracted services for those 2000 patients. Capitation encourages preventive care because the way to maintain a profit margin is to have systems in place to keep patients healthy at the lowest cost possible (Barbeiro 2017). In capitation, providers are responsible for effectively managing resource utilization. Some may argue that the drawbacks of capitation are possible undertreatment by increasing workload and reducing quality of care. Capitation may incentivize professionals to reduce services and defer care beyond the contract period (Kyeremanteng et al. 2019). Referrals or specialty consultations not provided within a contracted group are typically reimbursed to subcontracted providers. To help manage utilization and control costs associated with these external services, many managed care organizations incorporate structured programs—such as second opinions—within capitated or per-member-per-month (PMPM) payment arrangements (KFF 2025; CEBP 2022). These arrangements allow organizations to align incentives while overseeing service volume and expenditures. Capitation contracts are often renegotiated within short timeframes, particularly when actual utilization is lower than projected for the covered population (Tummalapalli et al. 2022).

2.3 Diagnosis-Related Payments

Diagnose-related payments are similar to fee-for-service mechanisms, where the amount reimbursed is linked to a diagnosis. This mechanism has been implemented in many countries worldwide. In 1983, the U.S. Health Care Financing Administration

(HCFA) system introduced a patient classification system of diagnosis-related groups (DRGs) for reimbursing providers under Medicare, primarily for secondary and tertiary care facilities. Many countries have based their diagnosis-related payment systems on the HCFA system, but costs and reimbursements for services vary from one country to another. This type of reimbursement will vary depending on the financing structure of the healthcare system, whether it is a country with social health insurance or competitive private and public healthcare facilities. It is crucial that coding for this mechanism is accurate for each patient to ensure proper reimbursement. However, standardizing fees is important for regions like Europe where cross-border movements of patients occur, and the aim is for comparable reimbursements (Woods and Murfet 2015). Variation of the fees in this system can occur as new drugs and technologies are introduced in the market. When new products or services are introduced, the DRG system may create a new category but also may increase the fee of the entire DRG which translates to higher costs for every patient classified under that specific group.

2.4 Relative Value Units

In addition to the use of DRGs for specialty and tertiary care, relative value units (RVUs) are the basic building blocks of U.S. physician and APN compensation from Medicare & Medicaid Services (CMS). Payment by CMS is based on a claim using a CPT® (Current Procedural Terminology) code. CPT® is copyrighted by the American Medical Association and is used in many countries. The CPT® provides a uniform language for coding medical services and procedures. In the U.S., each CPT® code has a RVU assigned to it. The RVU system does not determine the amount of compensation but provides a measure of the extent of provider work, clinical and nonclinical resources, and the expertise required to provide the service. The RVU measure is then added into a larger calculation of the Resource-Based Relative Value Scale (RBRVS) that includes the RVUs, the geographic practice cost indices, and a conversion factor, which is the amount by which each total RVU value is multiplied to obtain payment for a given service (AAPC 2025). The RBRVS system is frequently criticized for over-valuing procedures more than the cognitive work of primary care and other non-procedure-based specialties.

2.5 Pay for Performance

Pay-for-performance systems for reimbursement are linked to outcomes of quality of care and/or performance of providers. Pay for performance reimbursement aims to reduce costs and promote quality improvement. In contrast to fee-for-service systems, in which volume is important, pay for performance is an incentive system with the goal of achieving savings by improving patient outcomes through primary, secondary, and tertiary prevention actions. In this system, defining the outcome measurements that will determine the provider's performance is very important.

Providers obtain financial incentives for adherence to best clinical guidelines, which is thought not only to improve quality of care, but also clinical outcomes. The disadvantages of this system are that the provider reimbursement is dependent on adherence to prescribed care. Success with pay for performance will depend on the type of practice and the demographic and socioeconomic characteristics of their patient population. Monitoring and measuring outcomes can be time consuming and require significant financial investment (Weinstein 1997).

Salary and/or wages can also be paid out to employees when the employer is receiving reimbursement through insurance payments, population-based capitation, pay for performance, diagnosis-based payment, or self-pay by the client. The benefit of having a fixed salary for new APNs is that they do not have to worry about the number of patients or services required to secure a minimum salary. The disadvantage is that the income is fixed unless the salary is part of a bonus pay system. Unless negotiated, financial incentives for services provided and/or achieving certain outcomes will not be available. APNs can leverage their knowledge and experience to obtain more favorable salaries and benefits when negotiating their contracts. As an example, an NP in Chile recognized the value her previous RN knowledge and skill brought to a new NP specialty position and negotiated an 11% higher base rate for her salary along with a monthly productivity bonus.

3 Considerations for Negotiating Reimbursement for APN Services

Global variations in nursing, licensing, and credentialing, and the variations in APN education, role, titling, and scope of practices requires that APNs know their own practice environment as they negotiate reimbursement. Reimbursement for an APN could mean a salary, generated through indirect or direct billing of the APN services or the APN negotiating third-party payers for direct reimbursement, or the APN determining what they will charge clients for direct fee-for-service care (Wheeler et al. 2022). In countries that lack formal authority for APN practice, there often are nurses who have recognized their community's need for APN-level services and, working within their regulatory environment, use their knowledge and skills to meet the need (Weinstein 1997; Suzuki et al. 2022). Salaried positions under the supervision of physicians may be the first step in developing an APN career.

The first step in negotiating reimbursement for APN services is to understand the work environment. Will that be as a salaried employee within a large organization? If that is the case, before salary negotiations are completed, the APN should understand the process of billing for the APN services, whether direct or indirect within a fee-for-service, capitation, or pay-for-performance system. With indirect billing, there may be no record of APN-generated billables as they will be submitted without attribution to the APN. The risk of this approach is that the services and value of the APN work are hidden. Therefore, at the time of hire, the APN should consider how to track the value of their work outside of the billing system. However, if the

APN is negotiating a salary based on direct billing for the ANP services, the APN may negotiate for incentives based on productivity.

Regardless of whether an APN is negotiating a salary as an employee or setting up their own practice, the APN should consider the market in which the position is located and consider the following questions:

1. Which patient population will the APN provide services to?
2. Will the APN be working in a public or private practice?
3. Who pays for these services? How much is funded by the government or by third-party reimbursement? How much are patients paying out of pocket?
4. How much are other institutions charging for similar or same services in the same region?
5. What are salary ranges for nurses compared to advanced practice nurses in the country or in the region?
6. How much do APN think their services are worth?
7. How likely is the market going to change in the next few years? For example, is this a shrinking or growing population?
8. Are there potential partnerships? Is this tailored for one APN or a group of APNs?
9. What is an appropriate timeframe for a new negotiation for pay, either through bonus, pay for performance, or scheduled salary increases?
10. Are the compensation projections congruent with the APN current needs and future goals?

For APNs implementing a new role, defining a strategic plan can help to identify needs and gaps in the area's healthcare system, as well as identify and gather the support of interested parties (stakeholders). *The International Council of Nurses' Handbook on Entrepreneurial Practice* (Sanders and Kingma 2012) is a free guide to building a strategic plan. A strategic plan requires that the population to be served and the services that will be provided be defined along with outcomes. There are several outcomes that can be measured, such as increased number of patients evaluated in an office, decreased wait times, management of chronic conditions, decreased hospital stays, decreased readmissions, improved morbidity and mortality statistics, satisfaction with care, or other parameters. Depending on these outcomes, APNs can potentially calculate the revenue or cost savings generated by their services. Outcomes measurements are important not only to demonstrate value of the service but also helpful to negotiate future salary and/or other reimbursement adjustments. Figure 1 represents the steps anyone involved in preparing to negotiate reimbursement might go through.

As stated above, third-party reimbursement in many jurisdictions or institutions will be indirect (ascribed to physician, other provider, or institution), but there are many reasons (professional recognition, provider-specific data regarding outcomes and costs) to pursue direct reimbursement (ascribed to the APN). However, the process to achieve that level of professional recognition may be challenging. An excellent description of the nuances of the many-year effort for APNs in the U.S. to

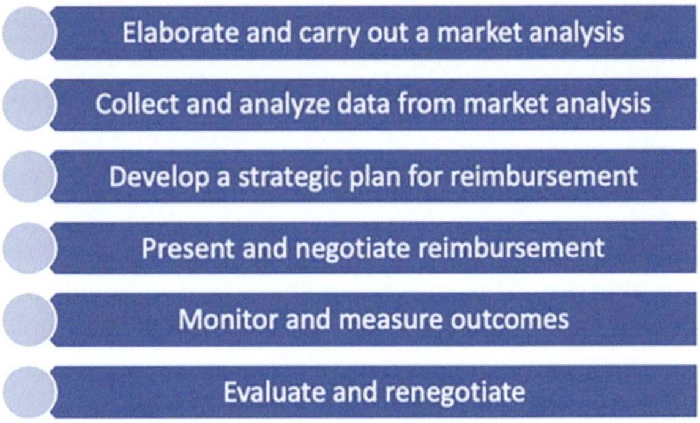
Elaborate and carry out a market analysis
Collect and analyze data from market analysis
Develop a strategic plan for reimbursement
Present and negotiate reimbursement
Monitor and measure outcomes
Evaluate and renegotiate

Fig. 1 Summary of steps in negotiation of reimbursement. (Developed from Sanders and Kingma 2012 and Weinstein 1997)

obtain direct reimbursement status is provided in a 2003 article (O'Brien 2003) entitled How Nurse Practitioners Obtained Provider Status: Lessons for Pharmacists. In challenging U.S. pharmacists to make the same effort to obtain direct reimbursement as the U.S. APNs the author, PharmD John Michael O'Brien, detailed the intense policy work, data keeping, and persistence that was required. The effort pertained to Medicare, the federal program to insure the elderly or disabled. Once the U.S. government recognized APNs for direct reimbursement, other third-party insurers across the U.S. followed suit.

In closing, reimbursement negotiations will vary depending on the country. If the APN role has not been established, differentiating the APN services from the traditional registered nurse role is important for reimbursement negotiation. Negotiating reimbursement in any reimbursement model can be difficult for some as nurses often do not ascribe an economic value on their services. Receiving market-based, equitable reimbursement for APN services is essential for the future of the profession (Naylor and Kurtzman 2010), allowing APNs to meet the global healthcare needs cited by the WHO.

References

American Association of Professional Coders (AAPC). What are relative value units (RVUs)? AAPC; 2025. https://www.aapc.com/resources/what-are-relative-value-units-rvus. Accessed 2 March 2025.

Barbeiro J. Starting a practice and practice management. In: Advanced Practice Nursing: Essentials for Role Development. 4th ed. Philadelphia: F.A. Davis Company; 2017.

Center for Evidence-Based Policy (CEBP). Payment model primer: capitated payments. Oregon Health & Science University; 2022. https://centerforevidencebasedpolicy.org/CEbP_PaymentModelPrimer_CapitatedPayments.pdf. Accessed 27 Aug 2025.

East LA, Arudo J, Loefler M, Evans CM. Exploring the potential for advanced nursing practice role development in Kenya: a qualitative study. BMC Nurs. 2014;13:1. https://doi.org/10.1186/s12912-014-0033-y.

Goodson JD, Bierman AS, Fein O, Rask K, Rich EC, Selker HP. The future of capitation the physician role in managing change in practice. J Gen Intern Med. 2001;16(4):250–6. https://doi.org/10.1046/j.1525-1497.2001.016004250.x. PMID: 11318926; PMCID: PMC1495203.

Johnson & Johnson. Unjani Clinic nurses: transforming healthcare in South Africa. Johnson & Johnson; 2018. https://nursing.jnj.com/nursing-news-events/nurses-leading-innovation/unjani-clinic-nurses-transforming-healthcare-in-south-africa. Accessed 2 May 2025.

KFF. Nurse practitioner services. KFF; 2023. https://www.kff.org/medicaid/state-indicator/nurse-practitioner-services/?currentTimeframe=1&sortModel=%7B%22colId%22:%22Location%22,%22sort%22:%22asc%22%7D. Accessed 2 Mar 2025.

KFF. 10 things to know about Medicaid managed care. KFF; 2025. https://www.kff.org/medicaid/10-things-to-know-about-medicaid-managed-care/. Accessed 27 Aug 2025.

Kyeremanteng K, Robidoux R, D'Egidio G, Fernando SM, Neilipovitz D. An analysis of pay-for-performance schemes and their potential impacts on health systems and outcomes for patients. Crit Care Res Pract. 2019;2019:8943972. https://doi.org/10.1155/2019/8943972. PMID: 31321097; PMCID: PMC6607710.

Naylor MD, Kurtzman ET. The role of nurse practitioners in reinventing primary care. Health Aff (Millwood). 2010;29(5):893–9. https://doi.org/10.1377/hlthaff.2010.0440. PMID: 20439877

O'Brien JM. How nurse practitioners obtained provider status: lessons for pharmacists. Am J Health Syst Pharm. 2003;60(22):2301–7. https://doi.org/10.1093/ajhp/60. PMID: 14652978.

Sanders L, Kingma M. Handbook on entrepreneurial practice: nurses creating opportunities as entrepreneurs and intrapreneurs. International Council of Nurses; 2012. https://www.icn.ch/sit1es/default/files/inline-files/2012_Handbook_entrepreneurial_practice_eng.pdf. Accessed 2 Mar 2025.

Suzuki M, Harada N, Honda K, Koda M, Araki T, Kudo T, et al. Facilitators and barriers in implementing the nurse practitioner role in Japan: a cross-sectional descriptive study. Int Nurs Rev. 2022;71(2):291–8. https://doi.org/10.1111/inr.12790. Epub 2022 July 15. PMID: 35839821.

Syengo M, Suchman AL. Team-based approaches to diagnosis: building a better diagnostic culture. Diagnosis (Berl). 2020;7(3):247–54. https://doi.org/10.1515/dx-2020-0022.

Tummalapalli SL, Estrella MM, Jannet-Khah DP, Keyhani S, Ibrahaim S. Capitated versus fee-for-service reimbursement and quality of care for chronic disease: a US cross-sectional analysis. BMC Health Serv Res. 2022;22(19):7313. https://doi.org/10.1186/s12913-021-07313-3.

Weinstein ML. CAPITATION: theory, practice, and evaluating rates for gastroenterology. Gastroenterol Clin N Am. 1997;26(4):773–84. https://doi.org/10.1016/S0889-8553(05)70332-0.

Wheeler KJ, Miller M, Pulcini J, Gray D, Ladd E, Rayens MK. Advanced practice nursing roles, regulation, education, and practice: a global study. Ann Glob Health. 2022; https://doi.org/10.5334/aogh.3698. PMID: 35755314; PMCID: PMC9205376.

Woods M, Murfet G. Australian nurse practitioner practice: value adding through clinical reflexivity. Nurs Res Pract. 2015:829593. https://doi.org/10.1155/2015/829593. PMID: 25705517; PMCID: PMC4325224.

World Health Organization (WHO). Health workforce. WHO; 2025. https://www.who.int/health-topics/health-workforce#tab=tab_1. Accessed 3 Mar 2025.

Health Policy for Education

Selected Policy Issues in Advanced Practice Nursing Education

Mary Ellen Biggerstaff, Lori Martin-Plank, Kathy J. Wheeler, Suzanne Hetzel Campbell, Sriyani Padmalatha Konara Mudiyanselage, Sujeewa Dilhani Mithreepala, Fathi Al Abri, Bonisile S. Nsibandze, Patricia B. Howard, Tracy Williams, Beatriz Rosana Gonçalves de Oliveira Toso, Rosimere Ferreira Santana, Maria Auxiliadora Rodrigues, and Ana Beatriz Serra Hércules

M. E. Biggerstaff (✉)
Pacific Lutheran University, Olympia, WA, USA
e-mail: biggerm@PLU.edu

L. Martin-Plank
University of Arizona College of Nursing, Pipersville, PA, USA

K. J. Wheeler
University of Kentucky College of Nursing, Lexington, KY, USA

S. H. Campbell
The University of British Columbia-Vancouver, School of Nursing, Easton, PA, USA

S. P. K. Mudiyanselage
Institute of Behavioral Medicine, The National Cheng Kung University, Tainan City, Taiwan

Department of Operation Theatre, National Hospital of Sri Lank, Colombo, Sri Lanka

S. D. Mithreepala
Department of Nursing, College of Medicine, National Cheng Kung University, Tainan, Taiwan

Department of Nursing, Faculty of Allied Sciences, University of Peradeniya, Peradeniya, Sri Lanka

F. Al Abri
Nursing Science, Oman College of Health Sciences, Muscat, Oman

B. S. Nsibandze
University of Eswatini, Faculty of Health Sciences, Kwaluseni, Eswatini

P. B. Howard
University of Kentucky College of Nursing, Louisville, KY, USA

K. J. Wheeler, M. Acorn (eds.), *Health Policy for Advanced Practice Nursing: A Toolkit for Implementation and Improvement*, Advanced Practice in Nursing,
https://doi.org/10.1007/978-3-032-03667-4_17

1 Introduction

Because the governance and operation of nursing schools and advanced practice nursing (APN) programs is extremely complex and dictated by multiple organizations and policies inside and outside of APN programs, this chapter can only address a few selected APN education policy issues. Topics are presented in the following order: Models of Delivery and Pedagogy, Admissions and Student Policy Issues, Resources for Learning, APN Faculty: The Duality of Practice and Teaching, and Funding of APN Education. Curriculum issues are covered in chapter "Exemplary Global Advanced Practice Nursing Curricula and Program Details", and credentialing and accreditation policy issues are covered in chapter "Credentialing and Accreditation of APN Education". Two exemplars are presented, one a partnership between a hospital-primary care system and school of nursing for the purpose of educating a staff of APNs, and the second, one country's attempt to create a consortium for the purpose of educating APNs.

2 Models of Delivery and Pedagogy

As advanced practice nursing develops globally, nurses in countries around the world are anticipating how to meet the unique education needs of advanced practice nurses (APNs) and how to adjust institutional pedagogy, the profession and practice of teaching and education, to meet these new challenges. This chapter discusses selected issues of APN education and policy that may affect the pedagogy, and what policy issues may flow from the pedagogy. By better understanding how policy can affect these specific pedagogical topics, nurses can better engage with its development to form and shape the future of nursing. This chapter discusses pressing issues including old and new teaching methods, simulation, distance/hybrid education, clinical education, interprofessional education (IPE), and artificial intelligence.

T. Williams
Norton Healthcare, University of Kentucky College of Nursing, Severna Park, MD, USA

B. R. G. de Oliveira Toso
Western Paraná State University, Cascavel, Brazil

R. F. Santana
Federal Fluminense University, Niterói, Rio de Janeiro, Brazil

M. A. Rodrigues
Rio de Janeiro State Council of Nurses, São Gonçalo, Rio de Janeiro, Brazil

A. B. S. Hércules
Epimed Solutions, Niterói, Rio de Janeiro, Brazil

2.1 Old and New Teaching Methods

Nursing educators have a long track record of successfully educating thousands of nurses annually. They also have a reputation for being innovative educators. For those reasons, nursing education is a blend of age-old, proven methods along with newer methods, those based on recent research and the movement toward student-centered learning. Traditional teaching methods pertain to brick-and-mortar education and mostly consist of teacher-centered education methods such as lectures and summative assessments (midterms, finals, papers, and other assignments graded at the end of teaching). Newer teaching methods consist of student-centered learning such as active learning, collaborative learning, differentiated learning (consists of presenting material in a variety of ways so as to address different learning styles; may be referred to as universal design for learning, VAK [visual, auditory, kinesthetic] learning, or multiple intelligences), experiential learning, flipped classroom (students familiarize themselves with materials before class discussions so they engage better in the discussion), formative assessment (assessing students while learning so as to adjust teaching to meet gaps in learning), gamification, inquiry-based learning, peer teaching, peer feedback, and personalized learning. Project based learning, problem-based learning or case-study learning, an education process many may consider a newer method, has been a longstanding part of nursing and APN education.

While the choice of teaching methods, those discussed above or those yet to be discussed below, may be up to the nursing faculty teaching a course, each has the potential to be a part of a larger policy decision by a program, school, accreditation agency, nursing council, or any agency that may affect nursing education and policy. For instance, a nursing program could decide to use problem-based learning or case studies throughout the curriculum, instituting a program-wide education policy. An administrator may want to reduce program costs by reducing technical support for technology-based education. In cases like these, faculty and interested parties (stakeholders) may need to be prepared to do whatever is required of them to positively affect the implementation or improvement of the policy.

Modern APN pedagogy increasingly relies on active student participation. This shifts the faculty role from a distributor of knowledge to a facilitator of learning. Policy must support curricula that empowers students to co-create their learning experiences, participate in program evaluation, and engage in peer-to-peer feedback, which mirrors the collaborative nature of the interprofessional healthcare team.

2.2 Simulation

Simulation is another example of pedagogy that has a long history of use in nursing but has once again come to the forefront. Simulation is a "technique for replacing or completing real-life experiences with guided experiences, which are a faithful imitation of the real world in a fully interactive way" (Koukourikos et al. 2021, p. 1). It can be focused on simple tasks or complex scenarios, and can include the following:

- High fidelity simulators, such as computerized manikins or immersive virtual reality platforms.
- Low fidelity simulators, such as static manikins or role playing.
- Standardized patients, for Structured Clinical Instruction Modules (SCIMs, formative). and Objective Structured Clinical Examinations (OSCEs, summative).
- Case studies.

The Covid-19 pandemic catalyzed a rapid global expansion in the use of simulation in nursing education, yet regulation and best practices remain underdeveloped. Establishing clear regulations is essential for defining the percentage of clinical preparation hours that can be substituted with simulation, as well as identifying best practices for its implementation (Smiley and Martin 2023). For instance, in Korea, the adoption of simulation in nursing education surged after the Korean Accreditation Board of Nursing Education proposed its use as a national standard (Park and Yu 2018). To navigate and shape these emerging standards, key organizations such as the International Nursing Association for Clinical Simulation and Learning (https://www.inacsl.org) and the Society for Simulation in Health Care (https://www.ssih.org) play a crucial role. Developing robust policies for nursing is critical for ensuring the effective and standardized use of simulation in nursing education globally.

2.3 Distance/Hybrid Education

Similar to the rapid advancement of simulation due to the Covid-19 pandemic, the rapid development of distance/hybrid education as an alternative to traditional, face-to-face education. These technology-based systems offer many advantages:

- Convenience, flexibility, and more equitable access to education.
- Students have more choice about types of programs to attend.
- Students can attend school without leaving their home or current work position.
- Communities are more likely to retain graduates if students can remain in their community to attend school.
- Local providers can precept APN students, perhaps developing professional relationships for the future.
- Programs can benefit from guest lectures and faculty from outside the physical limits of the school.
- Students have more opportunity to collaborate with students and faculty from outside the physical limits of the school.

Even though programs may be described as distance education or online education that title does not really describe the process for APN schooling. APN students will always have substantial face-to-face education in clinic with preceptors and school faculty. The didactic material can be exclusively taught by distance education or via hybrid or blended format, and can be synchronous and/or asynchronous.

However, the policy implications of distance education can be significant. Some of this is addressed in a following subsection of this chapter (resources/simulation) as well as in chapter "Exemplary Global Advanced Practice Nursing Curricula and Program Details" (curriculums and program details) and chapter "Credentialing and Accreditation of APN Education" (education credentialing). There is a strong need for nursing pedagogy policy to ensure quality, accessibility, and regulatory standards, and how to implement them while upholding basic standards of competency. Distance education has the possibility to expand nursing education to help address global nursing shortages, but it is important that it is equitable, so that students from diverse geographic and socio-economic backgrounds have equal access to these resources.

Distance education offers a vital pathway to help address the global nursing shortage, which remains a critical challenge for health systems worldwide. According to the State of the World's Nursing 2025 report, the global nursing workforce has grown to 29.8 million, yet a persistent deficit of 5.8 million nurses remains, with the most severe shortages concentrated in low- and middle-income countries (WHO 2025). With a large percentage of the current workforce expected to retire within the next decade, technology-based education is essential to scale up production and improve equitable access. However, as these programs expand, educators and interested parties (stakeholders) must ensure that the quality of distance-based APN programs remains on par with traditional face-to-face formats. That point could not be stated more clearly than by the statement made by the American Association of Colleges of Nursing, Alliance for Nursing Accreditation, and endorsed by more than a dozen US education, accreditation, and certification agencies, including the National Council of State Boards of Nursing (NCSBN) (AACN 2025, para 2–6):

> All nursing education programs delivered solely or in part through distance learning technologies must meet the same academic program and learning support standards and accreditation criteria as programs provided in face-to-face formats, including the following:
>
> - Student outcomes are consistent with the stated mission, goals, and objectives of the program.
> - The institution assumes the responsibility for establishing a means to assess student outcomes. This assessment includes overall program outcomes, in addition to specific course outcomes, and a process for using the results for continuous program improvement.
>
> Mechanisms for ongoing faculty development and involvement in the area of distance education and the use of technology in teaching-learning processes are established. Appropriate technical support for faculty and students is provided.
>
> When utilizing distance learning methods, a program provides learning opportunities that facilitate development of students' clinical competence and professional role socialization and establishes mechanisms to measure these student outcomes.
>
> When utilizing distance learning methods, a program provides or makes available resources for the students' successful attainment of all program objectives.
>
> Each accreditation and program review entity incorporates the review of distance-education programs as a component of site visitor/evaluator training.

The United Nations Educational, Scientific, and Cultural Organization (UNESCO 2025) does provide guidance to Distance Education, although not specific to clinical graduate education. It is available at https://unesco.org/en/digital-education/distance-learning-guidance.

2.4 Clinical Education

A foundational element of all nursing education is the clinical education nursing students experience, and this is true for APN students as well. Programs manage clinical education in a variety of ways. Some programs spread the clinical experience over multiple courses and multiple semesters/quarters. Some programs require students to complete the didactic coursework before completing clinical hours at the end of the program. Some programs devote a designated portion of clinical hours toward pharmacology (Wheeler et al. 2022). Faculty are expected to oversee the types of visits or patient experiences students log so each learns from a variety of clinical experiences representative of the APN type. Though an occasional program pays preceptors, most programs rely on the preceptor to volunteer their time, or the precepting is an expectation of their work. Some programs offer access to continuing education, access to online libraries, or a reduction on books via the school bookstore.

The clinical hour requirements vary according to country, specialty, and education track, and range from as low as 400 to as high as 1500 (Wheeler et al. 2022). Clinical hours education requirements are regulated by national governmental standards, program standards, and/or credentialing organizations. This variation may be an argument for competency-based education, where minimum hours may not be necessary, but specific competencies must be demonstrated (ICN 2020).

2.5 Interprofessional Education

The World Health Organization (WHO 2010) identifies interprofessional health collaboration in education as a needed component in improving the global health workforce and improving learning and health outcomes. Interprofessional education (IPE) is the pedagogical approach that occurs when two or more health professions learn in a collaborative environment. The goal is to develop knowledge, skills and attitudes that improve interprofessional team behaviors and competence long-term (Buring et al. 2009, p. 2). Like distance education and simulation, IPE can be done as a small component of a course or program, or extensively throughout a program.

While IPE is likely to be an increasing part of nursing education curriculum, policy decisions can help move this collaboration forward by including it in the accreditation process, ensuring nursing leadership is integrated into the design of these programs to foster mutual respect and optimal scope of practice for all health professionals (Herath et al. 2017). Resources are available for policy implementation, such as the WHO Framework for Action on Interprofessional Education & Collaborative

Practice. The WHO framework helps governments and institutions provide an assessment of the needs, designing programs so there is collaboration on curriculums and clinical education. The framework is available athttps://www.who.int/publications/i/item/framework-for-action-on-interprofessional-education-collaborative-practice

2.6 Artificial Intelligence and Education

The swift advancement of Artificial Intelligence (AI) into many aspects of healthcare and education has led educators to consider its many applications to curriculum (what content is taught) and pedagogy (how content is taught). As AI continues to evolve, its impact on nursing practices will be profound, necessitating corresponding adjustments in educational approaches. However, the regulatory framework for integrating AI into nursing education remains uncertain.

According to Davenport and Kalakota (2019), AI's healthcare applications encompass diverse domains such as machine learning (using data to create training models or predict treatment protocols; pathology detection; voice recognition), natural language processing (speech recognition; analysis of text; translation), rule based expert systems (clinical decision support; electronic health records), physical robots (surgical robots), and process automation (repetitive tasks such as prior authorization, updating patient records, or billing; image recognition to extract data). As these become imbedded into healthcare delivery systems throughout the world, nursing education will need to adjust the curriculum in order to prepare nurses and APNs for the healthcare delivery of the future. Nursing students and practitioners will need the necessary knowledge and skills to evaluate and seamlessly integrate AI technologies into person-centered nursing care. Urgent curricular reforms are imperative within nursing education programs across academic and clinical settings to ensure nurses and nursing students are adept at practicing safely and efficiently amidst the AI era.

The imperative is equally important in regard to AI and pedagogy, not only in terms of how faculty use AI but how students do as well. Faculty can leverage AI for assessments and grading, discussion prompts, feedback, plagiarism recognition, and content design. Any AI use that frees up faculty from repetitive and time-consuming routine tasks creates opportunities for more faculty-student contact. Nurse educators must embrace innovative pedagogies that incorporate AI to better support students at every educational level. But how students are allowed to use AI, and how they report its use is evolving as well. Leveraging its use for learning shows enormous potential but cannot be allowed to replace the deep learning required by clinicians.

Nations worldwide are swiftly formulating policy frameworks for AI implementation in education and healthcare. As of 2021, over thirty countries have unveiled national AI policy strategies (Schiff 2022). Advocacy approaches for the integration of AI vary by country; organizations must comply with national laws and ethical standards. The International Artificial Intelligence in Education Society offers valuable resources and guidance on integrating AI into educational contexts, available at https://iaied.org.

2.7 Policy Implications of Delivery Models and Pedagogy

Every issue discussed above applies to both nursing and APN education, so the policy processes are not new. As programs evolve and move to adopt new forms of pedagogy many of the policy processes described throughout the text apply here—assess for need, will, and resources; create a plan and assign tasks, implement the plan, evaluate the plan, revise the plan. As mentioned earlier, nursing educators are known to be innovators.

3 Admissions and Student Policy Issues

When it comes to nursing the dominant topic in the literature pertains to the shortage of nurses, and it is a universal problem, based on very complex issues (e.g., lack of investment in the profession, lack of nurse educators, diminishing enrollments, poor working conditions and nurse burnout, increased demand for healthcare, poor distribution, and lack of representation of the population). Since the supply of advanced practice nurses (APNs) relies on the supply of nurses, these issues affect the recruitment and education of advanced practice nurses (APNs). This chapter is a discussion of some of the issues that impact APN student admissions, including the policy implications if APN programs attend to diversity, equity, and inclusion (DEI).

Admissions policies must also evolve to reflect changes in student characteristics. Today's APN candidates are increasingly diverse, digitally native, and often balance professional roles with family responsibilities. To retain this new generation of learners, programs must offer modular, flexible pathways that recognize prior learning and accommodate the life-work balance of the modern nursing student.

3.1 Supply—Quality through Investment, Development, and Balance

One of the arguments often made against APN education is that the education of APNs has the potential to deplete an already limited supply of nurses. Obviously, the priority for a country or jurisdiction is to provide a sufficient supply of generalist nurses. However, for a country to meet Sustainable Development Goals (SDGs), there are other issues to consider. A nursing shortage impacts any country hoping to educate nurses for degrees beyond generalist nurse—educators, researchers, administrators, and advanced practice nurses (APNs). And each one of those has a unique role in meeting SDGs. For those countries where the APNs serve not only as clinicians but as educators, researchers, and administrators, the impact may be even more significant.

Aside from issues surrounding supply, APNs positively impact the nursing profession as a whole. As role models, APNs influence aspiring nurses. Their leadership abilities, expertise, and experience in research and policy has been shown to advance the entire nursing profession (Thejewel 2024). Interested parties (stakeholders) have a responsibility to invest in the development of generalist nurses as well as APNs.

3.2 Admission Processes—Quality through Rigorous Application Standards

APN schools customarily require the following for admission to the program: graduation from a nursing program (level may vary according to country); an active, unencumbered nursing license or registration (level may vary according to the country); and a certain grade point average or higher. Some programs may require letters of reference, personal essays, demonstrations of language and writing abilities, completion of certain courses (i.e., statistics), interviews, and some level of nursing experience. Most countries require at least two years of practice at the registered/generalist nurse level prior to acceptance into APN programs (Moore et al. 2024; Wheeler et al. 2022). For those applicants who do not meet the 2-year experience, part-time admission may be considered with clinical hours delayed until the experiential recommendation is met.

3.3 Diversity, Equity, and Inclusivity—Quality Through a Representative Workforce

Significant research is demonstrating underrepresentation of minorities as healthcare providers leads to worse health outcomes, from either gaps in care or limitations in culturally competent (culturally sensitive) care. Some of this may be culturally dictated (e.g., countries where women generally do not work outside the home or countries where women are banned from driving). Other reasons include limitations of funding and access to educational programs, deficiency of targeted recruitment techniques, and historical and systemic biases (Rossiter 2025, para 4).

Table 1 provides strategies that can be taken in order to recruit and retain representative members of the population, and assure ongoing contributions to the profession. For nursing, including advanced practice nursing, this work relies not only on what nursing schools do, but what was done to lay the foundation for the process (pre-admission) and what is done once students graduate and work within systems of care.

Table 1 Strategies to increase diversity, equity, and inclusivity in the nursing workforce

Strategy level	Strategy specifics	Strategy details	Strategy examples
Workforce strategies	Enhance educational access and support	Provide scholarship programs and financial aid	Scholarships and financial aid can be tailored and aimed to underrepresented groups.
		Develop and deliver preparatory and bridging programs	Remedial and bridging programs can be created that help students from underrepresented backgrounds build skills and confidence.
		Utilize inclusive admissions policies	Educational institutions can review and revise mission processes so they are equitable and inclusive (i.e., remove barriers related to standardized testing and/or rigid academic prerequisites).
	Strengthen recruitment and outreach efforts	Develop community engagement and partnerships	Educational and healthcare institutions can partner with schools, local leaders, and local organizations to raise awareness about nursing as a rewarding career (i.e., career fairs, informational meetings).
		Deliver targeted marketing and recruitment campaigns	Marketing about the impact of nurses from minority groups, societal impact of nursing, and potential for career opportunities can be provided via social media, local media, and community events.
		Develop and deliver pipeline programs and internships	Pipeline programs can be created to direct high school and college students through the process of becoming a nurse.
	Foster an inclusive workplace culture	Maintain mentorship and sponsorship programs	Healthcare organizations can implement mentorship programs that connect underrepresented individuals with experienced nurses.
		Provide cultural competence training	Cultural competence training can be provided via workshops, seminars, and continuing education.
		Adopt inclusive policies and practices	Institutions can adopt policies that promote diversity and inclusion (i.e., anti-discrimination policies, equitable hiring, support for work-life balance, career advancement).
	Encourage leadership and advocacy	Create and support leadership roles for individuals from underrepresented groups	Organizations can create leadership development programs for individuals from underrepresented groups.

Table 1 (continued)

Strategy level	Strategy specifics	Strategy details	Strategy examples
		Advocate for policy reform	Nursing organizations, advocacy groups, and policy makers can advocate for systemic changes at all levels (i.e., equitable access to education, monies for diversity programs, development of accountability processes).
		Lead research and data collection on DEI issues	Workforce research initiatives can be created to provide information on barriers faced by underrepresented groups and the success or limitations of diversity programs, thereby providing information so organizations can implement and adjust their practices.
Educational institution strategies	Attend to curriculum and pedagogy	Integrate diversity into curriculums	Curricula can be adjusted to represent community diversity, with content on cultural competence, health disparities, and social determinants of health.
		Apply student-centered teaching methods	Innovative teaching methods (collaborative learning, problem-based learning) can be provided in order to recognize and educate according to unique learning styles.
	Attend to faculty diversity and professional development	Recruit diverse faculty members	Programs can strengthen recruitment and retention of faculty from underrepresented groups.
		Provide continuous professional development	Programs can offer education on diversity, equity, inclusion, and unconscious bias, including how to support students from underrepresented groups.
Strategies for healthcare organizations	Create supportive work environments	Organize and support employee resource groups	Organizations can create employee resource groups to underrepresented groups, offering peer support, mentorship, and the means to provide a collective voice.
		Develop inclusive onboarding and training programs	Onboarding processes can be designed to welcome and integrate all new employees, with education on cultural competence, conflict resolution, and team building.
		Publish performance evaluation and advancement processes	Organizations can ensure that promotion and performance evaluation processes are transparent.

(continued)

Table 1 (continued)

Strategy level	Strategy specifics	Strategy details	Strategy examples
	Utilize technology and innovation	Make data driven decisions	Organizations can collect and analyze data on diversity initiatives, using data to validate accountability and/or improve initiatives.
		Use virtual mentorship and networking	Virtual platforms can connect individuals from underrepresented groups with mentors, bridging geographical and logistical divides.
Broader policy and system changes	Create national and local policy initiatives	Fund diversity programs	Governments and organizations can provide funding dedicated to diversity initiatives.
		Advocate for legislative reforms	Legislative reforms can be introduced by policymakers on a variety of measures that can reduce barriers and improve professional development (loan forgiveness programs, tax incentives for programs that meet diversity benchmarks, regulations that support recruitment transparency).
		Collaborate with professional organizations	Professional nursing organizations of all types can advocate for changes in standards and practices that affect diversity and inclusion.
	Build an inclusive future	Participate in long term strategic planning	Organizations can adopt long-term planning for diversity and inclusion.
		Support research on DEI and innovation	Educational and healthcare organizations can support studies that pertain to diversity and inclusion, informing decisions and strategies.
		Encourage and lead community partnerships	Educational and healthcare organizations can partner with local groups in order to understand local needs and adjust accordingly.

Adapted from Diversifying the Nursing Workforce: Strategies for Increasing Diversity and Inclusion, by Rossiter (2025) (https://blog.forthenurse.us/diversifying-the-nursing-workforce/)

4 Resources for Learning

In the development and delivery of an APN program, many resources are needed. This section will discuss specific resources for faculty, clinical experiences, simulation, and research for APN programs. Much of this is similar to resources used to educate generalist nurses but there are some unique features and unique policy needs for advanced practice. What will not be discussed are the resources all nursing programs use—educational materials and textbooks, learning management platforms or systems, and medical equipment.

4.1 Resources—Faculty

As there is a global nursing and nursing faculty shortage, APN programs face the same shortages. There are several areas that make this especially challenging. One of the struggles pertains to the expectation that nursing faculty have a 'terminal degree' in order to teach, in most cases, a PhD. The PhD requirement can be a significant barrier to the supply of faculty for APN programs. The PhD is a research doctorate. While APNs devote a portion of their schooling to research and the translation of research, the majority of their education is devoted to clinical issues and the delivery of care. What APN programs need are educators skilled in clinical issues and care delivery. The United States developed the Doctor of Nursing Practice (DNP), a clinical doctorate, to provide skilled clinicians with professionally recognized terminal degrees. Aside from the concern about faculty supply, there is another concern; programs that rely on research faculty to teach APN students must be careful not to be research heavy and light on clinical.

An added barrier pertains to the expectation that faculty who are APNs split time between teaching, practicing, and scholarly work (research, publication, presentations, policy work). Because these faculty are expected to practice a defined number of clinical hours per year for licensing, they must stay current with practice. However, even that is a potential barrier when schools of nursing and practice sites do not work together to create the means by which faculty can practice without 'adding' practice hours to an already demanding teaching and scholarly work schedule. This issue is discussed in greater detail later in the chapter.

4.2 Resources—Clinical Experiences

Identifying resources for clinical experiences is another area where programs exert considerable time and energy, especially since students need a variety of preceptors over their years in clinical. Programs recruit preceptors in many ways. Sometimes APN faculty work in large education and hospital systems, and there is an expectation that APNs within the same system will precept the APN students. Sometimes there are agencies that help find preceptors for programs, sometimes at a cost, sometimes not. And sometimes consortiums develop specifically so that multiple programs within a geographic area pair students with preceptors on a rotating basis. Some programs pay for preceptors, with the pay either going directly to the preceptor or the organization that employs the preceptor. For the most part, APN preceptors operate on a voluntary basis.

In building good relationships with mentors/preceptors, a clear outline of expectations, roles, outcomes, communication, and answers to frequently asked questions (FAQs) is important to establish. Several years ago, the American Association of

Table 2 NONPF[a]/AANP[b] Expectation checklist of preceptors (what faculty expect from preceptors)

Establishing clinical rotation	**Completed**
Review NP program policies regarding student placement guidelines.	
Communicate start date and time with student.	
Review documents related to the clinical course (welcome letter, clinical hour requirement, syllabus, course objectives, etc.) and seek clarification, if needed.	
Review family educational rights and privacy act (FERPA).	
Orientation	
Orient student to clinical site, clinical site policies, electronic medical record (EMR), and clinical team prior to student's patient experiences.	
Discuss course objectives, course requirements, student learning goals, and clinical experience expectations with the student.	
Discuss with student his/her experience/background.	
Outline appropriate tasks, patient cases, and caseload for each clinical day.	
Establish plan for student progression from observing to conducting visits with minimal intervention.	
Clinical experience	
Model clinical skills and professional/ethical behaviors for student learning.	
Be present to observe all student clinical activities.	
Include student as a pertinent part of the healthcare team and encourage interprofessional collaboration between student and other team members.	
Encourage learning using direct questioning methods and allowing reflection on feedback.	
Verify student clinical hours.	
Communication	
Guide, counsel, and encourage active student learning through clinical experiences.	
Communicate to faculty pertinent feedback regarding student performance and learning progression related to course expectations and requirements.	
Be available for virtual or face-to-face site visits.	
Evaluation	
Complete appropriate evaluation forms at intervals as outlined in course requirements.	
Discuss evaluation(s) with student providing constructive feedback on strengths, weaknesses, and a plan for improvement.	
Participate in faculty-initiated plans of remediation, if necessary.	
Completion of clinical rotation	
Submission of all documents as outlined in the course.	

Reprinted from "A Checklist for Faculty and Preceptor to Enhance the Nurse Practitioner Student Clinical Experience," by Pitts et al. (2019). Reprinted with permission from Wolters Kluwer Health, Inc.

[a]*NONPF* National Organization of Nurse Practitioner Faculties

[b]*AANP* American Association of Nurse Practitioners

Nurse Practitioners and the National Organization of Nurse Practitioner Faculties collaborated on a document to define two checklists to describe the expectations and responsibilities of both preceptors (Table 2) and faculty (Table 3) in clinical placements. The intent of the publication was to establish a standardized process for these experiences. Although the checklist was developed for nurse practitioners, it is adaptable for all forms of APN precepting in any location.

Table 3 NONPF[a]/AANP[b] expectation checklist of faculty (what preceptors expect from faculty)

Establishing clinical rotation	**Completed**
Communicate start date and time with preceptor/clinical site point of contact.	
Identify preceptor's preferred method of communication.	
Send documents related to the clinical course (welcome letter, preceptor handbook, clinical hours requirement, syllabus, course objectives, etc.) to preceptor/clinical site point of contact via mail or email.	
Provide preceptor/clinical site point of contact with student's credentials and clinical clearance paperwork.	
Discuss course objectives, course requirements, student learning goals, and clinical experience expectations with the preceptor.	
Orientation	
Provide the contact number/information to the clinical faculty responsible for the student.	
Discuss the purpose, frequency, length, and number of site visits with the preceptor.	
Offer face-to-face or online orientation opportunities addressing adult learning/teaching strategies and how to serve as an effective preceptor.	
Clinical experience	
Assume primary responsibility of the student throughout the clinical experience.	
Assess students clinical skills, knowledge, and competencies throughout clinical experience and assess for appropriate progression as it relates to course and clinical objectives.	
Support students in connecting knowledge obtained in academic setting with their clinical experiences.	
Review and confirm student clinical hours.	
Communication	
Engage in open communication with preceptor regarding student performance and learning progression related to course expectations and requirements.	
Schedule virtual or face-to-face site visits.	
Evaluation	
Collect and review evaluation forms completed by the preceptor at intervals, as outlined in course requirements.	
Collect and review preceptor evaluation forms completed by the student.	
Discuss evaluation(s) with student providing constructive feedback on strengths, weaknesses, and a plan for improvement.	
Initiate plans of remediation based on evaluations, if necessary.	
Completion of clinical rotation	
Review final evaluation submitted by preceptor, as outlined in the course.	
Send the preceptor and/or clinical site a thank you letter and/or token of appreciation, per program and/or university policy (including but not limited to continuing education credits, monetary compensation, adjunct faculty positions, access to school library resources).	
Provide the preceptor with documentation of preceptorship for national certification renewal or dossier.	
Provide the preceptor with feedback about preceptorship performance based on student evaluation(s).	

Reprinted from "A Checklist for Faculty and Preceptor to Enhance the Nurse Practitioner Student Clinical Experience," by Pitts et al. (2019). Reprint with permission from Wolters Kluwer Health, Inc.

[a]*NONPF* National Organization of Nurse Practitioner Faculties
[b]*AANP* American Association of Nurse Practitioners

New programs will not have graduates and previous mentors to rely on so must establish new relationships with APNs, physicians, or physician assistants (when appropriate) from the community. The benefits of interdisciplinary practice and gaining an outside nursing lens on patient care are positive aspects, while managing hierarchical power differentials and encouraging independence of APN students may be a challenge. At the same time, faculty will want to ensure that an understanding and application of the nursing process is not lost when the students work with those from other professions.

Hopefully, individuals and organizations who precept students are aware of the benefits of precepting students. Preceptors may recognize the intrinsic motivation and professional duty of educating the next generation, and it can be a worthy recruitment strategy when APN students stay at the site after graduation (Campbell and Hawkins 2007). Nursing faculty can provide support to preceptors through good communication, sharing insight on standards of evidence-based practice, and possibly working collaboratively on research, publications, and presentations.

However, sometimes specific incentives may be needed to recruit and retain good preceptors. Incentives may include sponsoring an APN preceptor appreciation day or celebration, presenting an annual award to recognize the best APN preceptor, providing access to library services, or offering discounts to bookstores or continuing education programs. In addition, if the school of nursing hosts lectures, research toolkit webinars, and events, it is important to invite preceptors and help them feel part of the school. Well-prepared students are the best incentive to preceptors, and often, that preparation lies in the use of simulation resources (Campbell and Hawkins 2007).

4.3 Resources—Simulation

Simulation-based education (SBE) has become standard pedagogy for APN programs, just as it has for general nursing education. SBE allows learners to translate their acquired knowledge to practical applications of realistic situations in a safe environment, building confidence for the learner, and providing opportunities for student evaluation. Simulated learning can be for a range of clinical skills, from very simple to very complex, and can apply to the use of low-fidelity mannequins, high-fidelity mannequins, partial task simulators, virtual reality, standardized patients, hybrid simulation, and some forms of e-learning. Even case studies are a form of SBE.

A significant benefit of SBE is its ability to educate the principles of evidence-based practice (EBP) via clinical scenarios, then provide the means to evaluate student competency. To do this, faculty must apply current EBP guidelines as part of the scenario (included in checklist) and discuss during debriefing episodes or second-run of scenarios. Transfer of learning can be evaluated in clinic on evaluation tools and with preceptors. Despite obvious benefits of SBE the process requires resources, and therefore careful consideration.

Table 4 Common enablers and inhibitors to the application of simulation-based education to APN education

Enablers	Inhibitors
Generational learners	Resources/equity
Cost efficiency/quality	Faculty competency
Need for competency-based movement	Gaps in the literature
Standardization	Resistance to change
Increasing expectations of employers/public	Lack of standardization/outcomes measures
Limited resources	Multiple regulatory body expectations
Need to address complexity of care	Workload allocation

Reprinted from "A Call to Action: Building Evidence for Use of Simulation in Nurse Practitioner Education," by Jeffries et al. (2019). Reprinted with permission from Wolters Kluwer Health, Inc.

4.3.1 Enablers and Inhibitors to the Use of Simulation

For APN programs, the degree of application of SBE depends on many factors. Common issues faced in the integration of simulation pedagogy in health sciences curricula are related to the lack of research demonstrating its impact, identifying its best use, and defining how learning through this method translates into evidence-informed practice and clinical practice, including outcomes on patient safety and quality of care. Recognition of simulation as substitution for clinical hours remains controversial and limited. Table 4 is a summary of common enablers and inhibitors to the application of SBE to APN education as defined by Jeffries et al. (2019). Each needs to be considered when implementing or improving SBE in APN schooling (Table 4).

4.3.2 Evolution of Simulation-Based Research and Education

Despite difficulties, it is key that APN faculty build capacity for facilitation of simulation (Watts et al. 2021). Curriculum mapping of what is being taught throughout courses and programs is the first step, then deciding what parts would benefit from SBE, how delivery of SBE would unfold, and what resources would be needed. Senvisky et al. (2023 para 2) summarize SBE costs in their article on financing and funding a simulation center as "stuff, staff, and space" and provide valuable advice for APN programs enriching their education through SBE. What follows is a discussion of resources to consider:

- *Equipment (stuff)*: depends on the fidelity of the environment, for example, an intensive care unit or operating room set-up requires more financial output and decision making such as will the oxygen and suction features work? High-fidelity vs. low-fidelity cost differences are worth considering (often much can be accomplished with sufficient suspension of disbelief). The use of simulated patients depends on the resources. Some APN programs partner with medical programs and share the cost of standardized patients (trained actors); other lower-resource programs use retired healthcare providers and patients to simulate healthcare conditions with which they are familiar. This requires more training time, active pre-briefing and debriefing of the simulation patients, and the burden often falls on the simulation faculty.

- *Faculty and support staff (staff)*: faculty to teach, tech and other support staff, faculty development and release time, including workshops and conferences.
- *Laboratory (space)*: space to house equipment, run scenarios, hospital-like, clinic-like, home-like. Decisions about placement of beds, areas for debriefing, extent of available equipment for learner use.

Aside from decision-making about the purchase and maintenance of simulation laboratories and equipment, potential student, and faculty subscriptions to simulations in a variety of forms (virtual reality, augmented reality, immersive experiences created with CHAT-GPT [Chatbot Generative Pre-trained Transformer]), and decisions related to staffing there are other issues to resolve. Decisions must be made about how the technology will be incorporated, and its unique issues of delivery and pedagogy are key. Another decision is whether it will be used in a formative manner (for learning and increasing skills) and/or in a summative/evaluative or high-stakes manner to assess competencies and program completion.

Simulation for distance/hybrid education requires additional specific planning. Residency Intensives involve bringing learners to campus, usually at the start and completion of the course to perform OSCEs (Objective Structured Clinical Examinations) and SCIMs (Structured Clinical Insights Modules). These can be done before, during, or after clinicals, depending on the timing of the Intensive. Aside from student evaluation all the way through the program, they can be used for program evaluation, preceptor feedback, learner portfolios (ePortfolio, Google Portfolio), and journal completion. Scaffolding must be planned, so the learning and evaluations build according to curriculum and clinicals. In parts of Canada, students are required to pass OSCEs prior to sitting for the NP licensing exam.

The following is a list of issues to consider in planning resources for SBE implementation and improvement:

- *Standard setting*
  - Healthcare Simulation Standards of Best Practice™ Operations, available from https://www.inacsl.org/healthcare-simulation-standards-ql OR https://www.nursingsimulation.org/article/S1876-1399(21)00099-2/fulltext
  - Healthcare Simulation Standards of Best Practice™ (all), available from: https://www.inacsl.org/healthcare-simulation-standards-ql.
- *Building faculty capacity and competency*
  - Pedagogical capacity can be built through curriculum mapping, bringing faculty together to collaborate, discuss issues, share experiences, and plan. Instructional design experts can assist in development and delivery.
  - Faculty Competency Rubric, available from https://www.healthysimulation.com/tools/evaluating-healthcare-simulation/facilitator-competency-rubric/.
  - Canadian Certified Simulation Nurse Educator of the Canadian Nurse Educators Institute (required by Canadian Association of Schools of Nursing), available at https://cnei-icie.casn.ca/our-programs/certification-programs/simulation-certification-program/. Textbook available at https://www.casn.ca/2023/12/simulation-in-canadian-nursing-education/.

  - Society for Simulation in Healthcare (SSH) provides simulation education certification, Certified Healthcare Simulation Educator, available at https://www.ssih.org/chse. Dictionary, available at https://www.ssih.org/healthcare-simulation-dictionary.
  - International Nursing Association for Clinical Simulation and Learning (INACSL) website, available at https://www.inacsl.org, provides numerous educational programs and other resources—standards, a journal, grants, and instruments.
  - A Guide for the Assessment of Clinical Competence Using Simulation edited by Vincent-Lambert and Bogossian (2017), available at https://static1.squarespace.com/static/555fc773e4b02c9d26ef2348/t/59e50596bce1762a6dd8d6c7/1508181421406/UJUQ_U21_SimulationGuide_Handbook_B5_ONLINE.pdf
- *Accessing, creating, and evaluating scenarios*—building scenarios requires careful planning, with attention to EBP as described above.
  - Multiple software programs are available through an Internet search to teach APN students a variety of skills, including physical assessment.
  - CyberPatient™—database of patients and symptoms that learners can access and are evaluated on. The initial focus was for medical students, but allied professions are being incorporated. Available at https://cyberpatient.ca
  - SSH, mentioned above—multiple resources, including a dictionary (provides consistency) and tools for evaluation. Available from https://www.ssih.org/chse.
  - Evaluation—The Evaluating Healthcare Simulation website provides multiple tools for simulation evaluation, available at https://www.healthysimulation.com/tools/evaluating-healthcare-simulation/.
  - Repository of Instruments used in Simulation Research—Simulation, available at https://www.inacsl.org/repository-of-instruments.

4.4 Resources—Research

APN programs devote a portion of their curriculum to research, particularly how to evaluate it and how to translate it into practice. APN culminating projects (scholarly projects, capstones), especially at the DNP level, tend to focus on practice, policy, and education with a variety of research methodologies (Cheng et al. 2016; Nye 2021). The focus of these culminating projects often incorporates the role of the APN, knowledge translation, system changes, and leadership. In the United States, scholarly projects tend to be quality improvement projects (Tovar et al. 2020).

Research concentrations and resources should align with the clinical and policy focus of APNs. Programs need to provide the following:

Library access, preferably online and resource-rich (interested parties [stakeholders] and librarians will need to decide which libraries and journals to access as there are associated costs).

- Access to a statistician. An excellent article on basic research statistics is Vandever's Introduction to Research Statistical Analysis: An Overview of the Basics (available at https://pmc.ncbi.nlm.nih.gov/articles/PMC10324782/).
- Access to databases and training on how to extract resources and data, including the use of reference management systems such as Covidence (https://www.covidence.org/).
- Instructions on the use of technology in research and writing, for such things as citations, reference storage, and retrieval. Students will need parameters of if/how to use artificial intelligence (AI) and how to cite use.
- Access to additional resources, such as Joanna Briggs Institute (https://jbi.global/), Sigma Theta Tau Repository (https://www.sigmarepository.org/sigma/).
- Where appropriate, access to human subject research approval and institutional review boards (IRBs).
- Access to publications through reputable publishers such as Elsevier and Springer, with available discounts to promote the advancement of advanced practice nursing research.

5 APN Faculty: The Duality of Practice and Teaching

When APNs begin to teach, there is an expectation they will continue direct clinical practice—at least a few hours or a shift or two weekly. For most APNs, this is not unreasonable; most APNs chose to be APNs because they wanted to stay close to patients. However, the process of teaching and maintaining a clinical practice can be challenging since faculty are also expected to publish, present, engage in research, and participate in APN policy making as well as teach. Within this context, schools of nursing face a persistent shortage and challenge to find faculty who can fulfill the dual expectations of teaching and scholarship while maintaining direct patient care and clinical leadership. The State of the World's Nursing 2025 report notes that faculty shortages are a primary bottleneck in expanding the workforce, with many countries reporting educator vacancies (WHO 2025). This section is a discussion of the issues involved in the duality of maintaining a clinical practice while teaching in APN programs. It provides an analysis of faculty practice models, the benefits of clinically engaged faculty, and the best methods for interested parties (stakeholders) to create sustainable faculty practice models that benefit everyone involved in the process. This section will not address issues related to adjunct faculty or guest lecturers; these are individuals who are full-time or nearly full-time APN clinicians willing to teach or contract for specific or limited content and do not receive the benefits or bear the responsibilities of full-time faculty.

5.1 APN Faculty: Meeting the Obligations of Direct Clinical Practice While Teaching

There are a number of reasons APN faculty are expected to continue to practice while teaching, not the least of which is that the most commonly adapted theory of advanced practice nursing, Hamric's 1996 Model of Advanced Nursing Practice, considers direct clinical practice a foundational competency. Of course, there are other expected competencies within the model, but each is in support of direct clinical practice. These include leadership, guidance and coaching, evidence-based practice, consultation, collaboration, and ethical decision-making (Arslanian-Engoren 2023). All the models of advanced practice nursing emphasize direct clinical practice, and the benefits are worthwhile:

1. *For the clinician.* Maintaining direct clinical practice allows the APN to stay up-to-date clinically, which is critical in the quickly evolving healthcare world that exists today. Aside from keeping the clinician up-to-date clinically, it assures credibility in the eyes of students but also with administrators and policymakers. Clinical practice also allows the APN to maintain practice hours that are often required by credentialing and certification bodies. It is possible that salaries may be improved since the remuneration is customarily higher for clinicians than educators (Huckstadt and Hayes 2013).
2. *For the academic institution and students.* Because the APN is functioning in the real-world, students are exposed to faculty who understand and are knowledgeable about current clinical situations. This applies to clinical scenarios but also to rapidly advancing technology used in clinic. Having knowledgeable and informed faculty improves the quality of the students who graduate, hopefully improving certification test scores. The resulting improved community standing improves program reputation, resulting in more student applications and increased appeal for faculty to apply. Faculty who practice often serve as preceptors for APN students, easing the recruitment process that programs experience. Often these clinicians participate in research programs based in clinical sites, leading to mutually beneficial relationships between clinic.
3. *For the clinical site.* Clinical sites benefit because faculty bring an added perspective and level of experience to practice. As they are exposed to recent research, they continuously bring the most recently updated clinical information to the site. When faculty are exposed to clinical issues, they also have the potential to recognize and assist with quality improvement projects and clinical educational innovation.

Despite these benefits, maintaining dual responsibilities presents significant challenges for the APN faculty. Maintaining an active clinical practice while meeting the academic demands can lead to role strain, especially when the faculty are expected to teach a full load, conduct research, and actively participate in community service (Gazza 2019). This may lead to burnout and disengagement with the role. Additionally, many institutions prioritize research, grants, and teaching activities rather than clinical activities which in turn leads the clinical faculty to miss leadership and professional growth opportunities (DeNisco and DeNisco 2023). Other challenges may include: limited administrative support, lack of protected clinical hours, and unclear policies, which will make it difficult to sustain the role.

5.2 Implementing Faculty Practice Models

To counter the above difficulties, schools of nursing have developed faculty practice models to provide guidance. Huckstadt and Hayes (2013, para 4) define "faculty practice as a contractual agreement with defined and clear boundaries that puts patient care as the focus. It consists of a collaborative partnership between practice and teaching that benefits both roles." Nursing programs are accustomed to working out various contract forms—memorandums of understanding (MOUs), affiliation agreements, or collaborative agreements—with clinical sites for nursing student rotations and for research collaborations. Multiple resources are available detailing the components and process of brokering these types of agreements.

There are a number of ways in which faculty practice models unfold. The process depends on the split of teaching and clinical hours and whether or not the clinical position is inside or outside the faculty position. For instance, some programs appoint faculty under a Clinical Title Series, where the faculty member splits time between teaching and practice, are often not offered tenure, and may or may not be expected to meet scholarly work requirements like other appointments (professor, associate professor, assistant professor). Below is a discussion of faculty practice models and the things that need to be considered by all interested parties (stakeholders) in the process. A more thorough discussion is available from the National Organization of Nurse Practitioner Faculties (2023), available at https://cdn.ymaws.com/www.nonpf.org/resource/resmgr/publications_/faculty_practice_toolkit_202.pdf.

5.2.1 The Clinical Practice Is Outside the Faculty Position

In these instances, the teaching workload is usually reduced to allow time for the APN to work in some clinical setting. Often, these are arranged when the faculty maintains connections with a previous employer and agrees to work a specified, but limited, number of hours or shifts per week. The clinical setting pays the APN directly, usually in a per diem manner and with limited benefits, if any. The APN program, recognizing the benefits of practicing faculty, usually pays a customary salary, including typical benefits. Sometimes programs do not reduce the workload but expect the APN to work clinically in order to maintain competence, certification, and credentialing standards. This is not desirable or sustainable if faculty are expected to work a full-time teaching position and provide added direct clinical hours as well. However, some faculty choose to do this and like the arrangement because of the added income.

5.2.2 The Clinical Practice Is Inside the Faculty Position and a Recognized Component of the Position

In these instances, as above, the teaching workload is reduced to allow time for the APN to work clinically a given number of hours or shifts per week. The school contracts with the entity, whether that entity is somehow affiliated with the school (e.g., a clinic or hospital affiliated with the school) or operates independently of the school. The triad of APN, school, and clinical setting must come to terms over salary split, benefits, clinical timing, workload, and issues such as malpractice insurance coverage. To protect everyone, these terms are usually defined and then agreed on by all parties (see below).

5.2.3 Issues to Consider When Creating and Sustaining Faculty Practice Positions

To avoid confusion and any potential problems the involved parties should discuss dimensions of work time equivalency and work time split, salary splits, benefit splits (including human resource structure), evaluation processes (including how clinical practice applies toward faculty scholarship), malpractice/indemnification, credentialing, practice agreements (if required), medical billing processes, any legal and regulatory requirements, and student involvement (NONPF 2023). For collaborative faculty models to succeed, the academic institution should prioritize clear communication, mutual benefits, and formal agreements. This can be done by aligning clinical expectations with the workload, ensuring a joint evaluation strategy is in place as well as formally supporting the credentialing, scheduling, and malpractice coverage of the APN.

6 Funding of APN Education

Quality nursing education remains a key component of ensuring that healthcare delivery is provided in a manner that speeds recovery, maintains health, or provides a peaceful death. The progress of nursing education has improved significantly in the past few decades and continues to expand exponentially. This has led to increasing healthcare and patient demands being placed on registered nurses, all advanced practice nurses (APNs), and nurse educators. The advent of medical technology, a highly educated nursing workforce, increased specialization, and the need for universal healthcare coverage are some of the important factors that drive the need for advanced practice education.

Advanced nursing practice cadres commonly include the clinical nurse specialist, nurse practitioner, and certified nurse anesthetist. In some jurisdictions, the nurse-midwife is also a nursing-based advanced practice role; however, its positioning is context-dependent and may exist as a separate profession elsewhere (ICN 2025). Advanced practice nursing education does not come cheap for the prospective candidate. Hence, funding options are necessary to understand for nurses to make financially informed decisions in terms of graduate program selection and enrollment. The purpose of this chapter is to explore the funding mechanism for nursing education globally and to provide insight into how an individual interested in APN education might finance their education.

6.1 Significance of Funding for APN Education

The significance of funding APN education is closely tied to the benefits of having an APN in the healthcare multidisciplinary team as well as the overall healthcare system landscape. When funding is made available for APN education, it indirectly supports the strengthening of the existing healthcare workforce. In rural, underserved, and specialized healthcare settings, there is a critical shortage of healthcare workers, and APNS can fill the gaps in primary care, maternal health, and chronic disease management. Funding for APNs ensures that a steady pipeline of qualified health professionals is made available to meet the national health goals. With regards to Universal Health Coverage (WHO 2025), access to quality healthcare remains the goal for every healthcare delivery system. Investing in APN education yields improved population health, increased gender equity in leadership, and strengthened national economic growth through a more strong workforce. Therefore, financial support of APN education promotes equity in education, which subsequently leads to equity in care—especially in marginalized communities. Furthermore, studies have shown that APNs significantly contribute to reduced hospital admissions (Mileski et al. 2020), improvement in patient satisfaction, and better chronic disease control (Htay and Whitehead 2021) and reduced healthcare costs (Horton et al. 2025), therefore, investing in their education is a direct investment in population health.

The identification of funding streams for advanced practice nursing education can prove to be a dauting undertaking. As nurses pursue advanced nursing degree programs, more funds are required to meet the financial requirements of these advanced degrees. Nurses are encouraged to be lifelong learners so that they maintain competence in clinical skills and knowledge (Jantzen 2022). Patient health status and demographics are changing accompanied by increased disease burden and more skilled and competent nurses are required to provide nursing care to patients.

Lifelong learning and ensuring competency are cornerstones of nursing practice (Bindon 2017). Continuous Professional Development (CPD) is defined as an ongoing, planned process that builds on and enhances existing education, experience, and skill for the benefit of the nurse/midwife, patient, and the nursing profession (Note: Where midwifery is regulated as a distinct profession, ICM standards apply; "nurse-midwife" is used here only to describe nursing-based advanced practice roles) (Wheeler et al. 2022). Proponents for CPD points have a foundation that to maintain competency, nurses need to engage in several activities that will add to their existing knowledge and improve practice (Jantzen 2022). In many countries, renewal of practice licensure is dependent on the evidence that the nurse has successfully engaged in continued professional development relevant to their specialty area.

Licensing and credentialing provide immediate proof that a nurse can provide competent nursing care. Renewal of certification requires evidence that the nurse has engaged in knowledge acquisition within the field of specialization and is still competent to provide safe and competent nursing care. According to the American Nurses Credentialing Center (n.d.), continued learning can be proven through completing activities in professional development including academic courses, continuing education publications or research, practice hours, preceptorship, and assessments. Lifelong education drives professional development and retention. Therefore, career advancement opportunities tied to funded education can improve retention in public health systems, thus promoting specialization, reducing burnout, and attrition of healthcare workers.

With regards to leadership, nurses are skilled in leading healthcare teams. However, recently, the magnitude of leadership required of nurses, since the multidisciplinary healthcare team is continuously evolving, is expanding (National Academies of Sciences, Engineering, and Medicine; National Academy of Medicine; Committee on the Future of Nursing 2020–2030 2021). As such, nurses need to be adequately prepared for these roles. The roles of nurses have evolved to include the reduction of health disparities, in order to achieve health equity (National Academies of Sciences, Engineering, and Medicine; National Academy of Medicine; Committee on the Future of Nursing 2020–2030 2021) and universal healthcare. Some of these responsibilities are in nursing leadership. By itself, leadership is not a traditional focus of nursing education, which makes it a prime area for educational funding to support skill development for nurses beyond the clinical space. APNs bring advanced clinical skills, leadership, and decision-making capacity. Funding for APN education is a critical lever for closing this gap by preparing nurses for high-level decision-making and policy advocacy (WHO 2025).

The nursing profession is considered dynamic, hence there is the expectation that it must respond effectively to novel diseases. As seen during the Covid-19 pandemic, new diseases transform the way nursing is practiced requiring advanced critical thinking skills, efficient problem-solving skills, and cutting-edge clinical nursing skills. Specific to the Covid-19 impact, nursing education and schools of nursing faced challenges in terms of finances, abrupt increase in online learning, and disruption to clinical learning opportunities (Leaver et al. 2022). New diseases require that nursing schools adapt curricula to drive changes in future nursing practice. In many contexts, including across Africa, APNs are increasingly taking on expanded roles through task-sharing. To ensure safety and efficacy, well-funded APN programs are essential to align these clinical responsibilities with formal education and recognized scopes of practice.

While the fourth Industrial Revolution introduces advanced connectivity and data analytics, the *ICN 2025 definitions* reaffirm that the core of APN practice remains a *patient-centered approach.* Funding for APN education ensures that nurses can lead the integration of technology while maintaining a dedicated focus on the holistic, culturally safe, and individual needs of the patient (ICN 2025). Professions are making attempts on how to stay relevant and adapt in the world of advancing technology. This holds true for the nursing profession. The decision-making processes of nursing rely heavily on the availability of information at the point of care (Garcia-Dia 2020). Clinical reasoning is driven by the smooth availability of patient records and other forms of patient data. Hence advancement of medical technology presents a valid reason for nurses to pursue advanced degrees while keeping abreast with the latest technologies that seek to promote patient care.

As mentioned previously, the future of nursing practice is evolving; therefore, educating nurses for the future remains imperative. The work toward creating a healthcare system that is equitable requires nurses to impact knowledge, skills, and experience to younger generation of nurses through mentoring and support.

6.2 Financing Nursing Education in Different Settings

This section will explore the advanced practice nursing funding opportunities in selected geographical settings. Commonly, the funding paradigms used encompass government funding, private funding, grants and scholarships, and personal savings.

6.2.1 Kingdom of Eswatini, Africa

The African continent faces a mirage of challenges for health and nursing education. The health sector has experienced a nearly collapsed situation during the height of HIV and AIDS, and its impact on the population. Increase in morbidity due to opportunistic infections and other almost "neglected" diseases such as noncommunicable diseases including diabetes mellitus, hypertension, and cancers placed a huge burden on the healthcare sector. Recently, the devastating effects of COVID-19 also contributed to the critical shortage of nursing personnel. Skillful nursing workforce shortages have always been a challenge for the African continent, particularly Sub-Saharan Africa. Development of models that seek to improve the quality, quantity, and relevance of nursing education has been to the forefront (Bvumbwe and Mtshali 2018).

Advanced practice nursing (APN) education is a cornerstone of health system strengthening, yet in Eswatini, financial barriers continue to limit access to postgraduate nursing programs. While undergraduate nursing education receives some government support, funding for advanced practice pathways remains fragmented and underdeveloped. This section examines existing funding models, identifies systemic gaps, and proposes strategic interventions to expand access and sustainability.

In the Eswatini context, the Government policy for scholarships reserves funding only for basic nursing education, which is a 4-year bachelor's degree. The advanced practice nursing cadres available in the country include Family Nurse Practitioners (FNP), Nurse-Midwives, and Nurse-Anesthetists. All these specialties—with the FNP and Advanced Midwifery offered at Masters' level—are not funded by the Eswatini Government, and their scholarships are extremely rare. The absence of a dedicated funding stream for APNs reflects a broader policy gap in recognizing advanced nursing roles within national health workforce planning. However, this presents an opportunity to integrate APN funding into strategic health initiatives such as Universal Health Coverage and the Human Resources for Health Strategy Plan (2024–2030) (EMH 2025).

Many aspiring APNs rely on personal savings, family support, or informal loans to finance their education. This model places a heavy financial burden on students and may deter qualified candidates from pursuing advanced practice roles. The current typical practice is that prospective candidates fund themselves through their personal savings and study part-time. This requires careful financial planning on the part of the candidate and also limits participation in academic work such as virtual seminars and or classes and conference attendance. This type of model for the Eswatini setting reinforces socio-economic disparities with regard to access to education. Another funding option that may be available is Donor and Non-Governmental Organization-Funded Scholarships. International donors and NGOs occasionally support nursing education through project-based grants. These programs often focus on specific health priorities—such as HIV/AIDS, maternal health, or community-based care—and may include APN training components. The limitation with this type of funding is that they are typically short term and dependent on external funding cycles and may rarely cover the duration of the training program.

Employer-Sponsored Education is another funding model that is provided mostly by private healthcare institutions that wish to upskill their current nursing workforce to APN level. This type of funding is mostly accompanied by agreements that focus on exchange for service commitment post-graduation. This model of funding fosters internal capacity building and retention whilst aligning education with workforce needs. The barrier with this form of funding is that it is limited to well-resourced health institutions, while rural institutions often lack the capacity to fund their healthcare workers.

Regional and International Fellowships programs offered by the African Union, SADC, or Commonwealth provide limited but valuable opportunities for APN education. These fellowships promote academic mobility and regional collaboration with the advantage of exposure to best practices and regional networks. The challenge remains that these are highly competitive and not widely accessible to most candidates for APN education.

6.2.2 South Africa, Africa

The shortage of nurses at baccalaureate and advanced degrees has been highlighted in South Africa along with the nursing education outputs which do not meet the service demands (Bvumbwe and Mtshali 2018). The Department of Health (DOH) National Strategic Direction for Nursing and Midwifery Education and Practice (2020/21–2025/26) was launched, which sets priorities in nursing education and training along with resources in nursing, legislation and policy, and nursing human resources for health. Human resource for health, as is in other countries, is a critical element in the South African nursing landscape. There exists an absolute shortage—with regards to numbers of nurses and a relative shortage—with regards to skill mix of nurses in the country. For instance, advanced clinical specialist nurse cadres trained at master's level are difficult to retain in SA. The Strategic Direction for Nursing and Midwifery Education and Practice states that there is a need for training, qualification, employment, and retention of nurses with the appropriate skill mix required to meet the healthcare demands of the population (DHSA 2022).

Multiple paradigms for nursing education funding exist in South Africa. The Government of South Africa identifies areas of skills needed and sets those as priority areas for study, which are usually funded. For the most part, nurses fund their studies from personal savings or co-payment with support from their employers. Independent agencies with interest in healthcare also fund nursing education in South Africa.

South African universities typically offer postgraduate bursaries for nursing and public health students and research grants, which are tied to faculty-led projects along with work-study programs or teaching assistantships for postgraduate students. Supervisor-linked bursaries, which are another form of financial assistance for postgraduate students, do not provide full scholarship coverage but are designed to offload some financial burden for students. These are often supported by national funding bodies like the National Research Foundation (NRF) and Health and Welfare Sector Education and Training Authority (HWSETA).

Employer and Provincial Health Department Sponsorships represent another funding model implemented in South Africa. Some provincial health departments sponsor nurses for advanced training in exchange for service commitments. Typically, the focus of study is determined by the provincial health department based on the healthcare needs of the province. These programs are especially active in rural health initiatives and maternal care.

6.2.3 United States (U.S.)

In the U.S., funding for nursing education is in several forms. Funding begins with the nursing institution. Schools of nursing are funded through some government funding, and grants funding. From these funds, schools may decide that they are in a position to issue competitive scholarships for candidates wishing to study toward an advanced practice nursing degree. Schools of nursing receive grant awards from the Health Resources and Services Administration to enhance nursing education programs and increase the number of faculty and student enrollment.

The American Rescue Plan signed in 2021 identified key elements specific to investments in the nursing workforce. Amongst other grants available, the rescue plan catered to funding for primary healthcare providers, scholarships, and loan repayments for nurse practitioners, nurse-midwives, and other health professionals (Reinecke 2022).

Grants and scholarships are also available for certain cadres of nursing. To illustrate, in 2023, the U.S. Health and Human Services announced a $100 million investment in the nursing workforce, primarily for APN programs. An additional $30 million went to the Advanced Nursing Education-Nurse Practitioner Residency and Fellowship Program and $26 million more went to loans and loan cancellations to help nursing schools encourage more people to become faculty (Cerutti 2023).

Despite the described support, most APN students borrow substantially in order to attend the school of their choice. For instance, the average student loan debt for nurse practitioner graduates is well over $150,000 (Lockert 2024).

6.2.4 United Kingdom (U.K.)

The United Kingdom has developed a robust and strategically aligned funding framework to support APN education. Through centralized coordination, employer engagement, and flexible learning pathways, the U.K. model offers valuable insights for students who wish to pursue APN studies as well as for other countries seeking to expand and sustain APN training. This section explores the UK's funding mechanisms and identifies key elements that could inform the approach to financing advanced nursing education. Beginning in 2017/18, there were reforms in relation to educational funding for nurses in the U.K. (Department of Health and Social Care 2016) with the intention of keeping healthcare courses accessible for all. Multiple grants exist in the U.K. for funding of nursing education, including postgraduate nursing education. The grants range from education grants to hardship grants to research and practice development grants (RCN Foundation n.d.).

The National Health Service England (NHSE) Funding provides substantial support for APN education through its Centre for Advancing Practice, which oversees standards, accreditation, and workforce development. The NHSE offers tuition funding, supervision grants, and top-up module funding. With regards to tuition funding, full tuition fees for MSc Advanced Practice programs are commonly covered for up to 3 years duration, where the funds are disbursed directly to Higher Education Institutions (HEIs). With supervision grants, the employers receive a determined amount of money per annum (£2500–£6000 per annum) to support workplace-based learning. Even though this money does not directly support the student's financial burden, it does support the education through ensuring that the student receives structured mentorship, academic support, and protected time for study. Lastly, funding for Top-Up Modules provides financial support for up to 100 credits to students who wish to convert a Postgraduate Diploma (PGDip) to a full MSc. However, credits beyond 100 must be funded by the employer or student. This flexible model supports career progression and academic mobility.

Apprenticeship pathway. The Advanced Practice Apprenticeship represents a cost-effective route where tuition is funded through the Apprenticeship Levy. The Advanced Practice Apprenticeship offers a cost-effective, alternative route to APN qualification, funded through the Apprenticeship Levy. This model allows nurses to earn while they learn, with tuition and supervision costs covered by employer contributions. It is particularly effective in widening access and reducing financial strain on individual learners.

University-based scholarships and loans. UK universities (e.g., University of Edinburgh, King's College London) offer institutional scholarships and bursaries for domestic and international students, including access to postgraduate student loans for eligible UK residents. Many APN programs are accredited by the Royal College of Nursing (RCN), ensuring professional recognition and alignment with workforce standards.

Regional Coordination and Strategic Alignment. Regional Faculties for Advancing Practice such as North West Faculty play a critical role in coordinating funding, workforce planning, and program implementation. These funding bodies ensure that APN education aligns with local health priorities, such as mental health, primary care, and rural service delivery.

6.2.5 Australia

Australia has developed a multifaceted approach to funding Advanced Practice Nursing (APN) education, combining government investment, institutional support, and regional collaboration. These funding mechanisms aim to strengthen clinical expertise, promote workforce sustainability, and align nursing education with national health priorities. This section explores Australia's APN funding landscape and identifies transferable strategies for nurses wishing to pursue APN education.

The Australian Government budget of 2022–23 allocated some investments toward health and care workforce to ensure that a skilled and professional workforce is available. With this, part of the government funding was reserved for establishment of university departments on rural health (DHA 2022). Scholarships and support for nurses are aimed at upskilling nurses, including nurse practitioners.

The following national and institutional funding mechanisms exist for Australian nurses:

Government health workforce programs. Australia's federal and state governments provide targeted funding to support APN education, particularly in areas aligned with national health priorities. These include postgraduate scholarships and bursaries for nurses specializing in rural health, mental health, and Indigenous health, Clinical training subsidies that fund supervised practice and mentorship during APN programs and Workforce development grants awarded to healthcare institutions to upskill nursing staff through accredited advanced practice pathways. These mechanisms ensure that APN education is both accessible and strategically aligned with service delivery needs.

University-based support. Australian universities play a critical role in financing APN education through Merit-based scholarships for both domestic and international students, Research assistantships and teaching fellowships linked to faculty-led projects and Flexible payment plans and student loans, including access to the government-backed HECS-HELP scheme for eligible residents. This institutional support enhances academic mobility and reduces financial barriers for aspiring APNs.

Regional and international funding opportunities. Australia's membership in the Asia-Pacific Network for Global Change Research (APN) opens additional funding avenues for collaborative research and capacity-building in health systems (www.apn-gcr.org/core-activities/regional-research). The Collaborative Regional Research Programme (CRRP) Funds multi-country research projects focused on sustainability, health resilience, and policy innovation. The grants emphasize actionable science and regional impact. The Scientific Capacity Development Programme (CAPaBLE) supports individual and institutional capacity-building initiatives and prioritizes early-career professionals and projects that strengthen science-policy linkages.

Employer-sponsored education. Australian healthcare institutions frequently sponsor nurses for APN training, especially in rural and remote areas. This model typically involves Service-linked scholarships, where nurses commit to working in underserved regions post-graduation and Internal funding for tuition and supervision, aligned with workforce retention strategies. This approach ensures that APN education directly contributes to addressing local health service gaps.

6.3 Steps Governments and Policymakers Might Take to Finance APN Education

For government and policymakers to address funding gaps and empower prospective APNs, the following strategies might be taken:

- Centralized Funding Portal: Create a national database of scholarships, bursaries, and fellowships accessible to nursing students.
- Targeted Scholarships: Develop funding programs for priority areas such as rural health, mental health, and maternal care.
- Multi-Sectoral Collaboration: Encourage partnerships between government, NGOs, private sector, and academic institutions to co-fund APN education.
- Policy Integration: Advocate for the inclusion of APN education in national health and education budgets, linked to strategic goals like SDG 3 (Good Health and Well-being).
- Mentorship and Guidance: Establish mentorship programs to help students navigate funding options and application processes.

6.4 Steps an Individual Might Take to Understand and Finance APN Education

Whether an individual is dreaming of becoming a clinical nurse specialist, nurse educator, or nurse practitioner, funding the advanced practice journey is possible—with the right strategy. Before any individual registers for an APN program, there are many things they must research and consider in order to plan wisely. The following are suggestions (Warren Institute n.d., paras 1–10) to help with the process:

Compare programs and program costs. Program costs do vary, particularly between private and public institutions and between traditional and hybrid/distance education programs. Some programs require full-time attendance, while others allow part-time attendance with the advantage of allowing students to work part-time while in school. Costs to consider include tuition, book fees, living expenses, transportation costs, and other miscellaneous costs associated with advanced education such as research funds, data, and technology requirements—laptop, software, networking, and costs associated with conference attendance. For students who plan to study internationally, consider visa fees, which are often overlooked but very crucial as well as considerations for exchange rate fluctuations, which can have an impact on budget if payment is in foreign currency.

Compare costs to expected salaries. Take time to review the total costs of educational investment to be undertaken. Review the current trends of employability of graduates in the preferred specialization along with the salary scale. Understanding costs of schooling, potential for employability, and return on investment may affect choice of program and school.

Investigate grants and scholarships. These are forms of financial aid that do not require repayment. Customarily, they are offered to students with high academic achievement or who have performed certain types of service such as military or community and, if ongoing, may require maintenance of certain academic standards. Use centralized databases, explore university and government websites, and leverage professional networks to identify funding opportunities. Sign up for scholarship alerts on scholarship portal, commonwealth scholarships, DAAD scholarships, track cycles, eligibility, documents required, and application deadlines.

Investigate government loans. Government loans are generally offered at lower interest rates than private loans and may be directed at specific professions, such as nursing.

Investigate private loans. Private loans are available from financial institutions, generally at higher interest rates than government loans. Take time to review these along with repayment plans to determine the feasibility of applying for one.

Investigate employer tuition programs. Employers often offer tuition coverage. Not only is this good for the nurse-employee but may also be good for the employer, who may be able to retain the employee when the advanced schooling is completed. Sometimes the arrangements are contracted so that the employee agrees to work an agreed number of years after graduation and employment as an APN. Thus, it is a good idea to talk to the employer early to identify whether they offer study leave or tuition, ability to return to work in a specialized role after graduation, and the availability of mentorship for APN candidates.

Investigate other forms of financial aid. A variety of other forms of financial aid are available from loan repayment programs for future service/employment, professional organizations, or private donors. The application should have a strong emphasis on the societal impact of the degree.

Explore regional and international partnerships. Consider applying for collaborative research grants or fellowships that support APN education through cross-border initiatives. Engage with networks such as APN (Asia-Pacific Network), SADC, or Commonwealth programs. Review testimonials from successful applicants to understand the application process.

Seek mentorship and peer guidance. Connect with current APN students or alumni to gain insights into funding pathways and application strategies. Join professional associations or online forums that share funding alerts and success stories. Join platforms such as LinkedIn, Facebook or WhatsApp groups that circulate funding opportunities.

Align educational goals with national health priorities. Target programs and funding streams that support priority areas such as rural health, maternal care, mental health, or infectious disease management. This alignment increases eligibility and relevance for strategic funding.

Prepare a strong application portfolio. Develop a compelling personal statement that highlights professional goals, community impact, and alignment with funding criteria. Secure references from current supervisors or mentors who can attest to your clinical and leadership potential.

6.5 Policy Implications of Funding APN Education

Expanding funding for APN education globally is not only a matter of financial investment—it is a strategic imperative for health equity, workforce development, and national resilience. By diversifying funding models and empowering prospective nurses to access financial support, countries can cultivate a skilled cadre of APNs capable of transforming healthcare delivery. The comparative analysis of APN funding models across Eswatini, South Africa, the United Kingdom, and Australia reveals a consistent theme: access to advanced nursing education is deeply influenced by awareness, preparation, and strategic engagement with funding opportunities. For prospective APN students, navigating this landscape requires proactive planning and informed decision-making.

7 Exemplar I: An Academic-Practice Partnership (Kentucky)

With the ongoing need to develop and enhance workforce programs that targeted specific organizational needs, an academic practice partnership was forged between Norton Healthcare (NHC) in Louisville, Kentucky, and the University of Kentucky College of Nursing (UKCON) located in Lexington, Kentucky (one hundred miles away). The intent of the program was to develop and graduate advanced practice nurses (APNs) and executive leadership nurses with Doctor of Nursing Practice (DNP) degrees. Although there are some master's degree programs available in the United States, for those wanting education as APNs or as Executive Leaders, most now do so via DNP programs (available as post-baccalaureate, post-master's, and even direct entry). This particular three-year BSN to DNP program was focused on educating existing experienced NHC BSN staff utilizing multiple delivery models (i.e., in person, virtual) with all learning experiences (i.e., didactic, experiential, clinical practicum) to be conducted on NHC campuses. Appropriate DNP staff employed within NHC would be used in adjunct faculty roles in the classroom and in the clinical rotations. The focus of the initial cohorts included Nurse Practitioner specialties in Family Health, Pediatrics, Women's Health, Acute and Critical Care, and Behavioral and Mental Health. A focus on Executive Leadership was added in cohorts (both BSN to DNP and MSN to DNP) as the program evolved.

The seven-year program yielded 95 DNP graduates (78 in APRN roles and 17 in Executive Leadership roles). Unique attributes of this academic practice partnership included:

- Equality of strength of both partners in commitment, resources, focus, and support.
- Mutual interdependence with mutual risk and mutual reward to both parties.
- Full transparency and accountability for results on both ends.
- Open, honest, and frank communication among and between the principals.
- Clarity of expectations, goals, and outcomes partnership was driving.
- Flexibility and adaptability of partners to changing needs, resolving issues, or addressing concerns.
- Resilience of partner principals when meeting resistance and overcoming barriers wherever it arose.
- Commitment to research (clinical and program).
- Focus on a reality-based curriculum that connects practice and change.
- Defined return on investment (ROI) for partners, faculty, staff, and participants.

While the program was underway and after completion, three publications explained the project, details of implementation, and the sustained impact of the accomplishment. In March/April 2017, Howard and Williams published An Academic-Practice Partnership to Advanced DNP Education and Practice, available at https://www.sciencedirect.com/science/article/pii/S8755722316301259. The article discussed the following:

- Multiple position statements and publications of the American Association of Colleges of Nursing from 2004 to 2015 regarding the need to transform advanced practice nursing in order to prepare nurses for the complexities of healthcare anticipated in the future.
- The literature review of education partnerships completed prior to discussions and planning.
- The request for proposals (RFPs), proposal response, alignment of goals between partners and according to the American Association of Colleges of Nursing education standards, and memorandum of agreement and partner responsibilities.
- The evaluation plan.

In December 2017, Williams and Howard published An Academic-Practice Partnership Model to Grow and Sustain Advanced Practice Nursing, available at https://www.jstor.org/stable/26813938. In addition to some of the material included in the above article (RFP, partner characteristics), this publication discussed the following:

- Implementation processes such as student selection according to NHC needs and maintenance of standing UKCON standards, logistics of scheduling, coordination of clinical sites and clinical preceptors, payroll processes, and academic advising.

- Evaluation of outcomes from development and application of a logic model. According to the Center for Disease Control (CDC), a logic model is a visual representation of the inputs (resources), activities, outputs, outcomes, impacts, and moderators for a program. (CDC 2024).
- Alignment of NHC system goals and DNP student project ideas.

In July 2021, Howard et al. published Sustained Impact of an Academic-Practice Partnership, available at https://www.sciencedirect.com/science/article/abs/pii/S8755722321001198. Aside from reviewing the conceptual framework, the literature review, partnership implementation, student enrollment and employment, and the evaluation logic model, the article discussed the sustained effects of the program, specifically (p. 1001):

- Specifics of the diffusion of graduates throughout the NHC enterprise (52 BSN-DNP Primary Care Nurse Practitioners, 3 BSN-DNP, Psychiatric Mental Health Nurse Practitioners, 23 BSN-DNP, Adult-Gerontology Acute Care Nurse Practitioners, 10 BSN-DNP Executive Leadership Graduates, 7 MSN-DNP Executive Leadership Graduates).
- System responses and programs for patients (protocols for research and DNP project implementation, development of an APN orientation and transition to practice program, strategically placing graduates in leadership positions leading to development of numerous programs benefitting patients and the nursing workforce [succession planning for nurses, mentoring bedside nurses, implementing evidence-based practice into patient care], growth of DNP prepared nurses at NHC [from 15 at program inception to 201 at end of program], multiple new and expanded patient specific programs (bariatric surgery post-operative care, behavioral health and neurology, breast health, cognitive and dementia care, infectious disease, pediatric orthopedic transition care, sickle cell anemia, trans-aortic valve replacement), and growth of the care delivery model (increased providers, increased roles in acute care and inpatient care [intensivists; cardiology, neurology, pulmonary teams], increased roles in primary care [immediate care centers, prompt care clinic in oncology], and increased roles in behavioral health [child/adolescent services for emergency settings, behavioral health services in outpatient settings].

The described academic-practice partnership was unique, theoretically based, and thoughtfully implemented. Viewed as successful, the project created opportunities for nurses to move to APN and leadership roles while also preparing a healthcare system for a demanding, ever-changing medical world. Among the many important aspects of planning and implementation shared above, the following were viewed as critical to sustaining the impact of the partnership (p. 1002):

- Share a vision of leadership.
- Formalize contractual agreements.

- Plan and implement according to agreed-on models and frameworks.
- Plan and dedicate support resources.
- Maintain ongoing open communication.

8 Exemplar II: A Consortium Proposal (Brazil)

In Brazil, so far, advanced practice nursing, existing for more than half a century in developed countries, has not been implemented. The discussion about its adoption in the country began approximately ten years ago, with visits to other health services in countries where this practice already exists, and the development of research and publications on the subject through literature reviews.

The Federal Council of Nurses (COFEN in Portuguese), in 2016, established the Advanced Nursing Practices Committee, with representative members modified over time, is still working until today. The goal of the committee is to support APN development, implementation, and future evaluation in the country through research studies, in addition to producing guidelines encompassing professional training, regulation, and practice.

In addition, the Brazilian Ministry of Health (BMH) established a Working Group (WG) focused on APN. The valorization of nursing, specialized education, regulation of professional practice and labor relations were themes in meetings of the WG on APN, held by the BMH, through the Secretariat of Work Management and Health Education (SGTES in Portuguese), in August, 2023, in Brasília, with representatives of various institutions, to collectively think about expanding the scope of practices in the category and regulating the nursing profession.

From the perspective of professional education for the qualification of nursing workers at the master's and doctorate levels, there is the CAPES/COFEN Agreement, established since 2016. This is a proposal to contribute to overcoming the shortage of generalist and specialized clinical nurses to work in healthcare networks, helping to mitigate the problem of the population's access, also contributing to the achievement of best practices in health.

Furthermore, Brazilian nursing has appropriated this theme and has held discussions and advances in its understanding. Based on that, to implement this function in the country, appropriate training is needed for nurses who will perform as nurse practitioners (NP). In this sense, this chapter discusses the possible alternatives of education programs for nurses with a view to assuming the new function.

8.1 Master's Program Proposal

A new post-graduation program in Brazil, in any field of knowledge, needs to be proposed to a governmental agency called *Coordination of Superior Level Staff Improvement* (CAPES in Portuguese). This agency, almost every year, opens a call to new submissions, which are evaluated by a field committee, receiving their opinion to recommend or not the new program. Only after the agency's decision, published officially in a public ordinance, could such a new program finally be installed.

In 2022, five public universities presented education proposals to CAPES during the opening of the Call for New Course Proposals (APCN in Portuguese), to prepare nurses for being a nurse practitioner. These proposals covered different fields of knowledge, including two courses in the women's health area, two in the chronic conditions care, and one in the format of an association among six Brazilian universities targeted at Primary Health Care (PHC).

This last one was called *Professional Master's Degree in Advanced Practice Nursing in Primary Health Care*. The purpose of the program was to educate nurses who work in Family Health Strategy (FHS)/Primary Health Care (PHC) in a variety of Brazilian municipalities, especially those with difficulties in accessing graduate education, far from large centers, in the presential modality for 60% of the activities and online for 40% of them. The integration of partnerships between academic institutions and public health managers of the municipalities was a goal, since PHC, as the regionalization of the Brazilian Unified Health System (SUS in Portuguese), is their responsibility.

The proposal joined six federal and/or state, public and free of tuition universities, from three regions of Brazil, namely: in the southern region, the Western Parana State University (Paraná State—proposal coordinator); and the universities associated with the proposal are the following ones: in the midwestern region—Federal University of Jataí (Goiás State); Federal University of Mato Grosso do Sul (Mato Grosso do Sul State); and Federal University of Goias (Goiás State); and in the northern region—State University of Roraima (Roraima State) and Federal University of Amazonas (Amazonas State).

In addition, the proposal established a partnership with foreign institutions, for its development, with tutoring and/or mentoring of Brazilian professors, conducted by the University of Miami (USA) and MacMaster University, School of Nursing, Hamilton, Ontario, Canada. This partnership for the development of competencies on APN of Brazilian professors would be operationalized through their access to online courses, auditing courses, practical monitoring of NP in their daily work, simulated learning, and exchange of professors.

The proposal followed the recommendations of the International Council of Nurses (ICN) regarding the nature of APN, added to the educational program, following these skills: 1) integrated research (practice-based evidence), education, and clinical management; (2) a high degree of professional autonomy and independence in practice; (3) experience with a large number of case management at advanced level; (4) the recognition of advanced clinical skills; (5) the ability to provide consulting services to other health professionals; 6) the ability to plan, implement, and evaluate programs; (7) the recognition of being the first point of contact for users/customers; (8) to have the authority to prescribe drugs and treatments; (9) to have the authority to refer clients to other professionals and admit patients to hospitals; (10) the official recognition of the APN title and specific policy legislation and/or regulatory mechanisms (ICN 2020).

The curricular structure of the professional program was composed of mandatory and elective subjects. One of the mandatory subjects focuses on 510 hours of practical activities in a FHS team, a traditional basic unit and/or outpatient clinics for chronic conditions care training. In total, the program had the intention to offer at least 72 credits, added by 10 credits for the thesis. The suggested modalities to present this thesis cover technological innovation, knowledge translation, education for practice in advanced activities, development of products, and technologies for care or management.

Unfortunately, in June 2023, based on the CAPES evaluation results, none of the proposals was deemed suitable for APN training by the current representatives of the Nursing Area coordination. The main arguments listed to deny the proposals varied according to the specificity of each program submitted. However, they converged on one aspect that determined the other evaluation criteria, described as follows: APN "is not related to the Nursing Area scope or to exercise of the profession, as the Advanced Practice Nursing is not yet regulated in the country".

8.2 Residency Programs Possibilities

The usual pathway in our country to submit a proposal for a new residency program is to send the project to be evaluated for the National Commission for Multiprofessional Residency in Health (COREMU in Portuguese). In Brazil, residency programs are considered the golden pattern to educate health staff, not only physicians. Usually, the programs follow national guidelines with 5.570 teaching hours, 20% of that theoretical studies and 80% learning in service practice guided by tutors/preceptors.

The Pan-American Health Organization (2018) considered this a way to educate NPs, linking the residency with master programs, which is also a possibility according to CAPES (BME 2024). Following this suggestion, a private national institution submitted a proposal to educate APNs for the national residency committee in 2024, supported by COFEN.

The residency in APN at this institution is a post-graduate program that aims to train nurses with specific skills and knowledge to work in areas of greater health complexity. The program offers a curriculum that includes both theory and practice, focused on developing leadership capacity, research, and interprofessional collaboration (Einstein Hospital 2025).

8.3 Awaiting Approval

At the submission of this chapter, the tendered proposal was waiting for approval. The implementation of the APN in Brazil is under process, and the propositions of education programs for NP are part of this stage, as expanding the scope of the nurse's role effectively responds to the goal of improving access to quality services and professionals. The intention of this advanced role is to provide nurses skills and competences to work autonomously focused on the clinical care, beyond the usual generalist practice of Brazilian nurses, producing qualified and risk-free care for the professional and the individuals under their care.

References

American Association of Colleges of Nursing (AACN). Alliance for nursing accreditation statement on distance education policies. 2025. .aacnnursing.org/news-data/position-statements-white-papers/alliance-for-nursing-accreditation-statement-on-distance-education-policies. Accessed 2 Jan 2025.

American Nurses Credentialing Center. Renew your certification. Author. n.d.. https://www.nursingworld.org/certification/renewals/. Accessed 4 Jan 2025.

Arslanian-Engoren C. Conceptualizations of advanced practice nursing. In: Traci MF, O'Grady ET, Phillips SJ, editors. Hamric and Hanson's advanced practice nursing: an integrative approach. 7th ed. St. Louis: Elsevier; 2023. p. 31–73. ISBN: 9780323777117.

Bindon SL (2017), Professional development strategies to enhance nurses' knowledge and maintain safe practice. AORN J 2017;106: 99–110. https://doi.org/10.1016/j.aorn.2017.06.002

Brazilian Ministry of Education (BME). CAPES ordinance number 290: residency program in integrated health to graduate studies (ResidPD). Author. 13 Sept 2024. https://cad.capes.gov.br/ato-administrativo-detalhar?idAtoAdmElastic=16304#anchor. Accessed May 2025.

Buring SM, Bhushan A, Broeseker A, Conway S, Duncan-Hewitt W, Hansen L, Westberg S. Interprofessional education: definitions, student competencies, and guidelines for implementation. AJPE. 2009;73(4):59. https://doi.org/10.5688/aj730459.

Bvumbwe T, Mtshali N. Nursing education challenges and solutions in Sub Saharan Africa: an integrative review. BMC Nurs. 2018;2018(17):3. https://doi.org/10.1186/s12912-018-0272-4.

Campbell SH, Hawkins J. Preceptor rewards: how to say thank you for mentoring the next generation of nurse practitioners. JAANP. 2007;19(1):24–9. https://doi.org/10.1111/j.1745-7599.2006.00186.x.

Center for Disease Control (CDC). Logic models 16 May 2024. https://www.cdc.gov/library/research-guides/logic-models.html. Accessed 2 Jan 2025.

Cerutti E. How the government aims to support growing demand for NP programs. 28 Aug 2023. https://www.beckershospitalreview.com/quality/nursing/how-the-government-aims-to-support-growing-demand-for-np-programs/. Accessed 3 Jan 2025.

Cheng A, Kessler D, Mackinnon R, Chang TP, Nadkarni VM, Hunt EA, et al. Reporting guidelines for health care simulation research: extensions to the CONSORT and STROBE statements. Adv Simul. 2016;1(1):25. https://doi.org/10.1186/s41077-016-0025-y.

Davenport T, Kalakota R. The potential for artificial intelligence in healthcare. Future Healthc J. 2019;6(2):94–8. https://doi.org/10.7861/futurehosp.6-2-94. PMID: 31363513; PMCID: PMC6616181

DeNisco SM. Clinical education: the role of the student, faculty, and preceptor. In: DeNisco SM, editor. Advanced practice nursing: essential knowledge for the profession. 5th ed. St. Louis: Jones and Bartlett; 2023. p. 237–54.

Department of Health and Social Care (UK). Plans for changing healthcare education funding. 21 Jul 2016. https://www.gov.uk/government/news/plans-for-changing-healthcare-education-funding. Accessed 4 Jan 2025.

Department of Health, Australia (DHA). How the 2022-23 budget is investing in the health and care workforce. Author. 2022. https://www.health.gov.au/sites/default/files/documents/2022/03/budget-2022-23-investing-in-the-health-and-care-workforce.pdf. Accessed 4 Jan 2025.

Department of Health, Republic of South Africa (DHSA). National strategic direction for nursing and midwifery education and practice 2020–2021 to 2025-2026. Author. 2022. https://knowledgehub.health.gov.za/elibrary/national-strategic-direction-nursing-and-midwifery-education-and-practice. Accessed 4 Jan 2025.

Einstein Hospital. Einstein multiprofessional residency. Author. 2025. https://ensino.einstein.br/pos-graduacao/residencia/residencia-multiprofissional. Accessed 4 Jan 2025.

Eswatini Ministry of Health (EMH). Annual budget performance report for financial year 2024–2025. Author. 2025. https://parliament.gov.sz/publications/parliament_reports/docs/ANNUAL%20REPORT%20HEALTH%202025.pdf. Accessed 3 Mar 2025.

Garcia-Dia MJ. Balancing care with technology. Nurs Manage. 2020;51(4):56. https://doi.org/10.1097/01.NUMA.0000657280.44223.10.

Gazza EA. Alleviating the nurse faculty shortage: designating and preparing the academic nurse educator as an advanced practice registered nurse. Nurs Forum. 2019;54(4):144–8. https://doi.org/10.1111/nuf.12307.

Herath C, Zhou Y, Gan Y, Nakandawire N, Gong Y, Lu Z. A comparative study of interprofessional education in global health care: a systematic review. Medicine (Baltimore). 2017;96(38):e7336. https://doi.org/10.1097/MD.0000000000007336. PMID: 28930816; PMCID: PMC5617683. https://www.ncbi.nlm.nih.gov/pmc/articles/PMC5617683/

Horton M, Dixon J, Turi E, Balusu C, Paikoff R, Maier CB, Poghosyan L. Advanced practice nurses in primary care and their impact on health service utilisation, costs and access globally: a scoping review. J Clin Nurs. 2025;34(5):1592–601. https://doi.org/10.1111/jocn.17614. Epub 2024 Dec 9. PMID: 39654015; PMCID: PMC12037310

Htay M, Whitehead D. The effectiveness of the role of advanced nurse practitioners compared to physician-led or usual care: a systematic review. IJNS Adv. 2021;3:100034. https://doi.org/10.1016/j.ijnsa.2021.100034.

Huckstadt A, Hayes K. Faculty practice models offer NPs better academic, clinical balance. Haymarket Media. 21 June 2013. https://www.clinicaladvisor.com/news/faculty-practice-models-offer-nps-better-academic-clinical-balance/. Accessed 3 Mar 2025.

International Council of Nurses (ICN). Guidelines on advanced practice nursing. Author. 2020. https://www.icn.ch/system/files/documents/2020-04/ICN_APN%20Report_EN_WEB.pdf. Accessed 4 Jan 2025.

International Council of Nurses (ICN). Renewing the definitions of 'nursing' and 'a nurse': final project report. Author. 2025. https://www.icn.ch/sites/default/files/2025-06/ICN_Definition-Nursing_Report_EN_Web_0.pdf. Accessed 20 Mar 2026.

Jantzen D. Getting grounded: educational foundation for nurses' lifelong learning. Dent Jpn. 2022;2022(39):34–40. https://doi.org/10.1016/j.profnurs.2021.12.009.

Jeffries PR, Bigley MB, McNelis AM, Cartier JM, William DB, Pintz C, Slaven-Lee P, Zychowicz ME. A call to action: building evidence for use of simulation in nurse practitioner education. JAANP. 2019;31(11):627–32. https://doi.org/10.1097/JXX.0000000000000335.

Koukourikos K, Tsaloglidou A, Kourkouta L, Papathanasiou IV, Iliadis C, Fratzana A, Panagiotou A. Simulation in clinical nursing education. Acta Inform Med. 2021;29(1):15–20. https://doi.org/10.5455/aim.2021.29.15-20. PMID: 34012208; PMCID: PMC8116070

Leaver CA, Stanley JM, Goodwin Veenema T. Impact of the COVID-19 pandemic on the future of nursing education. Acad Med. 2022;97(3S):S82–9. https://doi.org/10.1097/ACM.0000000000004528. PMID: 34789661; PMCID: PMC8855777

Lockert M. A guide to the average student loan debt for nurse practitioners. 6 May 2024. https://www.studentloanplanner.com/student-dept-nurse-practitioners/. Accessed 3 Jan 2025.

Mileski M, Pannu U, Payne B, Sterling E, McClay R. The impact of nurse practitioners on hospitalizations and discharges from long-term nursing facilities: a systematic review. Healthcare (Basel). 2020;8(2):114. https://doi.org/10.3390/healthcare8020114. PMID: 32354015; PMCID: PMC7348833

Moore KS, Lockwood EB, Lockwood CH, Mingzi L. Advanced practice nurses: a global overview of education. In: Rogers M, Lehwaldt D, Roussel J, Acorn M, editors. Advanced practice nurse networking to enhance global health. Switzerland: Springer Nature; 2024. p. 105–31.

National Academies of Sciences, Engineering, and Medicine, National Academy of Medicine, Committee on the Future of Nursing 2020–2030. Nurses leading change. In: Flaubert JL, Le Menestrel S, Williams DR, et al., editors. The future of nursing 2020–2030: charting a path to

achieve health equity. Washington, DC: National Academies Press (US); 2021. https://www.ncbi.nlm.nih.gov/books/NBK573918/.
National Association of Nurse Practitioner faculties (NONPF). 2023 faculty practice toolkit. 2nd ed. Author; 2023. https://cdn.ymaws.com/www.nonpf.org/resource/resmgr/publications_/faculty_practice_toolkit._202.pdf. Accessed 3 Mar 2025
Nye C. State of simulation research in advanced practice nursing education. In: Schneidereith T, editor. Ann Rev Nurs Res. 2021;39(1):33–51. https://doi.org/10.1891/0739-6686.39.33.
Pan American Health Organization (PAHO). Expanding the role of nurses in primary health care. Author. 2018. https://iris.paho.org/handle/10665.2/34968. Accessed 2 Jan 2025.
Park H, Yu S. Policy issues in simulation-based nursing education and technology development. HPT. 2018;7(3):318–21.
Pitts C, Padden D, Knestrick J, Bigley MB. A checklist for faculty and preceptor to enhance the nurse practitioner student clinical experience. JAANP. 2019;31(10):591–7. https://doi.org/10.1097/JXX.0000000000000310. https://pubmed.ncbi.nlm.nih.gov/31567777/. Accessed 7 July 2025
Reinecke P. 2021–22 Proposed federal policy changes related to nursing. 2022. https://campaignforaction.org/resource/2021-22-federal-policy-changes-related-to-nursing/. Accessed 4 Jan 2025.
Rossiter S. Diversifying the nursing workforce: strategies for increasing diversity and inclusion. ForTheNurse. 20 March 2025. https://blog.forthenurse.us/diversifying-the-nursing-workforce/. Accessed 2 Jan 2025.
Royal College of Nursing Foundation. Grants and funding. n.d.. https://rcnfoundation.rcn.org.uk/Grants-and-funding. Accessed 5 Jan 2025.
Schiff D. Education for AI, *not* AI for education: the role of education and ethics in national AI policy strategies. Int J Artif Intell Educ. 2022;32:527–63. https://doi.org/10.1007/s40593-021-00270-2.
Senvisky JM, McKenna RT, Okuda Y. Financing and funding a simulation center. In: StatPearls. Treasure Island (FL): StatPearls Publishing; 2023. PMID: 33760545. https://pubmed.ncbi.nlm.nih.gov/33760545/.
Smiley R, Martin B. Simulation in nursing education: advancements in regulation, 2014–2022. JNR. 2023;14(2):5–9. https://doi.org/10.1016/S2155-8256(23)00086-8.
Thejewel A. What is advanced nursing practice and why is it significant in the healthcare industry. 22 Jul 2024. https://mwtconsultancy.com/blog/advanced-nursing-practice-and-its-significant-in-the-healthcare-industry. Accessed 2 May 2025.
Tovar E, Ossege J, Farus-Brown S, Zonsius M, Morrow L. DNP program faculty and graduates' knowledge and use of QI and safety processes. Nurse Educ. 2020;45(1):11–6. https://doi.org/10.1097/NNE.0000000000000677.
United Nations Educational, Scientific, and Cultural Organization (UNESCO). Guidance on distance learning. 2025. https://www.unesco.org/en/digital-education/distance-learning-guidance. Accessed 2 Jan 2025.
Warren Institute. Six simple steps to financing your nursing education. n.d.. https://warreninstitute.org/is-absn-worth-it/. Accessed 3 Jan 2025.
Watts PI, Hallmark BF, Beroz S. Professional development for simulation education. Ann Rev Nurs Res. 2021;39(1):201–21. https://doi.org/10.1891/0739-6686.39.201.
Wheeler KJ, Miller M, Pulcini J, Gray D, Ladd E, Rayens MK. Advanced practice nursing roles, regulation, education, and practice: a global study. Ann Glob Health. 2022;88(1):42. https://doi.org/10.5334/aogh.3698. PMID: 35755314; PMCID: PMC9205376
World Health Organization (WHO). Framework for action on interprofessional education & collaborative practice. Author. 2010. https://www.who.int/publications/i/item/framework-for-action-on-interprofessional-education-collaborative-practice. Accessed 5 Jan 2025.
World Health Organization (WHO). State of the world's nursing 2025: investing in education, jobs, leadership and service delivery. Author. 2025. https://iris.who.int/handle/10665/376722. Accessed 10 Mar 2026.

Exemplary Global Advanced Practice Nursing Curricula and Program Details

Deborah C. Gray and Kathy J. Wheeler

1 Introduction

Advanced Practice Nursing (APN) is a highly specialized area of nursing around the world that includes specific protected roles such as nurse practitioner (NP), clinical nurse specialist (CNS), nurse anesthetist (NA), and advanced nurse midwife (NM), generally recognized under the umbrella term advanced practice nurse (APN). Overall, APN educational programs worldwide focus on developing advanced clinical skills, leadership, and research capabilities, along with an emphasis on collaborative evidence-based practice and patient-centered care. However, APN education and expected role competencies differ globally based on healthcare systems, regulatory requirements, educational frameworks, and specific country needs. The purpose of this chapter is to highlight several representative APN curricula from around the world and discuss critical APN educational content. It is hoped this information will be useful to interested parties (stakeholders) involved in APN development around the world.

D. C. Gray (✉)
Old Dominion University, Norfolk, VA, USA

Lucerne University of Applied Sciences and Arts, Lucerne, Switzerland

University of Botswana, Gaborone, Botswana
e-mail: dcgray@odu.edu

K. J. Wheeler
University of Kentucky College of Nursing, Lexington, KY, USA
e-mail: kjwheeler623@gmail.com

K. J. Wheeler, M. Acorn (eds.), *Health Policy for Advanced Practice Nursing: A Toolkit for Implementation and Improvement*, Advanced Practice in Nursing,
https://doi.org/10.1007/978-3-032-03667-4_18

2 Advanced Practice Nursing Curricula Background

Looking specifically at APN curricula, there are distinct similarities as well as differences in prerequisites, required courses, program structures, and expected competencies for each role, depending on the country as well as the individual educational institution. The key feature of all APN programs is a primary focus on advanced patient care skills and competencies. APN programs require advanced courses in clinical care, and most require advanced pathophysiology, advanced assessment, and advanced pharmacology, as well as supervised hands-on, role-specific patient care clinical hours. Other curricular contents such as role and/or patient-specific management, leadership, research, policy, and ethics are generally present in various forms depending on practice role, program educational level, and country-related factors (Xu et al. 2022; Nakamura 2024; Choi et al. 2022; Jokiniemi et al. 2022; Beauchesne et al. 2020; Christmals and Armstrong 2020; Jeffery et al. 2020; Zug et al. 2016).

Additionally, the majority of APN educational programs around the world are at the master's degree or post master's certificate entry to advanced practice level (Wheeler et al. 2022). This is particularly true across the globe for the NP and CNS, with the exception of a few countries, such as Botswana (which has both post RN certificate and master's level NP/APN programs) (Gray et al. 2023), Ghana (which has both bachelors and masters level NP/APN programs) (University for Development Studies 2025); University of Cape Coast (2025), and the United States (which has master's, post master's doctorate of nursing practice (DNP), post master's certificate, and DNP doctorate level programs) (NONPF 2018; NACNS 2019). However, the NA and NM roles have more educational variation with differing entrance to practice requirements in several countries, including post-basic RN certificate, bachelors, masters, and doctorate (IFNA 2022; AANA 2023; ICM 2021). Thus with regard to nurse anesthetists and nurse midwives, in many countries, the role is context dependent.

Furthermore, there are differing country or region-specific curricular requirements, sometimes across all APN roles, e.g., in Canada NP programs have a strong focus on primary health care and interprofessional collaboration (CASN 2012); in Australia programs have an emphasis on rural and remote healthcare, aligned with Australia's geographic needs (ANMAC 2019); in New Zealand programs emphasize cultural safety and the relevance of the Treaty of Waitangi in Aboriginal healthcare (NZNO 2020); in the European Union APN program structure varies between countries but there is a trend toward harmonization under frameworks like the Bologna Process (Collins and Hewer 2014; Janson et al. 2023); in Eswatini (previously Swaziland) there is an emphasis on health care management courses in addition to Family NP primary care skills to meet patient care and also health system-wide administration needs (Nsibanze 2024); and in Asian countries such as Singapore and others where APN roles are less developed (e.g., China, South Korea, Japan), curricula often address demographic shifts like aging populations or specific chronic disease management based on regional health priorities (Xu et al. 2022; Nakamura 2024; Choi et al. 2022; Jokiniemi et al. 2022).

3 Role Specific Curricula and Exemplars

3.1 Nurse Practitioner

When considering NP program curricula, it is important to consider the International Council of Nurses (ICN) APN Guidelines 2020 definition and scope of practice for the NP role.

> A Nurse Practitioner (NP) is an Advanced Practice Nurse who integrates clinical and biopsychosocial skills associated with nursing and medicine to assess, diagnose, and manage patients in primary healthcare settings and acute care populations as well as ongoing care for populations with chronic illness (Schober et al. 2020). The Nurse Practitioner possesses advanced health assessment, diagnostic and clinical management skills that include pharmacology management based on additional post-graduate education (recommended minimum standard Master of Science degree) and clinical education that includes specified clinical practicum to provide a range of healthcare services. The focus of NP practice is expert direct clinical care, managing healthcare needs of populations, individuals, and families, in primary health care or acute care settings with additional expertise in health promotion and disease prevention. As a licensed and credentialed clinician, the NP practices with a broader level of autonomy beyond that of a generalist nurse, advanced in-depth critical decision-making and works in collaboration with other healthcare professionals. NP practice may include but is not limited to the direct referral of patients to other services and professionals. NP practice includes integration of education, research, and leadership in conjunction with the emphasis on direct advanced clinical care (Schober et al. 2020).

While there is variation in NP curricula globally, NP programs by and large are consistent with the ICN definition and scope, and also prepare graduates with the NP competencies to fulfill the role in their country-specific setting (CASN 2012, ANMAC 2019, NONPF 2022, Ndirangu-Mugo et al. 2024, V&VN 2019, NMBI 2017, NZNO 2017, 18–19). For illustration and comparison, several examples of FNP and/or DNP curricula are provided.

3.1.1 Botswana: Master of Nursing Science and Post-Basic Diploma Certificate NP Exemplars

Botswana provides an interesting example of NP curricula at two different educational levels: a Master of Nursing Science at the University of Botswana (Table 1) (University of Botswana n.d.) and also a certificate program for post-basic diploma nurses initiated in 1983, at the Botswana Affiliated Health Training Institution (AHTIB) (Table 2) (University of Botswana and AHTIB 2008). Of note, Botswana is currently in the process of transitioning or phasing out its initial lower-level post-nursing diploma certificate program (Gray et al. 2023).

For comparison to the Master of Nursing Science and post-nursing diploma certificate FNP programs in Botswana, Ghana offers a Bachelor of Science NP program.

3.1.2 Ghana: Bachelor of Science NP Exemplar

Ghana offers a Bachelor of Science (BSc) Nurse Practitioner Program at the University for Development Studies (2025) (Table 3). This 3-year program trains

Table 1 Botswana: University of Botswana (UB) Family Nurse Practitioner Master of Nursing Science (MNS)

Year 1 Semester 1		Year 1 Semester 2		Year 1 Winter Semester		Year 2 Semester 1		Year 2 Semester 2		Year 2 Winter Semester	
Course Name	Cr	Course Name	Cr	Course Name	Cr	Course Name	Cr	Course Name	Cr	Course Name	Cr
Theoretical foundations of nursing	3	Health assessment in advanced practice nursing	4	Research dissertation 1	4	Children and adolescents primary health care (theory)	3	Research dissertation 3	6	*Internship 8 weeks* Integrated practice in the assessment and management of children and adolescents, adults and older adults, and sexual reproductive health practice	6
Research methods in nursing	3	Pharmaceutical interventions for advanced practice nurses	3			Children and adolescents primary care (practice)	3	Elective*	3		
Advanced pathophysiology	3	Adults and older adults primary health care (theory)	3			Sexual reproductive health and rights	3	*Note-elective course choices: Ethics and law in healthcare OR Advanced strategic leadership OR Counseling of persons with special needs OR Entrepreneurship			
Medical statistics	4	Adults and older primary health care (practice)	4			Research dissertation 2	6				

Entrance requirements to the master of nursing science degree Programme are:

A bachelor's degree in nursing, with at least a second class; second division or equivalent. Equivalent degrees from other recognized academic institutions will be considered on an individual basis. Candidates with a pass at the under-graduate level in nursing Programmes will be considered on an individual basis;

A current and active nursing license in Botswana or transferable in Botswana through the nursing and midwifery Council for Botswana;

A minimum of 2 years appropriate professional practice following the first degree, which may be acquired concurrently with part-time study. Professional practice for students who have obtained a pass in their undergraduate programs will be considered on an individual basis.

Adapted from University of Botswana materials

Table 2 Botswana: Affiliated Health Training Institution of Botswana (AHTIB) Post-Diploma Nurse Advanced Certificate/Diploma in Family Nurse Practitioner

Year 1 Semester 1		Year 1 Semester 2		Year 2 Semester 1		Year 2 Semester 2	
Course name	Credits	Course name	Credits	Course name	Credits	Course name	Credits
Health assessment (theory and practice)	4	Children and adolescents in health and illnesses (theory and practice)	5	Role development	3	*Internship* Primary Care of Children and Adolescents	5
Health promotion across the life span	3	Sexual and reproductive health (theory and practice)	5	Disease diagnosis and management in adults and older adults (theory and practice)	5	*Internship* Application sexual and reproductive health care	5
Family health (theory and practice)	3	Statistics	2	Research project	2	Internship Primary care of adults and older adults	5
Pathophysiology	3	Computer application in healthcare	2	Epidemiology	2		
Pharmacotherapeutics	3	Introduction to research (theory and proposal)	3				
Communications and study skills	2						
Entrance qualifications The minimum qualification shall be diploma in general nursing or its equivalent with a minimum of two years in nursing practice. The candidate must be registered with the nursing and Midwifery Council of Botswana and possession of a Botswana general certificate of secondary education or its equivalent with passes in English, mathematics, biology, and Physics/chemistry.							

Adapted from AHTIB materials

frontline Nurse Practitioners who are equipped with advanced knowledge, skills, and attitudes to provide comprehensive world-class healthcare. Nurse practitioners are trained at UDS with the key role of assessing, diagnosing, treating patients with acute and chronic conditions, and referring patients with complex conditions from the primary level of care to secondary level facilities in Ghana for further assessment and management (University for Development Studies 2025).

Table 3 Ghana: University for Development Studies Bachelor of Science (BSc)-NP Program

Description This program trains frontline Primary Care Nurse Practitioners who are equipped with advanced knowledge, skills, and attitudes to provide comprehensive world-class healthcare. Nurse practitioners are trained with the key role of assessing, diagnosing, treating patients with acute and chronic conditions, and referring patients with complex conditions from the primary level of care to secondary level facilities for further assessment and management. *Duration of Study* Three (3) years *Entry Requirements* An applicant to the 3-year BSc Nurse Practitioner program must be a Registered Nurse with Diploma (RGN), a State Registered Nurse (SRN) or Registered Mental Nurse (RMN) with Diploma, and Registered Community Health Nurse with Diploma. Candidates must be in good standing with the Nursing and Midwifery Council of Ghana with at least three (3) years post-registration work experience. International applicants must show evidence of registration with their home Professional Regulatory Bodies. Applicants from non-English speaking countries must also show evidence of English Language proficiency. University of Development Studies. (2025). Regular Undergraduate Studies: BSc Nurse Practitioner. https://uds.edu.gh/admissions/undergraduate-admissions		
BSc nurse practitioner curriculum		
Year 1 (level 200)		
1st trimester	**2nd trimester**	**3rd trimester**
Human growth and development Communication skills African studies Advanced nursing I Medical nursing I Surgical nursing I Pediatric nursing I Introduction French language Introduction to sign language Advanced nursing practical	Introductory information and communication technology Advanced nursing II Medical nursing II Surgical nursing II Pediatric nursing II Perioperative nursing and anesthesia Human anatomy I Human physiology I Advanced nursing practical	Field practicum
Year 2 (level 300)		
1st trimester	**2nd trimester**	**3rd trimester**

(continued)

Table 3 (continued)

Relational practice and therapeutic Communication Philosophy and principles of advanced nursing practice Human anatomy II Human physiology II Comprehensive health assessment Clinical pathology (general) Clinical microbiology Pharmacology and pharmacovigilance Health promotion, education, and advocacy Advanced nursing practical	Pharmacology and therapeutics Health assessment (medical laboratory) Nursing research Nutrition and dietetics Clinical pathology (systemic) Health Psychology for advanced nursing practice Medical biostatistics and data analysis Medical biochemistry Mental health in primary healthcare Health care law and ethics for advanced nursing Advanced nursing practical	Field practicum
Year 3 (level 400)		
1st trimester	**2nd trimester**	**3rd trimester**
Gender studies Public health nursing Mental health affiliation Obstetrics and gynecology Clinical medicine and medical nursing Nursing management, leadership, and health policies Emergency medicine Nursing seminar Maternal and child health Advanced nursing practical	Infectious diseases and emerging health problems Public health nursing (affiliation) Advanced nursing seminar Complementary and alternative medicine in primary care Obstetrics and gynecology (affiliation) Clinical surgery and surgical nursing Clinical pediatrics and pediatric nursing Specialists lectures Nursing informatics Advanced nursing practical	Project work (dissertation)

Adapted from materials from University of Development Studies, Ghana

Finally, the United States with the most experience and longest established programs for NPs is now providing not only Masters level programs, but encouraging Doctoral level education for NPs.

3.1.3 United States: Master of Science in Nursing and Doctor of Nursing Practice NP Exemplars

Since the inception of the first NP program 60 years ago, NP education in the United States has evolved to offer a broad range of specialties and over 500 Institutions offering NP programs, with the largest number of NP programs and NP graduates in the world (AANP 2025). Nationally board-certified NP practice concentrations include Family Nurse Practitioner (FNP), Pediatric Nurse Practitioner (PNP), Adult-Gerontology Primary Care Nurse Practitioner (AG-PCNP), Adult Gerontology Acute Care Nurse Practitioner (AG-ACNP), Psychiatric Mental Health Nurse Practitioner (PMHNP), Neonatal Nurse Practitioner (NNP), Women's Health Nurse Practitioner (WHNP), and Emergency Nurse Practitioner (ENP), with specialized curricula for each concentration (ANCC n.d.; AANPCB 2024). NP educational entry to practice program levels include masters, post-masters certificate, and more recently, the Doctor of Nursing Practice (DNP), attainable as BSN to DNP or MSN to DNP. While the majority of graduates in the USA are at the master's level, the current goal is a DNP for entry to advanced practice as an NP (NONPF 2018). The DNP degree was created in response to country and health care needs in order to expand the leadership and clinical skill set of the NP/APN, as well as enhance practice-based research competencies, given the trend in the USA to remove thesis research from master's level NP/APN curricula. DNP programs typically require either a previous bachelor or master's in nursing for admission with some curricular variation between the two entry levels (Moore et al. 2024). Two US examples are provided. One example is from Old Dominion University (ODU 2025), an FNP-DNP Program with a Master's Degree Step Out (Table 4). The master's degree is conferred at the end of semester five, and the graduate may sit for nationally approved FNP certification programs, then proceed to DNP education via two additional semesters of education. The other example is from the University of Kentucky (UKCON 2024), a Post BSN-DNP FNP Sample Plan of Study, an example of a continuous enrollment program (Table 5).

3.2 Clinical Nurse Specialist

In reviewing CNS program curricula, it is also important to consider the ICN APN Guidelines 2020 definition and scope of practice for the role.

> The CNS is a nurse who has completed a master's degree programme specific to CNS practice. The CNS provides healthcare services based on advanced specialised expertise when caring for complex and vulnerable patients or populations. In addition, nurses in this capacity provide education and support for interdisciplinary staff and facilitate change and innovation in healthcare systems. The emphasis of practice is on advanced specialised nursing

Table 4 Old Dominion University Post BSN FNP Master's-DNP Program with Master's Degree Step Out

MSN Year 1 **1st semester**	**Credits**
Ethical concepts and issues in advanced practice	3
Physical assessment for advanced practice nursing	3
Pathophysiology for advanced practice nursing	3
Population health and epidemiology	3
Total credits	**12**
Year 1 **2nd semester**	**Credits**
Pharmacology for advanced practice nursing	3
Advanced family nursing I: Management of acute illnesses	3
Evidenced-based research & theories	3
Health promotion & maintenance Health	2
Total credits	**11**
Year 1 **3rd semester**	**Credits**
Primary care approaches for children	3
Advanced family nursing I: MSN practicum (168 clinical hours supervised by NP/MD)	3
Family & community assessment	1
Aging in twenty-first century	3
Total credits	**10**
Year 2 **4th semester**	**Credits**
Primary care approaches for women	3
Advanced family nursing II: MSN practicum (224 clinical hours supervised by NP/MD)	4
Advanced family nursing II: Management of chronic illnesses	3
Total credits	**10**
Year 2 **5th semester**	**Credits**
Application of practice-based research methods	2
Advanced family nursing III: MSN practicum (168 clinical hours supervised by NP/MD)	3
Business of advanced practice nursing	3
DNP practicum I (112 practical hours with focus on practice in enhanced leadership, clinical skills, and evidence-based research)	2
Total credits	**10**
Note: Students receive their MSN degree and are eligible for FNP certification and licensure after completion of 5th semester with the successful completion of all FNP role-specific courses.	
Year 2 **6th semester**	**Credits**
DNP roles and responsibilities for transforming practice	3
Research proposal development and database management	4
DNP practicum II (112 practical hours with focus on practice in leadership, evidence-based practice and clinical diagnostics, teamwork, and evidence-based research)	2
Total credits	**9**
Year 3 **7th semester**	**Credits**

(continued)

Table 4 (continued)

DNP practicum III (168 practical hours with focus on practice in advanced evidence-based practice, program evaluation, and team leadership in health care research, business, quality, and technology)	3
Leadership in complex systems and organizations	3
Informatics and healthcare technology	3
Total credits	**9**
Year 3 **8th semester**	**Credits**
DNP practicum IV (168 practical hours with focus on team and organizational leadership, expert clinical practice, health care innovation, evidence-based research, and program development and evaluation)	3
DNP research completion	3
Advocacy & Health care public policy for advanced practice	3
Total credits	**9**
Total credits 80 including 1120 practical hours	

Adapted from Old Dominion University materials

> care and a systems approach using a combination of the provision of direct and indirect clinical services… [Further, an APN CNS differs from a specialized nurse in that]… the scope of practice for the CNS extends beyond the generalist and specialised nurse in terms of advanced expertise, role functions, mastery of a specific specialty with an increased and expanded level of practice that includes broader and more in-depth accountability…CNSs evaluate disease patterns, technological advances, environmental conditions and political influences. In addition, they interpret nursing's professional responsibility to serve the public's need for nursing services. CNSs function as expert clinicians in a specialty and are leaders in advancing nursing practice by teaching, mentoring, consulting and ensuring nursing practice is evidence-based/evidence-informed (Schober et al. 2020).

CNS educational programs vary by country, and curricula are often grouped around competencies in several focal areas including clinical care, system leadership, advancement of nursing practice, and evaluation and research. Some countries (e.g., New Zealand and the USA recommend or mandate CNS programs to require additional advanced pathophysiology, pharmacology, and assessment similar to NP curricula but overall, most programs typically contain CNS-specific competencies and curricular content focused on competencies that are different from the NP (CNSSNZ 2021, APRN Consensus Work Group and NCSBN APRN Advisory Group 2008). The majority of countries with CNS programs allow nurses considerable choice in clinical courses and self-determination in their specialization. Additionally, the flexibility of thesis and non-thesis CNS Masters curricula is available.

3.2.1 Canada: Master of Science CNS Exemplar

In Canada, master's programs for the CNS role were established in the 1970s. The early scope of practice for the CNS role focused on education and leadership; however over time, it also transitioned into supporting the implementation of evidence-based practice. Most CNS Advanced Practice Nurses in Canada, as in most countries, work in acute care, such as inpatient units and hospital-based clinics as a

Table 5 University of Kentucky, continuous post BSN-DNP FNP sample plan of study

Year	Fall	Credits	Spring	Credits	Summer	Credits
Year 1	Gathering, analyzing & using educational data	3	Applications of advanced health assessment[a]	3	Nursing leadership in health care	3
	Advanced physiology & pathophysiology	3	Advanced pharmacology for advanced[a]	4	Quality and safety in nursing & health care	3
	Research methods in advanced practice nursing	3	Evaluating evidence for research and evidence-based practice[a]	3	Primary care of children and childbearing families[a]	3
	Doctor of nursing practice seminar	1	APRN seminar I[a]	3		
	Total credits	**10**	**Total credits**	**13**	**Total credits**	**9**
Year 2	Applied biostatistics for outcome evaluation[a]	3	Protection of human subjects[a]	1	Informatics & healthcare technologies for advanced nursing practice	2
	Proposal development[b]	2	APRN seminar III[a]	3	Complex systems leadership and innovation	2
	APRN seminar II[a]	3	Clinical[a]	3	Economical & financial aspects of clinical & population-base health care delivery systems	3
	Clinical[a]	3	Application of biostatistics & epidemiology for strategic decision making[b]	3		
	Clinical hours	**180**	**Clinical hours**	**180**	**Clinical hours**	
	Total credits	**11**	**Total credits**	**10**	**Total credits**	**7**
Year 3	Population health assessment, planning & policy	3	Problems in advanced practice nursing	3		
	Pro seminar in contemporary health & nursing policy issues	3	DNP project[a]	2		
	Problems in advanced practice nursing	4				
	DNP project[a]	2				
	Clinical hours	**360**		**300**		
	Total credits	**12**		**5**		

Adapted from University of Kentucky College of Nursing materials
[a]Prerequisites or co-requisites apply
[b]Multiple prerequisites, including graduate statistics

Table 6 McGill University Master of Science (MSc) in Advanced Nursing Curriculum, Research Stream (Thesis)

Year 1 (24 Credits) Fall term	Year 1 Winter term	Year 2 (24 Credits) Fall term	Year 2 Winter term
Applied statistics for nursing	Knowledge translation in healthcare	Research project 2	Research project 3
Research methods in nursing	Professional issues in nursing	Advanced clinical reasoning	Applied knowledge translation in healthcare 2
Seminar in nursing	Teaching & Learning in nursing	Health equity	Policy leadership in nursing
Clinical in family systems nursing 1	Research project 1		Advanced practice practicum (either clinical or teaching specialization)
Total credits 12	**Total credits 12**	**Total credits 12**	**Total credits 12**
Program Total 48 credit hours			

Adapted from McGill University materials

- Clinician—providing expert care by conducting detailed assessments, creating care plans, and intervening in complex situations.
- Consultant—using expertise in their clinical specialty to support all interested parties (stakeholders) (e.g., regulated nurses, policy makers, and other healthcare providers) and promote positive client outcomes.
- Educator—educating clients, nurses, students, and other health-care providers on the use of evidence-based practice.
- Researcher—ensuring that their practice applies evidence-based care most effectively while being a leader in every aspect of research.
- Leader — promoting the advancement of their specialty and providing clinical leadership as an agent of change in their practice (CNSAC 2019; CNA 2014, 2016, 2025; Kilpatrick et al. 2013).

Multiple universities across Canada offer the Master in Nursing with a pathway to CNS. McGill University (McGill University 2025) offers two CNS programs, one as a Research Stream (Thesis) (Table 6) and the other as Knowledge Translation (Non-thesis) (Table 7).

3.3 Advanced Practice Nurse

In some countries, particularly those where advanced practice nursing is developing, there is an APN role (Moore et al. 2024) that combines elements of both the NP and CNS roles. Often, jurisdictions and institutions need a clinician who can bridge care between primary care and specialty care while also maintaining patient education, holistic care, and system improvement. According to the ICN definition:

Table 7 McGill University Master of Science (MSc) in Advanced Nursing Curriculum, Knowledge Translation (Non-thesis)

Year 1 (24 Credits) Fall term	Year 1 Winter Term	Year 2 (24 Credits) Fall term	Year 2 Winter term
Applied statistics for nursing	Knowledge translation in healthcare	Applied knowledge translation in healthcare 1	Applied knowledge translation in healthcare 2
Research methods in nursing	Professional issues in nursing	Advanced clinical reasoning	Applied knowledge translation in healthcare 2
Seminar in nursing	Teaching & Learning in nursing	Health equity	Policy leadership in nursing
Clinical in family systems nursing 1	Selected APN complementary course		Advanced practice practicum (either clinical or teaching specialization)
Total credits 12	**Total credits 12**	**Total credits 12**	**Total credits 12**
Program Total 48 credit hours			

Adapted from McGill University materials

> An Advanced Practice Nurse is a generalist or specialized nurse who has acquired, through additional graduate education (minimum of a master's degree), the expert knowledge base, complex decision-making skills and clinical competencies for Advanced Nursing Practice, the characteristics of which are shaped by the context in which they are credentialed to practice. The two most commonly identified APN roles are NP and CNS (Schober et al. 2020).

3.3.1 Singapore: Masters in Nursing APN Exemplar

Singapore is an example of a country with the hybrid APN role. Nurses are educated and certified in the APN role to practice in varied advanced clinical contexts based on their education preparation and experience. They have advanced clinical knowledge, skills, and professional attitude from a range of disciplines including advanced nursing practice, clinical medicine, social sciences, and public health. APN curricula in Singapore are at the master's level and build capabilities in the five competency domains specified by Singapore Nursing Board (SNB): patient care, clinical knowledge, interpersonal and communication skills, practice-based learning and improvement, and professionalism (SNB 2023).

The APN Masters in Nursing (MN) program (Table 8) at the National University of Singapore (NUS) is currently the only APN program in the nation. It is an 18-month program, delivered across 3 semesters, and offers 2 pathways in either Adult Health (AH) or Paediatrics (Paed). It includes 40 Units of theoretical courses, 1200 hours of clinical attachments (30 Units), and a summative OSCE at the end of the MN program. Upon successful completion of the MN program, graduates are then eligible to apply for APN provisional license with the SNB to continue with a 12-month Integrated APN Internship before receiving full licensure as an APN in the country (National University of Singapore n.d).

Table 8 National University of Singapore Alice Lee Centre for Nursing Studies, Master of Nursing

Year 1 January–July	Unit	Hrs	Year 1 August–December	Unit	Hrs	Year 2 January–May	Unit	Hrs
Integrated clinical decision making and management I (AH) *OR* Integrated clinical decision making and management I (Paed)	8	260	Integrated clinical decision making and management II (AH) *OR* Integrated clinical decision making and management II (Paed)	8	260	Evidence-based practice	4	130
Clinical pharmacology and pharmacotherapeutics I	4	130	Adult care across care continuum (AH) *OR* Paediatric care across care continuum (Paed)	8	260	Clinical practicum III (16 weeks)	16	640
Professional development and ethical healthcare	4	130	Clinical pharmacology and Pharmacotherapeutics II	4	130			
Clinical practicum I (10 weeks)	10	400	Clinical practicum II (4 weeks)	4	160			
Totals 26,920 24,810 20,770 **Totals units = 70** **Total hours = 2500**								
NUS MN entrance requirements: Bachelor's degree in nursing from a SNB accredited program with a minimum GPA of 3.2. Full registration and valid practicing certificate with the SNB and at least 5 years continuous clinical practice as a registered nurse. Advanced diploma/post-graduate diploma in a clinical specialty for acute care (critical care and emergency) and mental health care applicants. Strong recommendation from chief nurse, director of nursing, and head of respective department. Meets minimum health requirements stipulated by the Ministry of Health Singapore.								

Adapted from National University of Singapore Alice Lee Centre for Nursing Studies materials

3.4 Nurse Anesthetist

According to the ICN Guidelines on Advanced Practice Nursing-Nurse Anesthesia:

> A Nurse Anesthetist is an Advanced Practice Nurse who has the knowledge, skills and competencies to provide individualised care in anesthesia, pain management, and related anesthesia services to patients across the lifespan, whose health status may range from healthy through all levels of acuity, including immediate, severe, or life threatening illnesses or injury (Stewart et al. 2021).

Although the master's degree is the standard for NA education, nurse education for NAs lacks uniformity around the world (Björkman Björkelund et al. 2021). This reflects the many factors that impact the ability to deliver much-needed anesthesia to patients in every corner of the world—sufficiency of supply of generalist nurses willing and able to take on the education and responsibilities of nurse anesthesia, sufficiency of supply of educational and financial resources for nurse anesthesia education, and a supportive regulatory framework.

The International Federation of Nurse Anesthetists (IFNA 2022) has published three model curriculums, a Bachelor's degree program (Table 9), a post-basic nursing certificate (Table 10), and a Master's degree program (Table 11).

Table 9 International Federation of Nurse Anesthetists (IFNA) Model Curriculum, 36 Month Bachelor's Degree Nurse Anesthesia Program (Full Time)

First Year 1st Semester	First Year 2nd Semester	Second Year 3rd Semester	Second Year 4th Semester	Third Year 5th Semester	Third Year 6th Semester
Roles, ethical and legal issues of nurse anesthesia	Pathophysiology II	Research theory	Advanced principles of anesthesia III	Economics and organization	Review
Basic science	Pharmacology I	Advanced principles of anesthesia II	Bachelor's thesis project	Bachelor's thesis project	Clinical practice VI
Anatomy & physiology	Pharmacology II	Clinical practice III	Clinical practice IV	Clinical practice V	
Pathophysiology	Basic principles of anesthesia				
Clinical practice I	Advanced principles of anesthesia I				
	Advanced principles of anesthesia I				
Minimum applicant prerequisites (IFNA, 2, Para 5) Qualification enabling students to enter a university or university of applied science, defined by the respective national authorities. To be determined by national legislation. Ability to speak and write the language of the institution.					
Course credits Due to the variation in credit systems around the world credit assignments can be left up to respective educational institutions. *Program location* Program can be located within an academic department or in a sponsoring department of a university with involvement of faculty in several different departments (IFNA, 2, Para 3). *Graduate competencies* The graduate competencies, as outlined in the IFNA standards https://ifna.site/app/uploads/2015/08/IFNA-STANDARDS-2016.pdf should be met at the end of the course (IFNA, 3, Para 1). Revised Spring 2019					

This material was adapted from the IFNA website, available at https://ifna site. Detailed information available there

Table 10 International Federation of Nurse Anesthetists (IFNA) Model Curriculum, 18–24 Month Certificate (Non-Degree) Nurse Anesthesia Program (Full Time)

First Year 1st Semester	First Year 2nd Semester	Second Year 3rd Semester	Second Year 4th Semester
Roles, ethical and legal issues of nurse anesthesia	Physiology I	Advanced principles of anesthesia II	Economics and organization
Basic principles of anesthesia	Pathophysiology I	Pathophysiology II	Nurse anesthesia review
Basic science	Advanced principles of anesthesia I	Pharmaco-therapeutics	Clinical practicum IV
Anesthesia pharmacology I	Advanced anesthesia pharmacology II	Advanced principles of anesthesia III	
Clinical practicum I	Research theory	Clinical practicum III	
	Clinical practicum II		

Minimum applicant prerequisites (IFNA, 2, Para 5)

Completion of a basic nursing education program of at least 36 months in length from an institution recognized or accredited by governmental or nongovernmental accreditation or quality assurance entity (if available).

Nursing experience of at least one (1) year, preferably in an acute care setting.

Ability to speak and write in the language of instruction.

Course credits

Due to the variation in credit systems around the world countries can use their own credit systems.

Program location

Program can be located in an academic department, in a sponsoring department of a university or hospital or some other recognized learning setting (IFNA, 2, Para 3).

Graduate competencies

The IFNA graduate competencies, except the research competencies (thesis), (see IFNA graduate competencies in the educational standards for preparing nurse anesthetists) should be met at the end of the course (IFNA, 3, Para 1).

Approved May 2014, Revised May 2016

This material was adapted from the IFNA website, available at https://ifna site. Detailed information available there

3.5 Advanced Nurse Midwife

An Advanced Nurse Midwife is a nurse who has successfully completed a post-basic or post-graduate midwifery educational program, acquired the requisite qualifications to be registered, and/or legally licensed to practise as a midwife (ICM 2021; ICNM UNPF WHO 2021) and in addition has attained additional advanced practice education and skills generally through a Master's degree program to practice at an advanced level of expertise and autonomy, incorporating professional leadership, education, research, and support of systems into their practice (Goemaes et al. 2016; NMBI 2018; NMBA 2020; ACNM 2021). While

Table 11 International Federation of Nurse Anesthetists (IFNA) Model Curriculum, 24 Month Master's Degree Nurse Anesthesia Program (Full Time)

First Year: 1st Semester	First Year: 2nd Semester	Second Year: 3rd Semester	Second Year: 4th Semester
Roles, ethical and legal Issues of nurse anesthesia	Pathophysiology I	Pathophysiology II	Master thesis project
Basic principles of anesthesia	Advanced principles of anesthesia I	Pharmaco-therapeutics	Economics and organization
Basic science	Advanced anesthesia pharmacology II	Advanced principles of anesthesia III	Nurse anesthesia review
Anesthesia pharmacology I	Research theory	Master thesis project	Clinical practicum IV
Physiology I	Advanced principles of anesthesia II	Clinical practicum III	
Clinical practicum I	Clinical practicum II		
Minimum applicant prerequisites (IFNA, 2, Para 5) Completion of a basic nursing education program of at least 36 months in length. Nursing experience of at least one (1) year, preferably in an acute care setting. An earned baccalaureate degree from an institution recognized or accredited by governmental or nongovernmental. accreditation or quality assurance entity (if available) Ability to speak and write in the language of instruction.			
Course credits Due to the variation in credit systems around the world, countries can use their own credit systems. *Program location* Program can be located within an academic department or in a sponsoring department of a university with involvement of faculty in several different departments (IFNA, 2, Para 3). *Graduate competencies* The IFNA graduate competencies (see IFNA graduate competencies as outlined in the educational standards for Preparing nurse anesthetists) should be met at the end of the course (IFNA, 3, Para 1). Approved May 2014, Revised May 2016			

This material was adapted from the IFNA website, available at https://ifna site. Detailed information available there

in many regions of the world basic midwifery is taught as part of entry level nursing training and is not considered advanced practice nursing. Additionally in some countries, midwifery may be regulated as a distinct profession. This chapter refers to Advanced Nurse Midwifery only where it is a legally defined nursing-based advanced practice role.

3.5.1 Republic of Ireland: Master of Science in Advanced Practice Nurse Midwifery

Advanced nursing and midwifery practice was first introduced into the Republic of Ireland following the report on the Commission of Nursing in 1998 (IAANMP 2025). With official title protected registration, scope of practice, and regulatory guidelines for Advanced Midwifery Practitioners and Advanced Nurse Practitioners, advanced practice is defined in the Republic of Ireland by the Nursing and Midwifery Board (NMBI) as a career pathway for registered nurses,

Table 12 University College Cork MSc in Advanced Practice (Nursing/Midwifery) Curriculum

Year 1 (60 credits)
Systematic approach to assessing and evaluating patients (10 credits)
Professional, ethical, legal and communication issues informing nurse and midwife prescribing and clinical practicum (10 credits)
Holistic approach to prescribing medicinal products and clinical practicum (10 credits)
Advanced research methods for healthcare professionals (10 credits)
Decision making, and advanced practice professional roles (10 credits)
Leadership, quality improvement and governance for advanced practice (10 credits)
Year 2 (50 credits)
Dissertation for advanced practice nursing (30 credits)
Advanced practice clinical practicum (20 credits)
Each 10-credit module involves 200 hours of engagement and can be divided between classroom, clinical skills instruction, online activity, and independent learning. There will be up to 40 hours of directed learning such as required reading, e-tivities, group activities per module. Students engage in self-directed independent learning as part of each module. In year 1, students complete 60 credits, and this includes preparation for registration as a nurse midwife prescriber of medicinal products with the nursing and midwifery Board of Ireland (NMBI). In year 2, students complete a dissertation under the guidance of allocated research supervisors. Clinical learning is supported through an individualized learning plan and assessed by a clinical supervisor in practice. Students must complete a minimum of 500 hours of supervised practice in preparation for registration as an advanced midwife practitioner with the NMBI.
Pre-requisites for admission
Applicants for the MSc in advanced practice (nursing/midwifery) must meet the following requirements: Have a minimum of a primary honors degree (NFQ, level 8, or equivalent) in nursing or midwifery or equivalent. Hold active registration on a division of the professional register maintained by the NMBI. The candidate must have three years' recent post-registration clinical experience in nursing/midwifery (within the past 5 years) with the equivalent of 1-year full-time experience in the specific area of practice.

Adapted from University College Cork materials

committed to continuing professional development and clinical supervision, to practice at a higher level of capability as independent, autonomous, and expert practitioners (NMBI 2018; NCNZ 2017).

The 2-year Master of Science in Advanced Practice (Nursing/Midwifery) at University College Cork (Table 12) is one of several master's level advanced nurse midwifery programs in Ireland, and is designed to prepare nurses and midwives to practice at a higher level of capability in independent, autonomous, and expert practice, that is innovative, flexible, and patient-centered. The program also prepares students for registration as a nurse midwife prescriber of medicinal products, and for their role as clinical and professional leaders with a commitment to the dissemination of evidence-based knowledge and the instruction of others (University College Cork 2025).

4 Defining Features of APN Content

All APN programs provide curriculums and instruction so that generalist nurses are formally educated in advanced skills under the close eye of faculty and preceptors, meeting carefully delineated criteria and competencies. Programs provide the following content either in specified courses and/or threaded throughout the curriculum.

4.1 Core Content and Clinicals

All APN program content builds on foundational nursing content and according to longstanding nursing theory and principles. Most programs also require nurse applicants to have substantial experience as a nurse (Wheeler et al. 2022). From that background, the core program content builds on what the discipline will need to function in the new role. Once foundational material that cuts across all the disciplines (advanced physiology/pathophysiology, advanced pharmacology, and advanced physical assessment) is provided, programs move to role-specific management and clinical courses. Since direct patient care is at the core of advanced practice substantial time is spent in clinical settings, under the guidance of an appropriate preceptor, such as an APN or a Physician, but closely monitored by program faculty.

4.2 Leadership, System, and Organization Management

Because there is such a tremendous need for leadership skills in systems of care and patient care requires tremendous system navigation and coordination, APN programs customarily provide content to address this specific need. APNs will often be the most highly educated nurses to work in a system. As such they are often tasked with management and leadership duties. Strengthening leadership skills is particularly important in cultures where nurses may not be valued or respected, out of misunderstanding, cultural and societal biases, lack of autonomy, or outdated stereotypes. APN leadership is additionally discussed in Chap. 7, and the content of two leadership courses are provided as exemplars, a master's level course and a DNP level course.

4.3 Research, Evidence-Based Practice, and Translation into Practice

An additional expectation of APNs is the ability to be a resource for clinical research at a variety of levels. As clinical leaders, they are expected to understand research, scan for new evidence, oversee or assist with translation into practice, monitor adherence to guidelines, analyze outcomes, and guide or participate in research teams (Clarke et al. 2021; Brunt and Morris 2023). All APN programs include this content but programs at a master and higher level include this content because these programs require theses, graduate projects, and quality improvement projects.

4.4 Healthcare Policy, Patient Advocacy, and Healthcare Finance

APNs need to understand health policy and healthcare finance because each uniquely impacts patient care and the systems that provide that care. Though the two issues are very different, they go hand-in-hand. All care delivery and any change in care costs either the patient, the organization, the community, or the government. As clinical leaders, APNs are often involved in policy and financial decisions. APNs also face a lot of barriers to practicing to their full scope of practice and education. APNs also take on the task of patient advocacy in many situations, working for policy change at multiple levels. For these reasons, APN programs include content on healthcare policy, patient advocacy, and healthcare finance. As knowledgeable clinicians and advocates, faculty often lead the way through support of professional organizations, service on boards that influence policy, engaging interested parties (stakeholders), and working with policy makers and legislators (Chilton 2015).

4.5 Quality and Safety

Quality and safety assurance in healthcare has been a function of nursing since nursing began, largely because nurses are uniquely positioned to view situations from a system-wide perspective, and they are the organizational backbone of hospital, clinic, and community care. As APNs enter systems of care that responsibility grows due to the nature of advanced care but also because healthcare is complex and constantly evolving. Programs either offer stand-alone quality and safety courses or the material is threaded throughout the curriculum. Regardless, the content is foundational to nursing and APN education.

In the United States, due to health system complexity and the recognition nursing is central to quality and safety in healthcare, US nursing responded in 2005 by producing the Quality and Safety Education for Nurses (QSEN) initiative (Dolansky and Moore 2013). Funded by the Robert Wood Johnson Foundation the initiative resulted in the QSEN Institute, two sets of QSEN Competencies (undergraduate and graduate), and multiple education and practice resources, available at https://www.qsen.org. The six competencies consisted of the following: person and family-centered care, teamwork and collaboration, safety, quality and improvement, evidence-based practice, and informatics. This framework has been used by multiple organizations and in numerous publications around the world (Sherwood 2021).

4.6 Communication and Informatic Technology

Nurses have the responsibility to gather, interpret, organize, and communicate healthcare information to patients, families, communities, and healthcare institutions (Johnson 2022). For that reason, schools devote considerable attention to that skill at every level of nursing. As a defining feature of nursing, APNs must be adept at communicating despite a rapidly changing information and technology landscape, which includes electronic medical records, online prescribing, online billing, decision tools, Internet resources, wearable/mobile devices, large data sets, telehealth, and artificial intelligence (Williamson 2025; Koo et al. 2024). Because of that and the responsibility APNs bear for health education and health promotion APN programs educate on communication and informatics in multiple ways—how to communicate with patients despite barriers such as low literacy, limited health literacy or differences of language use (Nursing Education Staff 2025, Wilandika et al. 2023, Dickens and Piano 2013, 67–69), how to compensate for resource limitations including digital/internet divides and electricity divides (LinkedIn 2025), and how to educate patients on how to access, use, and evaluate technologies safely (Williamson 2025).

4.7 Projects

Early APN programs in the US customarily required a thesis so students would be able to demonstrate their ability to research an issue and present the findings in a coherent, defensible, useful format. As these master's programs felt the pressure to increase clinical content, the thesis requirement was often abandoned, replaced by clinical content and a streamlined project. This was similar to medical education abandoning the requirement for a dissertation as was done many decades ago (B.J. Gooch, personal communication, March 2, 2025). However, as healthcare and system issues became more complex and DNP programs became the recommended APN entry to practice, schools felt the need to bring back a scholarly project, one that reflected system change, planning, implementation, and evaluation as recommended by the American Association of Colleges of Nursing (AACN 2015), an agency in the United States that sets educational standards for nursing programs. These scholarly projects were not intended to be dissertations, nor were they to be called either that or capstone projects. At present in the United States, the majority of scholarly projects, at 85.5%, are quality improvement projects or practice improvement in nature (Tovar et al. 2020).

Outside the US master's-level programs have continued to require a master's thesis, not only to demonstrate academic ability but to allow nurses to enter PhD programs should they choose to do so. The thesis can be a literature review, a developmental project, or empirical research but all must be reflect research-based abilities (Sulosaari et al. 2023).

5 Conclusion

This chapter highlights a range of representative curricula from around the world and discusses critical educational content for Advanced Practice Nursing, the highly specialized area of nursing that includes specific protected roles such as Nurse Practitioner, Clinical Nurse Specialist, Nurse Anesthetist, and Advanced Nurse Midwife, generally recognized under the umbrella term Advanced Practice Nurse. While there are many commonalities in preparing nurses to take on expected advanced roles in evidence-based patient-centered care, leadership, and research, there is also variation in APN education and expected specific role competencies globally based on healthcare systems, regulatory requirements, educational frameworks, and specific country needs. Notably, the key feature of all APN programs is a core focus on advanced patient care skills and advanced-level competencies. All APN programs require advanced courses in clinical care, and most require advanced pathophysiology, advanced assessment, and advanced pharmacology, as well as supervised hands-on, role-specific patient care clinical hours. Other curricular content including role or patient-specific management, leadership, research, policy, and ethics are generally present in various forms depending on the advanced practice specialty role, program educational level, and country-related factors. Looking specifically at curricula for the APN roles, this chapter explores APN education globally and provides exemplars demonstrating the distinct similarities as well as differences in prerequisites, educational level, and program structure, required program content, and expected competencies for each role, in various countries and educational institutions to provide both an overall view and guidance for those seeking to learn about or develop the APN roles.

References

American Academy of nurse Practitioners Certification Board (AANPCB). AANPCB certification. Author 2024. https://www.aanpcert.org/certs/index. Accessed 2 May 2025.

American Association of Colleges of Nursing (AACN). The doctor of nursing practice: current issues and clarifying recommendations report from the task force on the implementation of the DNP. Author. 2015. https://www.pncb.org/sites/default/files/2017-02/AACN_DNP_Recommendations.pdf. Accessed 2 May 2025.

American Association of Nurse Anesthetists (AANA). Education and stats. Author. 2023. https://www.aana.com/about-us/about-crnas/become-a-crna. Accessed 4 May 2025.

American Association of Nurse Practitioners (AANP). Historical timeline. Author. 2025. https://www.aanp.org/about/about-the-american-association-of-nurse-practitioners-aanp/historical-timeline. Accessed 3 May 2025.

American College of Nurse Midwives (ACNM). Definition of midwifery and scope of practice of certified nurse-midwives and certified midwives. Author. Dec 2021. https://midwife.org/wp-content/uploads/2024/10/Definition-of-Midwifery-and-Scope-of-Practice-of-Certified-Nurse-Midwives-and-Certified-Midwives.pdf. Accessed 3 May 2025.

American Nurses Credentialing Center (ANCC). Nursing certifications: our certifications. Author. n.d. 2019. https://www.nursingworld.org/our-certifications/#FilterForm. Accessed 1 May 2025.

APRN Consensus Work Group, National Council of State Boards of Nursing (NCSBN) APRN Advisory Committee. Consensus model for APRN regulation: licensure, accreditation, certification & education. NCSBN Jul 2008. https://www.ncsbn.org/public-files/Consensus_Model_Report.pdf. Accessed 3 May 2025.

Australian Nursing and Midwifery Accreditation Council (ANMAC). Fact sheet: advanced nursing practice and specialty areas in nursing. Author. 2019. https://www.nursingmidwiferyboard.gov.au/codes-guidelines-statements/faq/fact-sheet-advanced-nursing-practice-and-specialty-areas.aspx. Accessed 4 May 2025.

Beauchesne MA, Honig J, Sevilla S, Carryer J, Debout C, Ganz FD, et al. A snapshot of clinical educational experiences for advanced practice nurses worldwide. Nurse Pract. 2020;45(9):14–22. https://doi.org/10.1097/01.NPR.0000694700.16463.c7.

Björkman Björkelund K, Horton B, Riesen M, Yang H, Anang S. History of the IFNA education committee. In: Ouellette SM, Horton B, Rowles J, editors. The global voice for nurse anesthesia: history of the International Federation of Nurse Anesthetists. Carmel, Indiana: IFNA; 2021. p. 101–81.

Brunt BA, Morris MM. Nursing professional development evidence-based practice. Treasure Island (FL): StatPearls Publishing; 2023. https://pubmed.ncbi.nlm.nih.gov/36943994/. Accessed 4 May 2025

Canadian Association of Schools of Nursing (CASN). Nurse practitioner education in Canada: national framework of guiding principles & essential components. Author. 2012. https://casn.ca/wp-content/uploads/2014/12/FINALNPFrameworkEN20130131.pdf. Accessed 3 May 2025.

Canadian Nurses Association (CNA). Pan-Canadian core competencies for the clinical nurse specialist. Author. 2014. https://hl-prod-ca-oc-download.s3-ca-central-1.amazonaws.com/CNA/2f975e7e-4a40-45ca-863c-5ebf0a138d5e/UploadedImages/documents/Clinical_Nurse_Specialists_Convention_Handout_e.pdf. Accessed 4 May 2025.

Canadian Nurses Association (CNA). Position statements – Canadian Nurses Association. Author. 2016. https://www.cna-aiic.ca/en/policy-advocacy/policy-support-tools/position-statements. Accessed 4 May 2025.

Canadian Nurses Association (CNA). Clinical nurse specialists. Author. 2025. https://www.cna-aiic.ca/en/nursing/advanced-nursing-practice/clinical-nurse-specialists. Accessed 3 May 2025.

Chilton L. Guest editorial: nurse practitioners have an essential role in health policy. JNP. 2015;11(2):A19. https://www.npjournal.org/article/S1555-4155(14)00687-4/abstract

Choi SJ, Kim YH, Lim KC, Kang Y. Advanced practice nurse in South Korea and current issues. JNP. 2022;19(9):104486. https://doi.org/10.1016/j.nurpra.2022.10.015.

Christmals CD, Armstrong SJ. Curriculum framework for advanced practice nursing in Sub-Saharan Africa: a multimethod study. BMJ Open. 2020;10(6):e035580. https://www.npjournal.org/article/S1555-4155(14)00687-4/pdf

Clarke V, Lehane E, Mulcahy H, Cotter P. Nurse practitioners' implementation of evidence-based practice into routine care: a scoping review. Worldviews Evid-Based Nurs. 2021;18(3):180–9. https://doi.org/10.1111/wvn.12510. Epub 2021 May 27. PMID: 34042238

Clinical Nurse Specialist Association of Canada (CNSAC). Regarding CNS [Internet]. Author. 2019. https://cns-c-canada.ca/home/regardingcns/. Accessed 2 May 2025.

Clinical Nurse Specialist Society of New Zealand (CNSSNZ). Suggested educational pathways for CNS in NZ. Author. 2021. www.cnssnz.org/_files/ugd/e40465_9c3e5386800b4aa7966b7cc6a8fea6af.pdf. Accessed 8 May 2025.

Collins S, Hewer I. The impact of the Bologna process on nursing higher education in Europe: a review. Int J Nurs Stud. 2014;51(1):150–6. https://pubmed.ncbi.nlm.nih.gov/23928323/

Dickens C, Piano MR. Health literacy and nursing. AJN. 2013;113(6):52–7. https://journals.lww.com/ajnonline/Abstract/2013/06000/Health_Literacy_and_Nursing___An_Update.29.aspx

Dolansky MA, Moore SM. Quality and safety education for nurses (QSEN): the key is systems thinking. OJIN. 2013;18(3):Manuscript 1. https://doi.org/10.3912/OJIN.Vol18No03Man01.

Goemaes R, Beeckman D, Goossens J, Shawe J, Verhaeghe S, Van Hecke A. Advanced midwifery practice: an evolutionary concept analysis. Midwifery. 2016;42(42):29–37. https://doi.org/10.1016/j.midw.2016.09.004.

Gray DC, Kgositau N, Lubinda-Sinombe G. The nurse practitioner role and practice in Botswana. In: Thomas S, Rowles JS, editors. Nurse practitioners and nurse anesthetists: the evolution of the global roles. Switzerland: Springer Nature; 2023. p. 225–34. https://ouci.dntb.gov.ua/en/works/lDAL8Rg9/.

International Confederation of Midwives (ICM). Global standards for midwifery education. Author. 2021. https://internationalmidwives.org/resources/global-standards-for-midwifery-education/. Accessed 3 May 2025.

International Confederation of Nurse Midwives (ICNM), United Nations Population Fund (UNPF), World Health Organization (WHO). State of the world's midwifery. ICM. 2021. https://internationalmidwives.org/resources/state-of-the-worlds-midwifery-2021/. Accessed 3 May 2025.

International Federation of Nurse Anesthetists (IFNA). Approved non-physician anesthesia programs/schools. Author. 2022. https://ifna.site/ifna-accreditation-program/. Accessed 4 May 2025.

Irish Association of Advanced Nurse Midwife Practitioners (IAANMP). Position statement: | Advanced nurse practitioners. 2025. https://iaanmp.com/position-statement/. Accessed 4 May 2025.

Janson AL, Opheim R, Hellesø R. Advanced practice nurse education in its infancy: an exploratory study of Norwegian higher education institutions' program descriptions. Scand J Educ Res. 2023;68(4):779–91. https://doi.org/10.1080/00313831.2023.2185810.

Jeffery N, Donald F, Martin-Misener R, Bryant-Lukosius D, Johansen EA, Egilsdottir HÖ, et al. A comparative analysis of teaching and evaluation methods in nurse practitioner education programs in Australia, Canada, Finland, Norway, the Netherlands and USA. Int J Nurs Educ Scholarsh. 2020;17(1) https://pubmed.ncbi.nlm.nih.gov/32543454/

Johnson, J. AACN QSEN learning modules: health informatics. QSEN. 2022. https://www.aacnnursing.org/our-initiatives/education-practice/teaching-resources/qsen-learning-modules. Accessed 1 May 2025.

Jokiniemi K, Chair SY, Wong FKY, Bryant-Lukosius D. Advanced practice role delineation within Hong Kong: a cross-sectional study. Nurs Health Sci. 2022;24(3):679–89. https://pubmed.ncbi.nlm.nih.gov/35699666/

Kilpatrick K, DiCenso A, Bryant-Lukosius D, Ritchie JA, Martin-Misener R, Carter N. Practice patterns and perceived impact of clinical nurse specialist roles in Canada: results of a national survey. J Nurs Stud. 2013;50(11):1524–36. https://pubmed.ncbi.nlm.nih.gov/23548169/

Koo TH, Zakaria AD, Ng JK, Leong XB. Systematic review of the application of artificial intelligence in healthcare and nursing care. Malays J Med Sci. 2024;31(5):135–42. https://doi.org/10.21315/mjms2024.31.5.9. Epub 2024 Oct 8. PMID: 39416729; PMCID: PMC11477473

LinkedIn. What are effective communication strategies for patients with limited digital access? Author. 2025. https://www.linkedin.com/advice/1/what-effective-communication-strategies-patients-limited-fmabe#:~:text=Effective%20communication%20strategies%20for%20patients%20with%20limited%20digital%20access%20can,and%20tailoring%20the%20communication%20accordingly. Accessed 3 May 2025.

McGill University. Advanced practice nursing (APN) – courses of study. Author. 2025. https://www.mcgill.ca/nursing/programs/masters-programs/msca/advanced-practice-nursing. Accessed 1 May 2025.

Moore K, Lockwood E, Henderson C, Li M. Advanced practice nurses: a global overview of education. In: Rogers M, Lehwaldt D, Roussel J, Acorn M, editors. Advanced practice nurse networking to enhance global health. Switzerland: Springer Nature. 2024.p. 105–31. https://doi.org/10.1007/978-3-031-39740-0_6.

Nakamura M. The current state of Japan's nursing and advanced practice nursing education system. IJAP 2 2024;2(3):149–152. https://doi.org/10.12968/ijap.2024.0027

National Association of Clinical Nurse Specialists (NACNS). Statement on clinical nurse specialist practice and education, third edition. Author. 2019. https://nursing.lsuhsc.edu/Docs/Quality/2019-NACNS_CNS%20Statement_FINAL.pdf. Accessed 4 May 2025.

National Organization of Nurse Practitioner Faculties (NONPF). NP competencies. Author. 2022. https://cdn.ymaws.com/www.nonpf.org/resource/resmgr/competencies/nonpf_np_role_core_competenc.pdf. Accessed 1 May 2025.

National Organization of Nurse Practitioner Faculty (NONPF). The doctor of nursing practice degree: entry to nurse practitioner practice by 2025. Author. 2018. https://cdn.ymaws.com/www.nonpf.org/resource/resmgr/dnp/v3_05.2018_NONPF_DNP_Stateme.pdf. Accessed 4 May 2025.

National University of Singapore Alice Lee Centre for Nursing Studies. Master of nursing. n.d.. https://medicine.nus.edu.sg/nursing/wp-content/uploads/sitEs/2/2024/06/2024-MastEr-of-Nursing-E-Brochure_update-June24.pdf. Accessed 1 May 2025.

Ndirangu-Mugo E, Kimani RW, Onyancha C, Mutwiri BD, May B, Kambo I, Tallam E, Koech N, Mukuna A, Henderson C, Shumba CS. Scopes of practice for advanced practice nursing and advanced practice midwifery in Kenya: a gap analysis. Int Nurs Rev. 2024;71(2):276–84. https://doi.org/10.1111/inr.12947. Epub 2024 Mar 15. PMID: 38488333

New Zealand Nurses Organisation (NZNO). Competencies for the mātanga tapuhi nurse practitioner scope of practice. Author. 2017: p. 1–11. https://www.nursingcouncil.org.nz/common/Uploaded%20files/Public/Nursing/Nurse%20Practitioner/Competencies%20for%20matanga%20tapuhi%20nurse%20practioner%20scope%20of%20practice%20March%202017.pdf. Accessed 4 May 2025.

New Zealand Nurses Organization (NZNO). Position statement on advanced nursing practice. Author. 2020. https://www.nursingcouncil.org.nz/common/Uploaded%20files/Public/Nursing/Nurse%20Practitioner/Competencies%20for%20matanga%20tapuhi%20nurse%20practioner%20scope%20of%20practice%20March%202017.pdf. Accessed 3 May 2025.

Nsibanze B. Implementing the FNP role in Eswatini: successes and challenges. Presentation at: International Council of Nurses Nurse Practitioner Advanced Practice Nurse Network Conference; 12 Sept 2024; Aberdeen, Scotland.

Nursing And Midwifery Board of Australia (NMBA). Fact sheet: advanced nursing practice and specialty areas within nursing. Author. 2020. https://www.nursingmidwiferyboard.gov.au/Codes-Guidelines-Statements/FAQ/fact-sheet-advanced-nursing-practice-and-specialty-areas.aspx. Accessed 2 May 2025.

Nursing and Midwifery Board of Ireland (NMBI). Advanced practice (nursing) standards and requirements acknowledgement. Author. 2017. https://www.nmbi.ie/NMBI/media/NMBI/Advanced-Practice-Nursing-Standards-and-Requirements-2017.pdf?ext=.pdf. Accessed 3 May 2025.

Nursing and Midwifery Board of Ireland (NMBI). Advanced practice (midwifery) standards and requirements acknowledgements. Author. 2018; p. 12–18. https://www.nmbi.ie/NMBI/media/NMBI/Advanced-Practice-(Midwifery)-Standards-and-Requirements-2018-final_4.pdf?ext=.pdf

Nursing Council of New Zealand (NCNZ). Competencies for the nurse practitioner scope of practice. Author. 2017. https://nursingcouncil.org.nz/Public/NCNZ/nursing-section/Nurse_practitioner.aspx. Accessed 3 May 2025.

Nursing Education Staff. Nurse insights: how do nurses address language barriers? Author. 2025. https://nursingeducation.org/insights/addressing-language-barriers/. Accessed 5 May 2025.

Old Dominion University. Catalog. Author. 2025;82(1). https://catalog.odu.edu/. Accessed 4 May 2025.

Schober M, Lehwaldt D, Rogers M, Steinke M, Turale S, Pulcini J, Roussel J, Stewart D. International Council of Nurses guidelines on advanced practice nursing. 16 April 2020. https://www.icn.ch/system/files/documents/2020-04/ICN_APN%20Report_EN_WEB.pdf. Accessed 1 May 2025.

Sherwood G. Patient safety: sharing new evidence to confront a global crisis. J Nurs Res. 2021;26(1–2):3–5. https://doi.org/10.1177/1744987121992903.

Singapore Nursing Board (SNB). Singapore nursing board core competencies of advanced practice nurse. Author. 2023. https://isomer-user-content.by.gov.sg/78/164d803e-ce80-45ef-82d9-f8154ef89759/core-competencies-of-apn_2023.pdf. Accessed 3 May 2025.

Stewart D, Horton B, Madsen J, Rowles R, Akalu L, Debout C, Yang M. International Council of Nurses guidelines on advanced practice nursing nurse anesthetists 2021. International Council of Nurses; 2021. https://ifna.site/app/uploads/2021/05/ICN_Nurse-Anaesthetist-Report_EN_WEB.pdf. Accessed 3 May 2025

Sulosaari V, Blaževičienė A, Bragadóttir H, Bäckström J, Heikkila JJ, Hellesø R, et al. A comparative review of advanced practice nurse programmes in the Nordic and Baltic countries. Nurs Educ Today. 2023;127(104857):105847–7. https://pubmed.ncbi.nlm.nih.gov/37216703/

Tovar E, Ossege J, Farus-Brown S, Zonsius M, Morrow L. DNP program faculty and graduates' knowledge and use of QI and safety processes. Nurse Educ. 2020;45(1):11–6. https://pubmed.ncbi.nlm.nih.gov/31022071/

University College Cork. Nursing – advanced practice (nursing/midwifery). Author. 2025. https://www.ucc.ie/en/ckx24/#section1. Accessed 3 May 2025.

University for Development Studies. Regular undergraduate programmes. Author. 2025. https://uds.edu.gh/admissions/undergraduate-admissions. Accessed 1 May 2025.

University of Botswana. Master of nursing science. Author. n.d.. https://www.ub.bw/programmes/health-sciences/school-nursing/master-nursing-science-mnsc. Accessed 4 May 2025.

University of Botswana and Affiliated Health Training Institutions of Botswana (AHTIB). Curriculum for the advanced diploma in family nurse practitioner. Botswana ministry of Health 2008.

University of Cape Coast. Advance practice nursing. Author. 2025. https://ucc.edu.gh/programmes/master-science-advance-practice-nursing. Accessed 1 May 2025.

University of Kentucky College of Nursing (UKCON). Post BSN-DNP family NP sample plan of study: Full time. 2024. https://nursing.uky.edu/sites/default/files/2024-05/fnp-post-bsn-dnp-ft-2024.pdf. Accessed 2 May 2025.

Verpleegkundigen & Verzorgenden Nederland (V&VN) (Nurses & Carers Netherlands). Nurse practitioner professional competency framework. Colophon 2019. https://venvnvs.nl/wp-content/uploads/2019/06/2019-06-25-Nurse-Practitioner-Professional-Competency-Framework.pdf. Accessed 3 May 2025.

Wheeler KJ, Miller M, Pulcini J, Gray D, Ladd E, Rayens MK. Advanced practice nursing roles, regulation, education, and practice: a global study. Ann Glob Health. 2022;88(1):42. https://doi.org/10.5334/aogh.3698. PMID: 35755314; PMCID: PMC9205376

Wilandika A, Pandin MGR, Yusuf A. The roles of nurses in supporting health literacy: a scoping review. Front. Public Health. 2023;16(11):1022803. https://doi.org/10.3389/fpubh.2023.1022803. PMID: 37663836; PMCID: PMC10469320

Williamson K. The future of healthcare: a focus on informatics. American Hospital & Healthcare Management 2025. https://www.americanhhm.com/articles/the-future-of-healthcare-a-focus-on-informatics. Accessed 1 May 2025.

Xu C, Koh KWL, Zhou W. The development of advanced practice nurses in Singapore. INR. 2022;71(2):238–43. https://pubmed.ncbi.nlm.nih.gov/36409288/

Zug KE, Cassiani SHDB, Pulcini J, Garcia AB, Aguirre-Boza F, Park J. Advanced practice nursing in Latin America and the Caribbean: regulation, education and practice. Rev Lat-Am Enferm. 2016;24:e2807. https://pubmed.ncbi.nlm.nih.gov/27508923/

Credentialing and Accreditation of APN Education

Michelle Acorn, Barbara Bailey, and Kelly Kokus

1 Background and Context

Advanced practice nursing (APN) educational programs must be developed with many factors in-mind. These include regional and national scope of entry-to-practice competencies based on local and national regulations (CCRNR 2023; CNO 2024; CNA 2010, 2019). International perspectives such as global health workforce priorities and best practices may also be considered (ICN 2020; WHO 2025; Wheeler et al. 2022). APN education credentialing policies provide the necessary background and structure upon which APN programs may be established, regulated, and credentialed (CNA 2019; CASN 2015, 2025; CCAPR 2023).

The information in this chapter may be used by either individual APN leaders or educational institutions that provide APN education. The contents include consideration of local to global factors such as national nursing councils, regulatory bodies, accreditation and credentialing agencies, health organizations, and legislative ministries (CNA 2019; CCAPR 2023; CCNE 2024; CNO 2025; HEE 2017; EFNA 2025).

Several principles have guided the creation of this chapter. These include competency-based education, quality assurance, global alignment, diversity, equity, inclusion, access and anti-racism and oppression lens (AACN 2021; CASN 2025; ICN 2020).

APN educational programs must meet the appropriate clinical and leadership competencies as outlined by their regional and national regulatory nursing boards

M. Acorn (✉)
University of Toronto & Queen's University, Toronto & Kingston, ON, Canada
e-mail: michelleacorn@gmail.com

B. Bailey
University Health Network, Toronto General Hospital, University of Toronto, Toronto, ON, Canada

K. Kokus
Fanshawe College, London, ON, Canada

K. J. Wheeler, M. Acorn (eds.), *Health Policy for Advanced Practice Nursing: A Toolkit for Implementation and Improvement*, Advanced Practice in Nursing,
https://doi.org/10.1007/978-3-032-03667-4_19

(CCRNR 2023; CNO 2024; CNA 2010, 2019). These competencies must be measurable, and programs should routinely undergo evaluation by the appropriate overseeing regulatory body to ensure they are achieved (CCAPR 2023; CCNE 2024; CNO 2025; EFNA 2025). These programs should also consider a global perspective for the strategic directions for nurses and midwives as outlined by the World Health Organization (WHO 2025) and International Council for Nurses (ICN 2020).

Diversity, equity and inclusion (DEI), anti-racism and oppression are all factors that should be embedded within every component of APN education credentialing policy (AACN 2021; CASN 2025; ICN 2020). These factors have been considered and applied to each aspect of this chapter's recommendations.

2 Credentialing Recommendations

The chapter is divided into seven sections: educational standards; program credentialing; specialty certification; global competency framework alignment; cross-border recognition and mobility; quality assurance and evaluation metrics; and governance and accountability (CNA 2019; CASN 2012, 2015; CCAPR 2023; CCNE 2024; CNO 2025; HEE 2017; EFNA 2025; Gardner et al. 2016). DEI and an anti-racism and oppression lens are also considered and discussed within each section (AACN 2021; CASN 2025; ICN 2020) (Fig. 19.1).

2.1 Educational Standards

APN programs must consider a range of factors to become an accredited program. These include meeting various educational standards set out by their respective regional and national nursing regulators and associations (CCRNR 2023; CNO 2024; CNA 2019; CCNE 2024). International perspectives should also be considered and incorporated into educational standards to maintain global consistency in APN education and promote adherence to best practices, while supporting APN role development (AACN 2021; ICN 2020; WHO 2025). APN programs should strive to

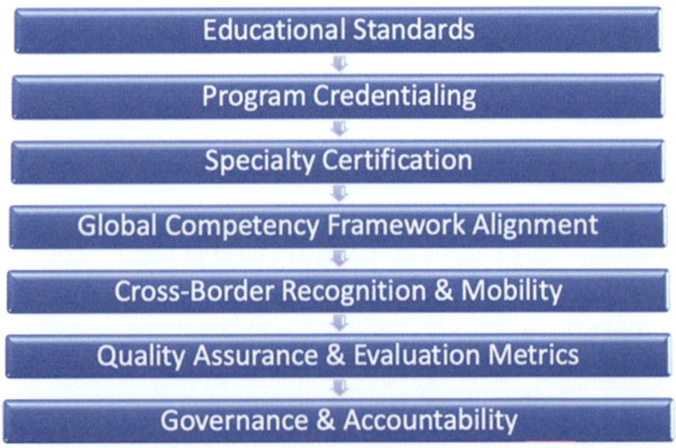

Fig. 19.1 Policy components of an APN education credentialing

be inclusive in both their access and admissions criteria. They should endeavor to provide support for nurses from diverse and underrepresented communities to access APN education programs (AACN 2021; CASN 2025). Table 19.1 presents the standard APN minimum educational program components. More details have been provided throughout the text.

Table 19.1 Minimum education standards for advanced practice nursing (APN) programs from a regional, national and global perspective

Minimum educational standards for APN programs	Local to Global (Regional, National & International)
Entry/admission requirements should include:	Active Registered Nurse (RN) license in jurisdiction of practice Bachelor's undergraduate degree in nursing or equivalent Two years of full-time clinical practice experience (or equivalent) within the last 5 years (CCRNR 2023; CNA 2010)
APN degree awarded:	In most high-income countries, APN programs are at the graduate level, resulting in either a Master's or Doctorate degree (CNA 2010, 2019; Wheeler et al. 2022) In low and lower-middle-income countries, APN programs are often at the undergraduate level and may or may not include additional certificate-level training (Wheeler et al. 2022)
Curriculum content should include:	Clinical (advanced health assessment, advanced pharmacology, advanced pathophysiology, clinical decision making) Research (including quality improvement and patient safety) and knowledge translation (presentations and publications) Leadership (including policy advocacy) Consultation and collaboration (interprofessional and intersectoral) Virtual care Health equity and social determinants of health Cultural competence and safety Indigenous health and cultural safety Ethics and professional practice Global health challenges and planetary health Mentorship and Teaching Skills (AACN 2021; CASN 2015, 2025; ICN 2020)
Clinical hours should include:	Minimally 500 supervised clinical hours Various clinical settings across sectors/system Consideration of equitable, rural and global health placement opportunities (CCRNR 2023; CNA 2010; CASN 2012; Gardner et al. 2016)
Faculty qualifications should include:	APN licensed faculty APN licensed preceptors Doctorally prepared faculty (PhD or DNP) Faculty with clinical expertise, leadership training, and development on cultural safety and humility, DEI, and anti-racism and oppression (CASN 2025; CCAPR 2023; EFNA 2025)
Accreditation:	Program must meet the eligibility criteria for accreditation through the relevant regional and national nursing associations, legislative and regulatory bodies (CCNE 2024; CNO 2025)

2.2 Program Credentialing

Credentialing in APN programs is fundamental to be able to practice at an advanced level in nursing. It is composed of a variety of key components, namely: institutional eligibility criteria; credentialing process; external peer review; site visit and evaluation; and post-approving monitoring. In this section, a breakdown of these components will be discussed. First, institutional eligibility criteria vary significantly globally. Most APN programs require a Bachelor of Science in Nursing (BSN) or equivalent, completion of prerequisite coursework including statistics and clinical nursing experience, a minimum of 2 years of relevant full-time (or equivalent to full time) registered nursing practice within the last 5 years (CCRNR 2023; CNO 2024; CNA 2010; CASN 2015).

The International Council of Nurses (ICN) advocates for standardized education (minimum of a master's degree, defined scope of practice, and regulatory recognition and autonomy (ICN 2020). However, APN credentialing can be hindered by unclear role definitions, limited educational programs, and political and institutional resistance (WHO 2025; Wheeler et al. 2022). Some high-income countries such as the United States (US), Canada, and the United Kingdom (UK) have well-defined APN frameworks, while low to middle-income countries may not, which highlights the importance of standardization (CNA 2019; ICN 2020; WHO 2025; Wheeler et al. 2022). The credentialing process for APNs is a formal systematic approach to ensure that a nurse has the education, qualifications, and experience to practice at an APN level and use the title APN (CASN 2015; CCAPR 2023). Importantly, this process protects the public and upholds professional standards (CCAPR 2023; CCNE 2024).

External peer review is a critical element of credentialing for APNs. This includes an objective, unbiased, third-party evaluation (CCNE 2024). The process can compose of direct peers or external to the institution. These reviewers often compile a report with recommendations, areas of improvement, and recognizing strengths (CASN 2015; CCNE 2024). It is important to consider what this process may look like globally. Many developing countries collaborate with international partners to perform external evaluations based on international criteria (ICN 2020; WHO 2025; Wheeler et al. 2022). Overall, this peer-reviewed process can contribute to the mobilization of APN credentials across the globe which leads to the importance of site visit and evaluation for program credentialing (CNO 2025; EFNA 2025).

It is imperative for academic institutions along with other clinical practice settings to support APN site visits as a part of their programs. External reviewers (clinicians, educators, regulators) often conduct these visits to ensure the program meets regional, national, and global accreditation standards (CCNE 2024; CNO 2025; EFNA 2025). The evaluation would include the following: observations in both academic and clinical settings, simulation labs, interviews (students, faculty, preceptors), and incorporating the integration of evidence-based practice frameworks (CASN 2012; CCNE 2024).

Post-approval monitoring is a crucial phase in the credentialing process of APN programs. Once a program has been formally accredited by a regulatory body, continued oversight ensures the program maintains quality standards, maintains public trust, and adapts to the ever-changing healthcare needs (CCAPR 2023; CCNE 2024). In countries such as the US, UK, or Canada, post-approval monitoring is standardized and typically mandated by national agencies (CNA 2019; CCNE 2024). Yet many low and middle-income countries are still developing formal post-monitoring mechanisms. The importance of global partners such as WHO and ICN are fundamental to the success and sustainability in the post-approval monitoring in those low-income countries (ICN 2020; WHO 2025).

2.3 Specialty Certification

Upon graduation, APNs may pursue certification in a clinical speciality. In order to be eligible to sit for a certification exam, candidates must have graduated from an accredited program, be a licensed registered nurse (RN), be in good standing, meet the number of clinical hours in a speciality area, submit transcripts and pay application and certification fees (CCRNR 2023; CNA 2010; CASN 2015; CCNE 2024). Although some certification processes are portfolio-based certification exams can be multiple-choice, clinical scenario based and are developed through rigorous efforts including regulators, faculty, clinicians input (CASN 2015; CCAPR 2023; CCNE 2024). Many areas of speciality exist such as Family Nurse Practitioner (FNP), Pediatric NP, Adult-Gerontology Primary/Acute Care NP, Psychiatric-Mental Health NP, Certified Nurse Midwife (CNM), Certified Registered Nurse Anesthetist (CRNA), and Clinical Nurse Specialist (CNS) (CASN 2015).

Canada is moving toward a single NP designation with the development of national NP standards in 2026 (CCRNR 2023; CNA 2019). This shift reflects an effort to improve consistency, mobility, and clarity in APN role nationwide. NP practice in Canada has been governed at the provincial and territorial levels resulting in role confusion and fragmented titles (CNA 2019). The Canadian Council of Registered Nurse Regulators (CCRNR) launched a NP regulation framework to harmonize NP regulation nationally (CCRNR 2023). This initiative is consistent with global trends toward role clarity and mobility in advanced practice nursing (ICN 2020; WHO 2025). Countries such as Australia and the UK have already moved toward a national standardization (ICN 2020; Gardner et al. 2016).

Specialty certification is a fundamental component of the credentialing verification process for APNs (CASN 2015; CCAPR 2023). Certification is typically given after passing a national board exam and completing a credentialing application. After certification, the verification process includes important steps, such as submitting confirmation of certification to employers, regulators, and it may be visible and searchable on public databases (CCNE 2024; CNO 2025). This comprehensive approach ensures that only certified APNs deliver care across the globe (ICN 2020; WHO 2025). In order to maintain and renew certification, APNs often complete continuing education hours or units (CEU). In some cases, re-examination is optional versus CEUs (CASN 2015; CCAPR 2023). Additionally, the integration with licensure and practice authority needs to be considered since APN certification is not only a credential but rather a mainstay of licensure, clinical practice, and public safety (CNA 2010; CCNE 2024; CNO 2025).

Through this process, APNs maintain their expertise required to provide autonomous, specialized evidence-based care (CNA 2010; ICN 2020).

Credentialing for APNs is a structured process designed to validate clinical expertise, and legal authorization to practice at an advanced level (CCRNR 2023; CASN 2015; CCAPR 2023). It is a multilayered system involving academic merit, licensure, speciality certification, and regulators (CCRNR 2023; CNO 2024; CASN 2015; CCNE 2024). Policy enforcement and compliance are fundamental to APNs, strong policy frameworks and enforcement mechanisms ensure the public is protected but also support APN professional integrity (HEE 2017). Importantly, they support the sustainability of the APN role across the health systems globally (ICN 2020; WHO 2025).

2.4 Global Competency Framework Alignment

Globally, the role and need for APNs continues to expand. The World Health Organization's (WHO's) 2025 State of the World's Nursing (SoWN) reported an increase of 12% since their last report, in countries that documented having established APN roles (WHO 2025). Furthermore, 13% of countries stated they were in the process of establishing the APN role (WHO 2025). Establishment of the role involves multiple steps including education, accreditation, certification, licensure, and registration (AACN 2021; ICN 2020; CASN 2015). Establishment of the APN role begins with the creation of APN education training programs that meet eligibility criteria for accreditation by the governing bodies in their respective countries (CASN 2015; CCNE 2024). Programs must also ensure their graduates meet the requirements for certification which may involve the completion of a registration exam to demonstrate knowledge of, and competence in, clinical and professional practice standards (CNA 2010; CASN 2015; CCAPR 2023). Once competence has been established through certification, APNs are eligible to apply for licensure, which authorizes them to practice and receive registration as an APN (CCRNR 2023; CNO 2024; CNA 2010). This process may vary, as some countries do not distinguish between certification and licensure (AACN 2021; ICN 2020).

Globally, minimum education standards for APNs vary. The ICN provides specific recommendations for several types of APNs (ICN 2020). For Nurse Practitioners (NPs), both the ICN and World Health Organization (WHO) recommend a postgraduate, master's level degree (ICN 2020; WHO 2025). The ICN acknowledges, however, that this may not be feasible in all countries globally (ICN 2020). Additionally, the ICN suggests a specific program focus and clinical practicum recommendations (ICN 2020). Programs should be tailored toward the type of APN and their corresponding clinical specialty area. The two main types of APNs are Clinical Nurse Specialists (CNS) and Nurse Practitioners (NP) (ICN 2020; CASN 2015). All NP programs should include clinical practicums. These practicums must include a minimum number of supervised clinical hours, which in most countries is set at 500 or more (CNA 2010; CASN 2015). Formal recognition of the education program is therefore viewed as essential by the ICN (2020). The WHO acknowledges the ongoing challenges presented by the variations in education and regulation between countries (WHO 2025). Inconsistent standards can lead to challenges in the recognition of APN education and training, along with barriers to international mobility, which will be discussed later in the chapter (ICN 2020; WHO 2025). APN programs, especially those in middle- and higher-income countries, should strive to achieve the minimum standards outlined by the ICN (2020).

The process of APN credentialing is directly connected to educational qualifications. Credentialing is a crucial mechanism in the regulation of APNs because it provides evidence of the successful achievement of knowledge, skills, and clinical experience, in alignment with professional APN practice standards (CASN 2015; CCAPR 2023). The credentialing process may vary globally, but often involves multiple key components including certification, registration, licensure, and authorization (CCRNR 2023; CNO 2024; CNA 2010, 2019; CASN 2015; CCAPR 2023). Emerging models of credentialing including macro-certifications and micro-credentialing are increasingly being used to achieve continuing education requirements (Southard 2021). Macro-certifications often involve broad credentials that are demonstrated through the achievement of formal qualifications, such as obtaining a degree or successfully completing a certification exam, for example, the Canadian Nurse Practitioner Examination (CCRNR 2023; CNA 2010). As of 2023, there were 28 recognized APN specialty certification programs worldwide (CCAPR 2023). Comparatively, micro-credentials are not as strictly standardized and involve acquiring specific knowledge on a topic such as wound care (Wheeler et al. 2022). These models also aid in achieving global standardization through the inclusion of educational standards to promote competencies and support workforce mobility (ICN 2020; HEE 2017; EFNA 2025; Gardner et al. 2016).

Regulation of APNs offers numerous benefits to the profession, to public safety, and role clarity. Title protection is a crucial component of both regulatory and credentialing systems. It is also a means of safeguarding the public from unqualified clinicians (ICN 2020; CCNE 2024). According to the ICN, title protection is a crucial component of policy, legislation, and credentialing in the regulation of APN practice (ICN 2020). Despite its importance, not all countries provide title protection. For example, in Canada, Clinical Nurse Specialists (CNS) programs still require standardization, and the title is not formally protected (CNA 2019).

Lifelong learning is a fundamental component of Advanced Practice Nurses' (APNs') practice. Usually, this involves the completion of continuing professional development (CPD) activities such as learning modules and courses (AACN 2021; ICN 2020; CASN 2015). The responsibility for ongoing education lies with both the APN and their regulatory body, whose role it is to ensure APNs are remaining current in their clinical practices (CNO 2024; CCNE 2024). The World Health Organization (WHO) recommends ongoing development of APN roles as a key policy priority for the years 2026–2030 (WHO 2025). The WHO suggests that further development of CPD opportunities including micro-credentialing may offer solutions for creating accessible options for ongoing professional education and development (WHO 2025; Southard 2021).

2.5 Cross-Border APN Recognition and Mobility

APN license mobility refers to an APN's ability to practice in multiple regions such as provinces or states by utilizing a single licensure in their original jurisdiction of practice. Portability, however, refers to the ease with which an APN can transfer their license between jurisdictions without requiring the completion of an additional licensing process and a subsequent new license. The mobility and portability of APN credentials is an ongoing area of discussion and exploration in both policy and literature (ICN 2020; WHO 2025; CNO 2025; EFNA 2025). Mutual recognition agreements, credential portability, and bridging programs that enable mobility across jurisdictions all have unique educational, regulatory, and legal considerations (ICN 2020; WHO 2025; CNO 2025; EFNA 2025).

In Ontario, Canada, the regulatory body of nurses, the College of Nurses of Ontario (CNO) launched an interjurisdictional nurse licensure initiative. This initiative enables both registered nurses (RNs) and Nurse Practitioners (NPs) to maintain registration in multiple Canadian provinces and territories while decreasing the duplication of regulatory requirements (CNO 2025).

In Europe, further advancements in cross-border recognition and mobility have been achieved as of 2025 under the European Union's Directive 2005/36/EC, also known as the Professional Qualification Directive. This directive was created so that working professionals, including nurses and APNs, can have their licenses recognized in multiple European countries. However, to comply with this directive, the APN's education must meet the minimum training requirements outlined in the directive (EFNA 2025).

Mutual recognition agreements between countries are a newer phenomenon in the literature. Presently, only two countries, Australia and New Zealand, have such an agreement. Over a decade ago, the countries developed cross-border Nurse Practitioner (NP) competency standards that extended to education authorization and clinical practice (Gardner et al. 2016).

Many countries continue to work toward increasing APN mobility. Nonetheless, achievement of APN mobility remains challenging. Variability amongst countries in education, clinical hours, scope of practice, professional autonomy, and competencies can create challenges when considering APN licensure mobility (ICN 2020; WHO 2025; Wheeler et al. 2022; CASN 2015). Other factors include language and cultural practices. For example, in Canada, NPs must complete a minimum number of clinical practice hours to graduate and can work independently and autonomously (CCRNR 2023; CNA 2010). In the UK however, there is no national requirement for a set number of completed clinical hours, and scope of practice is often determined by employers instead of through a centralized regulatory body (HEE 2017; EFNA 2025).

When considering an APN education credentialing policy, the International Council of Nurses (ICN's) frameworks for APN education and clinical practice should be utilized as a guiding framework (ICN 2020). These factors are crucial considerations for APNs future opportunities for mobility. APN mobility further highlights the need for international alignment on NP competencies (ICN 2020; WHO 2025; Gardner et al. 2016). This would ensure future ease in policy creation and implementation and portability of licensure across countries. Further data collection on practice barriers and employment outcomes relating to mobility of APNs is needed to direct future policies (WHO 2025; Wheeler et al. 2022; EFNA 2025).

2.6 Quality Assurance and Evaluation Metrics

There are many factors to consider when evaluating a program's effectiveness. These factors will be reflective of the country in which the program is located. Some high-income countries, such as the US, utilize graduate certification exam pass rates as a key indicator of the program's effectiveness. The US Commission on Collegiate Nursing Education (CCNE) mandates a minimum 80% certification exam pass rate to receive accreditation (CCNE 2024). In other high-income countries such as Canada, there is no required minimum exam pass rate. However, exam pass rates are closely considered when regulatory nursing bodies assess and approve programs (CCRNR 2023; CNA 2010; CASN 2015). In some countries where such exams do not exist, other metrics must be utilized (ICN 2020; WHO 2025).

Program evaluation must consider various factors such as faculty-to-student ratios, variety and categories of clinical rotations, and graduate employment rates. These factors can serve as key metrics. The Canadian Association of Schools of Nursing (CASN) and CCNE similarly recommend focusing more on diverse clinical experiences as they relate to patient populations and clinical settings (CASN 2015; CCNE 2024). Clinical placements should be reflective of graduates' future scope of practice and incorporate opportunities to engage in interdisciplinary collaboration in team-based care models (CASN 2015; CCNE 2024). They should also prepare students for independent and safe clinical practices in their area of specialty (CASN 2015; CCAPR 2023; CCNE 2024). In contrast, many European countries mandate structured clinical training programs that include specific clinical settings. Each European country is responsible for its own program regulatory standards; however, the European Higher Education Area (EHEA) follows the Bologna Process principles of competency-based education, academic transparency, and quality assurance (EFNA 2025).

In North America, the CCNE and the CASN Nursing do not mandate specific faculty-to-student ratios. Instead, both organizations recommend keeping the numbers low without providing specifics (CASN 2015; CCNE 2024). In Europe, several countries provide recommendations and regulations for faculty-to-student ratios in both didactic and clinical settings (EFNA 2025).

Graduate employment rates also serve as a crucial program evaluation metric. Both the CASN and CCNE direct graduate programs to maintain statistics on types of roles graduates work in, in addition to rates of employment (CASN 2015; CCNE 2024). CASN also recommends programs to gather stakeholder feedback from alumni and employers on additional topics including readiness for practice and employer satisfaction (CASN 2015). In Europe, additional data including time to employment is also considered (EFNA 2025).

Diversity, equity, and inclusion (DEI) and an anti-racism and oppression lens should be considered in all aspects of quality assurance and evaluation metrics. Programs must consider their effectiveness in preparing their graduates to address health systems disparities and provide culturally appropriate and safe care to various populations in the communities in which they serve (AACN 2021; CASN 2025; ICN 2020). Evaluation metrics should consider factors relating to DEI, and quality improvement projects should operate from a DEI framework (AACN 2021; CASN 2025).

Some strategies for implementation include DEI-focused curriculum audits by utilizing existing tools such as the American Association of Colleges of Nurses DEI toolkit (AACN 2021). Implementation of CASN's standards for Cultural Humility and Cultural Safety in nursing education may also be measured as a metric, along with alumni surveys in preparation and readiness to provide culturally safe care (CASN 2015, 2025). Lastly, data analysis of student demographics, specifically, rates of admissions and attrition, along with alumni surveys, should be considered (CASN 2015; CCNE 2024).

After collecting this data, programs can create measurable, outcome-based quality improvement projects, as informed by stakeholder feedback (CASN 2015). Programs can set their own goals for graduate employment rates, workplace settings, and employer feedback responses (CASN 2015; CCNE 2024). If a program's goals are not being met, a review of potential causes and strategies to address the factors can be created and implemented (CASN 2015).

2.7 Governance and Accountability

Advanced practice nursing education program governance can vary by geographical location. It often includes governance by regional or national regulatory bodies of nursing as well as national nursing education associations (CCRNR 2023; CNA 2019; CASN 2012; CCNE 2024). In some countries, government ministries may also be involved in APN education program operation, licensing, and funding (ICN 2020; WHO 2025; EFNA 2025). Academic institutions are responsible for ensuring adherence of internal policies to educational standards and ongoing assessment (CASN 2015; CCAPR 2023; CCNE 2024).

For the purposes of both public trust and internal quality improvement, APN programs should prioritize transparency by publishing their accreditation outcomes (CCNE 2024). Increasingly, distance-based and online APN programs are being developed to increase access and address workforce requirements (WHO 2025; Wheeler et al. 2022; EFNA 2025). Comparatively, regulations for these programs differ from standard in-person programs (ICN 2020; CCNE 2024). Many distance and online programs must consider cross-jurisdictional credentialing factors, especially around clinical placements (CCRNR 2023; CNO 2024, 2025). For example, a student may enroll in an online APN program based in one province, state, or country and then complete their clinical rotations in another (CNO 2025; EFNA 2025). Ultimately, each region's regulatory body is responsible for determining whether another jurisdiction's program is suitably accredited and meets the necessary requirements for licensure and certification in their own jurisdiction (CNA 2019; ICN 2020; CCNE 2024; EFNA 2025). Quality assurance for these digital and online programs must also be implemented virtually. This includes oversight of curriculum, faculty, and clinical rotations (CASN 2015; CASN 2012; CCNE 2024). While online programs may initially appear to improve equity and access, students from low or middle-income countries may be challenged to receive recognition of a program completed in a high-income country (WHO 2025; Wheeler et al. 2022; UNESCO 2020).

The International Council of Nurses (ICN) and the World Health Organization (WHO) offer comprehensive direction for APN education programs to ensure alignment with APN global standards, competencies, and global workforce planning (ICN 2020; WHO 2025).

Community stakeholder engagement is encouraged as an important means of ensuring accountability to the patients whom the APN graduates will serve. Engagement may include focus groups with community members from various socioeconomic and cultural backgrounds to ensure inclusive representation (AACN 2021; CASN 2025). Other engagement methods may include patient and organizational surveys from clinical placement sites. This provides the opportunity to collect feedback on the program's efficacy (CASN 2015).

3 Summary

APN education credentialing policies are instrumental in guiding APN education, training, and certification (CCRNR 2023; CNA 2019; CASN 2015; CCAPR 2023). This chapter reviewed key policy concepts including program standards, credentialing, and specialty certification (CNA 2019; CASN 2015; CCAPR 2023). Additional topics examined included quality assurance and evaluation metrics, cross-border recognition and mobility, alignment with global competency frameworks, and governance and accountability (AACN 2021; CASN 2025; ICN 2020; WHO 2025; CCNE 2024; CNO 2025; HEE 2017; EFNA 2025). The results include increased public protection, professional role clarity, and mobility (ICN 2020; WHO 2025; CNO 2025; EFNA 2025; Gardner et al. 2016). Looking to the future, innovative continuing professional development opportunities such as micro-credentialing will play an important role in global recognition and mobility (AACN 2021; ICN 2020; WHO 2025; Southard 2021).

References

American Association of Colleges of Nurses (AACN). Diversity, equity and inclusion—an AACN faculty toolkit. AACN; 2021. https://www.aacnnursing.org/diversity-tool-kit/contact. Accessed 4 Apr 2025.

Canadian Association of Schools of Nursing (CASN). Nurse practitioner education in Canada—national framework of guiding principles and essential components. CASN; 2012. https://casn.ca/wp-content/uploads/2014/12/FINALNPFrameworkEN20130131.pdf. Accessed 2 Apr 2025.

Canadian Association of Schools of Nursing (CASN). National nursing education framework. CASN; 2015. https://www.casn.ca/wp-content/uploads/2014/12/Framwork-FINAL-SB-Nov-30-20151.pdf. Accessed 5 Apr 2025.

Canadian Association of Schools of Nursing (CASN). Cultural humility and cultural safety standards for nursing education. CASN; 2025. https://www.casn.ca/wp-content/uploads/2025/02/CASN_Cultural_Humility_Safety_Standards_2024_EN.pdf. Accessed 4 Apr 2025.

Canadian Centre for Advanced Practice Research (CCAPR). Certification of specialty practice for advanced practice nursing roles—establishing evidence-informed recommendations. CCAPR; 2023. https://ccapnr.com/wp-content/uploads/2024/04/Certification-of-Specialty-Practice-for-APNs-Briefing-Note.pdf. Accessed 1 Apr 2025.

Canadian Council of Registered Nurse Regulators (CCRNR). National entry-level competencies for nurse practitioners. CCRNR; 2023. https://static1.squarespace.com/static/671142bd58709c1e559e8c2a/t/672fdb07719a981d7c5480b7/1731189512640/english-national-np-elcs-final-bibliography-updated-june-2024.pdf.

Canadian Nurses Association (CNA). Canadian nurse practitioner core competency framework. CNA; 2010. https://hl-prod-ca-oc-download.s3-ca-central-1.amazonaws.com/CNA/2f975e7e-4a40-45ca-863c-5ebf0a138d5e/UploadedImages/documents/Competency_Framework_2010_e.pdf. Accessed 4 Apr 2025.

Canadian Nurses Association (CNA). Advanced practice nursing—a pan-Canadian framework. CNA; 2019. https://hl-prod-ca-oc-download.s3-ca-central-1.amazonaws.com/CNA/2f975e7e-4a40-45ca-863c-5ebf0a138d5e/UploadedImages/documents/nursing/Advanced_Practice_Nursing_framework_e.pdf. Accessed 4 Apr 2025.

College of Nurses of Ontario (CNO). Entry-level competencies for nurse practitioners. CNO; 2024. https://cno.org/Assets/CNO/Documents/Standard-and-Learning/Practice-Standards/47010-np-etp-competencies.pdf. Accessed 4 Apr 2025.

College of Nurses of Ontario (CNO). Moving forward with labour mobility. CNO; 2025. https://www.cno.org/news/moving-forward-with-labour-mobility. Accessed 3 Apr 2025.

Commission on Collegiate Nursing Education (CCNE). Standards for accreditation of baccalaureate and graduate nursing programs. CCNE; 2024. https://www.aacnnursing.org/Portals/0/PDFs/CCNE/CCNE-Education-Standards-2024.pdf. Accessed 1 Apr 2025.

European Federation of Nurses Associations (EFNA). EFN advanced practice nursing (APN) implementation toolkit. EFNA; 2025. https://efn.eu/wp-content/uploads/2025/04/EFN-APN-implementation-toolkit.pdf. Accessed 4 Apr 2025.

Gardner G, Duffield C, Doubrovsky A, Adams M. Nurse practitioner competency standards: findings from collaborative Australian and New Zealand research. Int J Nurs Stud. 2016;63:54–62. https://doi.org/10.1016/j.ijnurstu.2016.08.0091.

Health Education England (HEE). Multi-professional framework for advanced clinical practice in England. HEE; 2017. https://www.hee.nhs.uk/sites/default/files/documents/multi-professional frameworkforadvancedclinicalpracticeinengland.pdf. Accessed 4 Apr 2025.

International Council of Nurses (ICN). Guidelines on advanced practice nursing. ICN; 2020. https://www.icn.ch/sites/default/files/2023-06/ICN_APN%20Report_EN.pdf. 2 Apr 2025.

Southard EP. Micro-credentials and badges in healthcare. Am Nurse J. 2021;16(10):19–20. Available from: https://www.myamericannurse.com/wp-content/uploads/2021/09/an10-Badges-920.pdf.

United Nations Educational, Scientific and Cultural Organization (UNESCO). Education in a post-COVID world: nine ideas for public action. UNESCO; 2020. https://unesdoc.unesco.org/ark:/48223/pf0000373717. Accessed 4 Apr 2025.

Wheeler KJ, Miller M, Pulcini J, Gray D, Ladd E, Rayens MK. Advanced practice nursing roles, regulation, education, and practice: a global study. Ann Glob Health. 2022;88(1):42. https://doi.org/10.5334/aogh.3698. PMID: 35755314; PMCID: PMC9205376.

World Health Organization (WHO). State of the world's nursing 2025—investing in education, jobs and service delivery. WHO; 2025. https://iris.who.int/bitstream/handle/10665/381329/9789240110236-eng.pdf?sequence=1. Accessed 5 Apr 2025.

Conclusion: Health Policy Implementation and Improvement

Pearls and Parting Words: Highlights of Policy Implementation and Improvement for Advanced Practice Nursing

Kathy J. Wheeler and Michelle Acorn

1 Toolkit Highlights

This toolkit explores multiple policy areas that are foundational to the primary goal of advanced practice nursing (APN) practice—to deliver high-quality, patient-centered, evidence-based care in cost-effective and efficient ways. When able to practice to the full scope of their education and experience, they also seek to improve systems of care, advocate for patients, and counter health disparities. At the same time, as educated and experienced professionals, they have the opportunity to shepherd the APN profession through leadership and sound policy development. Highlights of the toolkit include the following:

1. *Policy is everywhere.* For APNs, policy is everywhere, and a part of everything that impacts how APNs practice, are educated, and are governed. Where APNs practice, what they learn, how they learn it, how they consult and collaborate, what tests they order, what tests they interpret, what medications they order—these are just a few examples, but they are everywhere for an APN. That realization should underscore how APNs approach their day-to-day experiences, realizing it is they who must champion policy implementation and improvement if they are going to provide the care for which they are educated. While there are many participants involved in the creation and delivery of quality healthcare, APNs have a principal role to play in the process—spotting what works and what does not work, and spotting the gaps and opportunities. Once spotted hopefully they can work within the system to bring about needed change.

K. J. Wheeler (✉)
University of Kentucky College of Nursing, Lexington, KY, USA
e-mail: kjwheeler623@gmail.com

M. Acorn
University of Toronto & Queen's University, Toronto & Kingston, ON, Canada

K. J. Wheeler, M. Acorn (eds.), *Health Policy for Advanced Practice Nursing: A Toolkit for Implementation and Improvement*, Advanced Practice in Nursing,
https://doi.org/10.1007/978-3-032-03667-4_20

2. *Supportive policies for APNs serve the populace and the profession.* Barriers to practice, education, leadership, scholarship, and governance are everyday realities for APNs. Aside from frustrating the APN and healthcare systems, these barriers interfere with equitable, efficient, and effective care delivery. For APNs and policy makers to work to counter these barriers is not a selfish act by the APN or policy maker. Nonetheless, they are often portrayed that way. The reality is nurses and APNs work in incredibly difficult situations, with high workloads and limited resources, often in the presence of violence or risky situations. To practice, educate, lead, and govern without additional hindrance makes sense so APNs can provide the care that is needed.
3. *Nursing has always been a forward-facing profession.* Nursing is at the center of healthcare wherever nursing is needed, focused on the patient, ready to evolve, and eager to meet challenges. Nursing has been at the front of advancements in education, technology, telehealth, team care, system improvements, and implementation of evidence-based care. Leading the change can best be done when APNs and nurses are skilled at navigating policy implementation and improvement.
4. *Advanced practice nursing is good for nursing.* There are countless examples of APNs initially facing some opposition by nursing, followed by examples of improvements for the nursing profession overall once APNs are fully functioning within systems of education, practice, and governance. Multiple studies report improved patient outcomes, improved access to care, improvements in systems of care, improved mentoring, and increased numbers of faculty.
5. *Rarely is professional policy an either-or situation.* As professions evolve, there is always a concern that those professionals at the forefront of introduction of the profession might be abandoned in the evolutionary process. Nursing offers a big table, valuing experienced professionals and providing systems of legacy. Nonetheless, nursing must continue to invest in bridge education systems and must craft governance so professionals are not abandoned but can evolve to maintain quality and healthcare delivery.
6. *Policy work requires a lot of tools and takes a lot of time.* Rarely does a single policy initiative accomplish whatever was desired. Usually, the process is complicated, takes a lot of time, and requires multiple attempts. The need may not just be time and repeated attempts, but patience and the will to succeed. APNs and interested parties must be looking for new policy tools, new insights, evolving evidence, multiple mentors and policy champions, creativity, and leadership. Information about both failures and successes needs to be shared so APNs and policy leaders can learn.
7. *Policy work takes a team.* Just as healthcare delivery requires the collaboration of a well-coordinated, communicating team, the same is true of policy work. Building a team is an important part of the process and requires members to be educated and willing to reach out to administrators, legislators, and other team members.
8. *Organizations are critical to the APN policy process.* Because policy work is complicated and requires a lot of resources and time, organizations are extremely

important to the process. But, that also means APNs and interested parties need to invest in organizations so they have the resources they need to do the work they are asked to do. That investment includes time and effort, not merely money.

Hopefully, this toolkit will prompt APNs and those interested in improving healthcare around the world to undertake the policy implementation and improvement. The editors thank all the authors for the work and wisdom they provided to this project.

Kind regards,

Kathy Wheeler and Michelle Acorn

MIX
Papier aus verantwortungsvollen Quellen
Paper from responsible sources
FSC® C105338

If you have any concerns about our products,
you can contact us on
ProductSafety@springernature.com

In case Publisher is established outside the EU,
the EU authorized representative is:
Springer Nature Customer Service Center GmbH
Europaplatz 3, 69115 Heidelberg, Germany

Printed by Libri Plureos GmbH
in Hamburg, Germany